Clinical Kinesiology for Physical Therapist Assistants

Clinical Kinesiology for Physical Therapist Assistants

THIRD EDITION

Lynn S. Lippert, MS, PT
Program Director
Physical Therapist Assistant
Mount Hood Community College
Gresham, Oregon

 F. A. DAVIS COMPANY • Philadelphia

F. A. Davis Company
1915 Arch Street
Philadelphia, PA 19103

Printed in the United States of America

Last digit indicates print number: 10 9 8 7 6 5 4 3 2

Publisher: Jean-François Vilain
Developmental Editor: Christa A. Fratantoro
Production Editor: Stephen D. Johnson
Cover Designer: Louis J. Forgione

As new scientific information becomes available through basic and clinical research, recommended treatments and drug therapies undergo changes. The author(s) and publisher have done everything possible to make this book accurate, up to date, and in accord with accepted standards at the time of publication. The authors, editors, and publisher are not responsible for errors or omissions or for consequences from application of the book, and make no warranty, expressed or implied, in regard to the contents of the book. Any practice described in this book should be applied by the reader in accordance with professional standards of care used in regard to the unique circumstances that may apply in each situation. The reader is advised always to check product information (package inserts) for changes and new information regarding dose and contraindications before administering any drug. Caution is especially urged when using new or infrequently ordered drugs.

Library of Congress Cataloging in Publication Data

Lippert, Lynn, 1942– .
    Clinical kinesiology for physical therapist assistants / Lynn Lippert–3rd ed.
      p. ; cm.
    Includes bibliographical references and index.
    ISBN 0-8036-0453-X (alk. paper)
    1. Kinesiology. 2. Physical therapy assistants. I. Title.
    [DNLM: 1. Kinesiology, Applied 2. Movement. 3. Allied Health Personnel. 4. Physical Therapy. WE 103 L765c 2000]
    QP303 .L53 2000
    612.7′6–dc21

                                            00-020083
                                              CIP

To those who have given me help and encouragement when I needed it the most:

Mercedes Weiss, my mentor
Molly Dott Lippert, my mother
Ann McGregor Lewis, my coach
Sal Jepson, my friend
Dr. Angela Kaliashek and
Dr. Jo Anne Nelson, my
oncologist and my surgeon, skilled
wizards of medicine and my lifelines

Preface to the Third Edition

There are some changes and several new faces in this revision, however, the depth and scope of the text remains the same. It has been satisfying and rewarding to continually hear that one of the main strengths of the book is the simple, easy-to-follow descriptions and explanations.

The muscular system has been expanded to include an explanation of open and closed kinetic chain principles. The gait chapter now includes an explanation of many common pathological gait patterns. Several illustrations have been redrawn for greater clarity.

Five new chapters have been added. A chapter on basic biomechanics provides explanations and examples of the various biomechanical principles commonly used in physical therapy. Chapters describing the temporomandibular joint and the pelvic girdle have been added for those who want a basic description of those joints' structure and function. Normal posture and arthrokinematics, which were included in the *Kinesiology Laboratory Manual for Physical Therapist Assistants,* have been described and expanded upon in this revision.

There is not universal agreement within the physical therapy community regarding the scope of practice of the physical therapist assistant. It is generally felt that joint mobilization is not an entry-level skill. I do not disagree with this. However, PT assistants are exposed to and involved in patient treatments where these skills are utilized. For this reason, they need basic understanding of the terminology and principles, and this text provides them with this information.

This revision of *Clinical Kinesiology for Physical Therapist Assistants* is the result of many suggestions from educators, students, and clinicians. The profession needs good textbooks that cover many additional areas of physical therapist assistant education. I hope that by its fourth edition, this text will have its place on the bookshelf along with those yet-to-be-written texts.

Lynn S. Lippert

Preface to the Second Edition

Most of the people who write and lecture on anatomy agree on what is there and where it is, although they do not always agree on what to call it. Kinesiologists tend to agree that motion occurs, but they certainly do not agree on what muscles cause a motion or on the relative importance of each muscle's action in that motion.

In *Clinical Kinesiology for Physical Therapist Assistants,* the emphasis is on basic kinesiology. In describing joint motion and muscle action, I have focused on describing the commonly agreed-on prime movers, using the terminology most widely accepted within the discipline of physical therapy. Many textbooks exist that describe in greater detail various motions and muscles, in both normal and pathological conditions. For more in-depth analysis, the student should consult these books.

The idea of writing a kinesiology textbook for physical therapist assistant students has been around for several years. Somehow, time constraints and the pressures of other projects always got in the way. When educators gathered to discuss issues regarding physical therapist assistant education, lack of appropriate textbooks was always high on the list of problems. It became evident that if such textbooks were to exist, the physical therapist assistant educators were the ones who needed to write them.

Clinical Kinesiology for Physical Therapist Assistants is the result of those discussions. I hope that it is only the first of many textbooks that emphasize physical therapist assistant education.

Lynn S. Lippert

Acknowledgments

Someone told me that writing a revision was not as difficult as writing the original text. I now realize that everyone has his or her own definition of reality. While it is true that e-mail and the computer have made writing and communication much easier, it still takes much more time and energy than you would ever believe necessary.

As with previous editions, I have had a great deal of help from many people. Sal Jepson, now a veterinary medicine student, stopped palpating cows and other such activities to draw several illustrations. Joyce Shields drew the new illustrations in the hand chapter prior to heading off to pursue a degree in oriental medicine. Mary Rutt graciously took time from her very full life as a retired physical therapist to lend her hand and artistic skill to the majority of the new illustrations. Don Davis, my physics guru, continues to assure me that gravity makes everthing roll only downhill and keeps my thoughts in the world of physics and biomechanics accurate.

The folks at F. A. Davis have been great. Christa Fratantoro used her editorial skills to tactfully provide many useful suggestions without making it seem that I should return to WR 121 class. She also has an amazing ability to track me down anyplace in the continental U.S., and I suspect I could not hide even in the mountains of Nepal. Jean-François Vilain defines what an acquisitions editor should be. He has been most supportive and understanding especially during these difficult past two years.

Pam Levangie and Meryl Gersh have been very supportive colleagues, whose pearls of wisdom I respect greatly. Finally, this text would never have been written without the hundreds of students who have helped me learn how to become a more effective educator.

Thank you one and all, I wouldn't have wanted to do it without you.

Contents

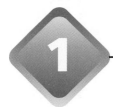

Basic Information

Descriptive Terminology

Types of Motion

Joint Movements (Osteokinematics)

Review Questions

By definition, **kinesiology** is the study of movement. However, this definition is too general to be of much use. Kinesiology brings together the fields of anatomy, physiology, physics, and geometry, and relates them to human movement. Thus, kinesiology utilizes principles of mechanics, musculoskeletal anatomy, and neuromuscular physiology.

Mechanical principles that relate directly to the human body are used in the study of **biomechanics.** Because we may use a ball, racket, crutch, prosthesis, or some other implement, their biomechanical interaction must be considered as well. This may involve looking at the *static* (nonmoving) and/or *dynamic* (moving) *systems* associated with various activities. Dynamic systems can be divided into kinetics and kinematics. **Kinetics** are those forces causing movement, whereas **kinematics** are those time, space, and mass aspects of a moving system. These and other basic biomechanical concepts will be discussed in Chapter 6.

This text will give most emphasis to the musculoskeletal anatomy components, which are considered the key to understanding and being able to apply the other components. Many students are subject to negative thoughts at the mere mention of the word *kinesiology.* Their eyes glaze over, and their brains freeze. Perhaps, based on past experience with anatomy, they feel that their only hope is mass memorization. However, this may prove to be an overwhelming task with no long-term memory gain.

As you proceed through this text, you should keep in mind a few simple concepts. First, the human body is arranged in a very logical way. Like all aspects of life, there are exceptions. Sometimes the logic of these exceptions is apparent, and sometimes the logic may be apparent only to some higher being. Whichever is the case, you should note the exception and move on. Second, if you have a good grasp of descriptive terminology and can visualize the concept or feature, then strict memorization is not necessary. For example, if you know generally where the patella is located and what the structures are around it, you can accurately describe its location using your own words. You do not need to memorize someone else's words to be correct.

By keeping in mind some of the basic principles affecting muscles, understanding individual muscle function need not be so mind-boggling. If you know (1) what motions a particular joint allows, (2) that a muscle must span a particular joint surface to cause a certain motion, (3) what that muscle's line of pull is, then (4) you will know the particular action(s) of a specific muscle. For example, (1) the elbow allows only flexion and extension. (2) A muscle must span the joint anteriorly to flex and posteriorly to extend. (3) The biceps brachii is a vertical muscle on the anterior surface of the arm. (4) Therefore, the biceps flexes the elbow.

Yes, kinesiology can be understood by mere mortals. Its study can even be enjoyable. There is also no natural or human-made law that says otherwise. A word of caution should be given: Like exercising, it is better to study in small amounts several times a week than to study for a long period in one session before the exam.

Descriptive Terminology

The human body is active and constantly moving; therefore, it is subject to frequent changes in position. The relationship of the various body parts to each other also changes. To be able to describe the organization of the human body, it is necessary to use some arbitrary position as a starting point from which movement or location of structures can be described. This is known as the **anatomical position** (Fig. 1–1A) and is described as the human body standing in an upright position, eyes facing forward, feet parallel and close together, arms at the sides of the body with the palms facing forward. Although the position of the forearm and hands is not a natural one, it does allow for accurate description. The **fundamental position** (Fig. 1–1B) is the same as the anatomical position except that the palms face the sides of the body. This position is often used in discussing rotation of the upper extremity.

Specific terms are used to describe the location of a structure and its position relative to other structures (Fig. 1–2). **Medial** refers to a location or position toward the midline, and **lateral** refers to location or position farther from the midline. For

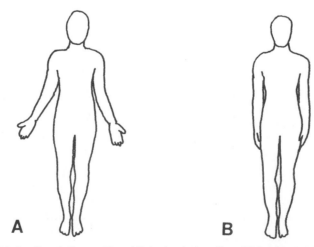

FIGURE 1–1.   Descriptive position. (*A*) Anatomical position. (*B*) Fundamental position.

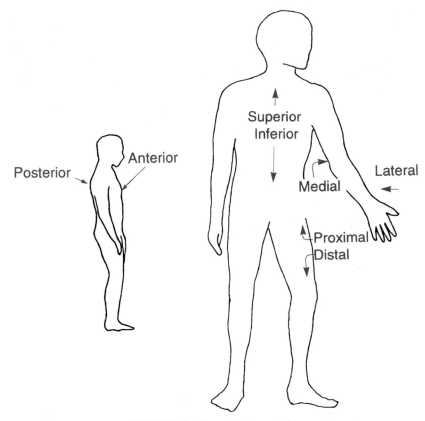

FIGURE 1–2.   Descriptive terminology.

example, the ulna is on the medial side of the forearm, and the radius is lateral to the ulna.

Anterior refers to the front of the body or to a position closer to the front than another. **Posterior** refers to the back of the body or to a position more to the back. For example, the sternum is anterior on the chest wall, and the scapula is posterior. **Ventral** is a *synonym* (word with the same meaning) of anterior, and **dorsal** is a synonym of posterior; *anterior* and *posterior* are more commonly used in kinesiology. *Front* and *back* also refer to the surfaces of the body, but these are considered lay terms and are not widely used by health care professionals.

Distal and **proximal** are used to describe locations on the extremities. *Distal* means away from the trunk, and *proximal* means toward the trunk. For example, the humeral head is located on the proximal head of the humerus. The elbow is proximal to the wrist but distal to the shoulder.

Superior is used to indicate the location of a body part that is above another or to refer to the upper surface of an organ or structure. **Inferior** indicates that a body part is below another or refers to the lower surface of an organ or structure. For example, the body of the sternum is superior to the xiphoid process but inferior to the manubrium. Sometimes people use cranial or cephalad (from the word root *cephal,* meaning "head") to refer to a position or structure close to the head. **Caudal** (from the word root for "tail") refers to a position or structure closer to the feet. For example, cauda *equina,* which means "horse's tail," is the inferior end of the spinal cord. Cranial and caudal are terms like dorsal and ventral that are best used to describe po-

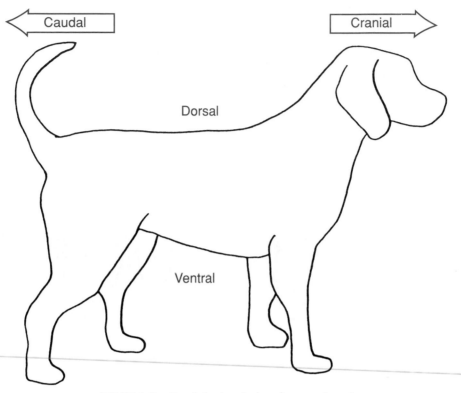

FIGURE 1–3. Descriptive terminology for a quadruped.

sitions on a quadruped (four-legged animal). Humans are bipeds or two-legged animals. You can see that if the dog in Figure 1–3 was to stand on its hind legs, dorsal would become posterior and cranial would become superior, and so on.

A structure may be described as **superficial** or **deep** depending on its relative depth. For example, in describing the layers of the abdominal muscles, the external oblique is deep to the rectus abdominis but superficial to the internal oblique. Another example is the scalp being described as superficial to the skull.

Types of Motion

Linear motion, also called *translatory motion,* occurs in more or less a straight line from one location to another. All the parts of the object move the same distance, in the same direction, and at the same time. If this movement occurs in a straight line, it is called **rectilinear motion,** such as the motion of a child sledding down a hill (Fig. 1–4). If the movement occurs not in a straight line but in a curved path, it is called **curvilinear motion.** Figure 1–5 demonstrates the path a diver takes, after leaving the diving board, until entering the water. Other examples of this type of motion are the path of a ball, a javelin thrown across a field, or the earth's orbit around the sun.

Movement of an object about a fixed point is called **angular motion,** also known as *rotary motion* (Fig. 1–6). All the parts of the object move through the same angle, in the same direction, and at the same time. They do not move the same distance. When a person flexes the elbow, the hand travels farther through space than does the wrist or forearm.

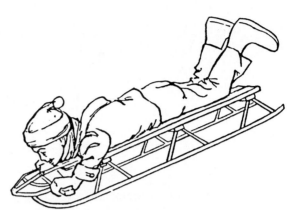

FIGURE 1–4. Rectilinear motion.

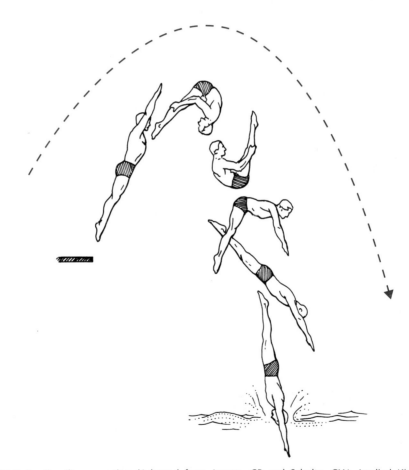

FIGURE 1–5. Curvilinear motion (Adapted from Jensen, CR and Schultz, GW. Applied Kinesiology, McGraw-Hill, New York, 1970, p 200, with permission.)

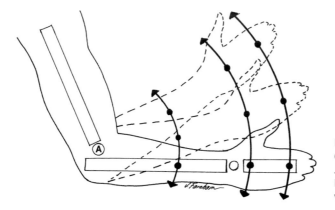

FIGURE 1–6. Angular motion. (From Norkin, CC and Levangie, PK: Joint Structure and Function, ed 2. FA Davis, Philadelphia, 1992, p 4, with permission.)

It is not uncommon to see both types of movement occurring at the same time, the entire object moving in a linear fashion and the individual parts moving in an angular fashion. In Figure 1–7, the person's whole body moves across the room in the wheelchair (linear motion), while individual joints, such as the shoulders, elbows, and wrists, rotate about their axes (angular motion). If the individual were walking, the whole body would be exhibiting linear motion, while the hips, knees, and ankles would be exhibiting angular motion. For the ball to travel in its curvilinear path, it must be thrown. Thus, the upper extremity joints of the person throwing the ball move in an angular direction.

Generally speaking, most movement within the body is angular; movement outside the body tends to be linear. Exceptions to this statement can be found. For example, the movement of the scapula in elevation/depression and protraction/retraction is essentially linear. However, the movement of the clavicle, which is attached to the scapula, is angular and gets its angular motion from the sternoclavicular joint.

Joint Movements (Osteokinematics)

Joints move in many different directions. As will be discussed, movement occurs around joint axes and through joint planes. The following terms are used to describe the various joints movements that occur at synovial joints (Fig. 1–8). **Synovial joints** are freely movable joints where most joint motion occurs. These joints are discussed in more detail in Chapter 3. This type of joint motion is also called **osteokinematics.** This deals with the relationship of bony movement, as opposed to **arthrokine-**

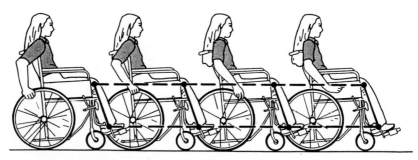

FIGURE 1–7. Combination of linear and angular motion. (From Hay, JG and Reid, JG: The Anatomical and Mechanical Bases of Human Motion. Prentice-Hall, Englewood Cliffs, NJ, 1982, p 116, with permission.)

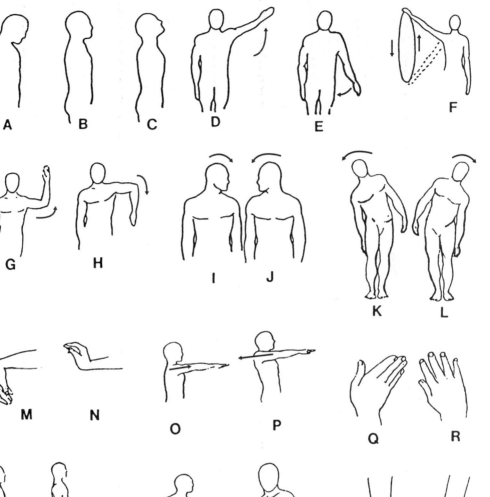

FIGURE 1–8.   Joint motions.

A	Flexion	I	Rotation (l)	Q	Ulnar deviation
B	Extension	J	Rotation (r)	R	Radial deviation
C	Hyperextension	K	Lateral bending (r)	S	Pronation
D	Abduction	L	Lateral bending (l)	T	Supination
E	Adduction	M	Flexion	U	Horizontal abduction
F	Circumduction	N	Extension	V	Horizontal adduction
G	Lateral rotation	O	Protraction	W	Dorsiflexion
H	Medial rotation	P	Retraction	X	Plantar flexion

matics, which deals with the relationship of joint surface movement. This will be discussed in more detail in Chapter 21.

Flexion is the bending movement of one bone on another, causing a decrease in the joint angle. Usually this occurs between anterior surfaces of articulating bones. However, with the knee and toes, the posterior surfaces approximate each other, causing flexion. The hip can be viewed as flexing on the trunk when the lower extremity is the moving component. When the lower extremities are fixed and the trunk becomes the moving component, the trunk flexes. Actually, whether flexion represents an increase or decrease in joint angle will depend upon your point of reference. As described above, flexion begins at 180 degrees (full extension) and moves toward zero degrees; thus it is a decrease in the joint angle. However, when performing a goniometric measurement of elbow flexion, one would begin in anatomical position (full extension), which is considered zero. The amount of flexion increased toward 180 degrees. In this case, flexion would represent an increase in the joint angle.

Conversely, **extension** is the straightening movement of one bone from another causing an increase of the joint angle. This motion usually returns the body part to the anatomical position after it has been flexed. Hyperextension is the continuation of extension beyond the anatomical position.

Abduction is movement away from midline of body, and adduction is movement toward the midline. Exceptions to this midline definition are the fingers and toes. The reference point for the fingers is the middle finger. Movement away from the middle finger is abduction. It should be noted that the middle finger abducts (to the right and to the left) but adducts only as a return movement from abduction. The point of reference for the toes is the second toe. Similar to the middle finger, the second toe abducts to the right and the left but does not adduct except as a return movement from abduction.

Circumduction is the combination of all of these motions in a sequence in which the distal end of the extremity (or part) makes a wide circle in the air, the sides tapering to the proximal end, which makes a narrow circle. For example, if the shoulder were to adduct, flex, abduct, then extend in that order, the hand would make a circle in the air and the whole upper extremity would make the shape of a cone.

Rotation is movement of a bone or part around its longitudinal axis. If the anterior surface moves toward the midline, it is called medial rotation. This is sometimes referred to as *internal rotation.* Conversely, if the anterior surface moves away from the midline, it is called lateral rotation, or *external rotation.* The trunk also rotates, but to either the right or left side. If the right shoulder moves forward toward the left, it is "*left* rotation," and so on.

The following are terms used to describe motions specific to certain joints. **Inversion** is moving the sole of foot inward at the ankle, and **eversion** is the outward movement. **Protraction** is movement along a plane parallel to the ground and away from the midline, and **retraction** is movement in the same plane toward the midline. Protraction of the shoulder girdle moves the scapula away from the midline as does protraction of the jaw, whereas retraction in both of these cases returns the body part toward the midline, or anatomical, position.

In anatomical position the forearm is in **supination.** The palm is facing forward, or anteriorly. In **pronation,** the palm is facing backward, or posteriorly.

Flexion at the wrist may be called **palmar flexion,** and flexion at the ankle may be called **plantar flexion.** Extension at both joints may be called **dorsiflexion.**

When the shoulder joint is flexed to 90 degrees and then adducted, it is called **horizontal adduction.** If the shoulder is abducted from this 90-degree position, it is called **horizontal abduction.**

Terms more commonly used to refer to wrist adduction and abduction are *ulnar* and *radial deviation.* When the hand moves medially from the anatomical position toward the ulnar side, it is **ulnar deviation.** When the hand moves laterally, or toward the radial bone side, it is **radial deviation.**

When the trunk moves sideways, the term **lateral bending** is used. The trunk can laterally bend to the right or to the left. If the right shoulder moves toward the right hip, it is called *right lateral bending.* The term *lateral flexion* is sometimes used to describe this sideward motion. However, because this term is easily confused with *flexion,* it will not be used.

REVIEW QUESTIONS

Using descriptive terminology, complete the following:

1. The sternum is _____ to the vertebral column.

2. The calcaneus is on the _____ portion of the foot.

3. The hip is _____ to the chest.

4. The femur is _____ to the tibia.

5. The radius is on the _____ side of the forearm.

6. Using examples other than those used in this chapter, identify an object in linear motion and one in angular motion.

7. Looking at a spot on the ceiling directly over your head involves what joint motion?

8. Putting your hand in your back pocket involves what shoulder joint motion?

9. Picking up a pencil on the floor beside your chair involves what joint motion?

10. Putting your right ankle on your left knee involves what type of hip rotation?

11. What is the only difference between *anatomical* position and *fundamental* position?

12. If you place your hand on the back of a dog, that is referred to as what surface? If you place your hand on the back of a person, that is referred to as what surface?

13. When a football is kicked through the goal posts, what type of motion is being demonstrated by the football? By the kicker?

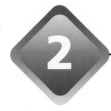

Skeletal System

Functions of the Skeleton

The skeletal system, which is made up of numerous bones, is the rigid framework of the human body. It gives support and shape to the body. It protects vital organs such as the brain, spinal cord, and heart. It assists in movement by providing a rigid structure for muscle attachment and leverage. The skeletal system also manufactures blood cells in various locations. The main sites of blood formation are the ilium, vertebra, sternum, and ribs. This formation occurs mostly in flat bones. Calcium and other mineral salts are stored throughout all osseous tissue of the skeletal system.

Types of Skeletons

The bones of the body are grouped into two main categories: axial and appendicular. The axial skeleton forms the upright part of the body. It consists of approximately 80 bones of the head, thorax, and trunk (Fig. 2–1). The appendicular skeleton attaches to the axial skeleton and contains the 126 bones of the extremities (Fig. 2–2). There are 206 bones in the body. Individuals may have additional sesamoid bones, such as in the flexor tendons of the great toe and of the thumb.

Table 2–1 lists the bones of the adult human body. The sacrum, coccyx, and hip bones are each made up of several bones fused together. In the hip bone, these fused bones are known as the *ilium, ischium,* and *pubis.*

Composition of Bone

Bones can be considered organs because they are made up of several different types of tissue (fibrous, cartilaginous, osseous, nervous, and vascular), and they function as integral parts of the skeletal system.

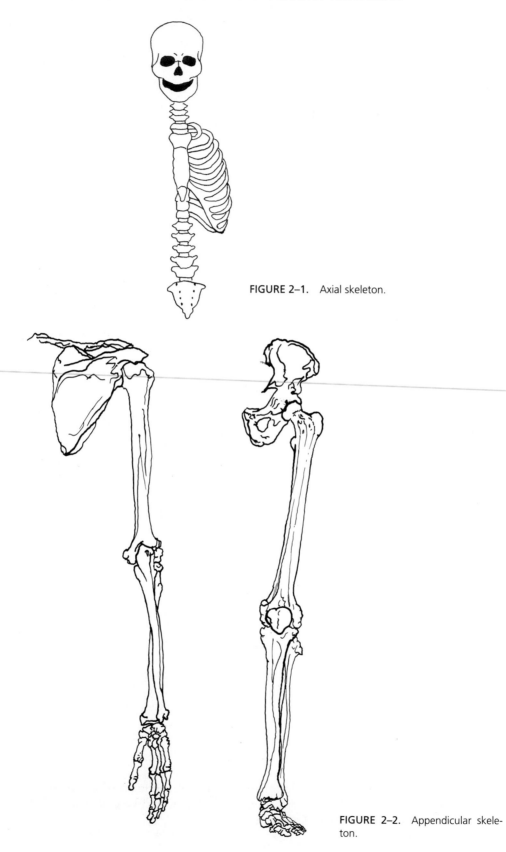

FIGURE 2–1. Axial skeleton.

FIGURE 2–2. Appendicular skeleton.

TABLE 2–1	**BONES OF THE HUMAN BODY**		
	Single	**Paired**	**Multiple**
	Axial Skeleton		
Cranium (8)	Frontal	Parietal	None
	Sphenoid	Temporal	
	Ethmoid		
	Occipital		
Face (14)	Mandible	Maxilla	None
	Vomer	Zygomatic	
		Lacrimal	
		Inferior concha	
		Palatine	
		Nasal	
Other (7)	Hyoid	Ear ossicles (3)	None
Vertebral column (26)	Sacrum (5)*	None	Cervical (7)
	Coccyx (3)*		Thoracic (12)
			Lumbar (5)
Thorax (25)	Sternum	Ribs (12 Pairs)	None
		True: 7	
		False: 3	
		Floating: 2	
	Appendicular Skeleton		
Upper Extremity (64)	None	Scapula	Carpals (8)
		Clavicle	Metacarpals (5)
		Humerus	Phalanges (14)
		Ulna	
		Radius	
Lower Extremity (62)	None	Hip (3)*	Tarsals (7)
		Femur	Metatarsals (5)
		Tibia	Phalanges (14)
		Fibula	
		Patella	

*Denotes bones that are fused together.

Bone is made up of one-third *organic* (living) material and two-thirds *inorganic* (nonliving) material. The organic material gives the bone elasticity, whereas the inorganic material provides hardness and strength, which makes bone opaque on an x-ray.

Compact bone makes up a hard, dense outer shell. It always completely covers bone and tends to be thick along the shaft and thin at the ends of long bones. It is also thick in the plates of the flat bones of the skull.

Cancellous bone is the porous and spongy inside portion called the *trabeculae,* which means "little beams" in Latin. They are arranged in a pattern that resists local stresses and strains. These trabeculae tend to be filled with marrow and make the bone lighter. Cancellous bone makes up most of the articular ends of bones.

Structure of Bone

The **epiphysis** is the area at each end of the diaphysis, and this area tends to be wider than the shaft (Fig. 2–3). In adult bone the epiphysis is osseous, but in growing bone the epiphysis is cartilaginous material and is called the **epiphyseal plate.** Here growth occurs through the manufacturing of new bone. On an x-ray, a growing bone will show a distinct line between the epiphyseal plate and the rest of the bone. Because this line does not exist in the normal adult bone, its absence indicates that bone growth has stopped.

The **diaphysis** is the main shaft of bone. It is made up mostly of compact bone, which gives it great strength. Its center, the **medullary canal,** is hollow, which, among other features, decreases the weight of the bone. This canal contains marrow and provides passage for nutrient arteries. The **endosteum** is a membrane that lines the medullary canal. It contains **osteoclasts,** which are mainly responsible for bone resorption.

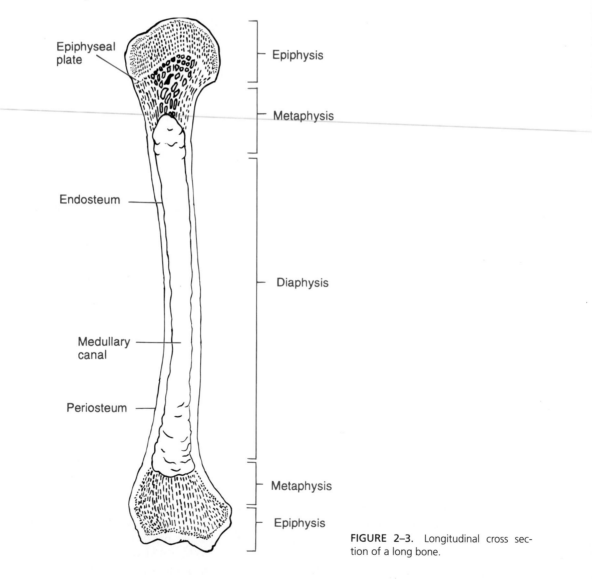

Epiphyseal plate

Endosteum

Medullary canal

Periosteum

Epiphysis

Metaphysis

Diaphysis

Metaphysis

Epiphysis

FIGURE 2–3. Longitudinal cross section of a long bone.

In long bones, the flared part at each end of the diaphysis is called the **metaphysis.** It is made up mostly of cancellous bone and functions to support the epiphysis.

Periosteum is the thin fibrous membrane covering all of the bone except the articular surfaces that are covered with hyaline cartilage. The periosteum contains nerve and blood vessels that are important in providing nourishment, promoting growth in diameter of immature bone, and repairing the bone. It also serves as an attachment point for tendons and ligaments.

Types of Bones

Long bones are so named because their length is greater than their width (Fig. 2–4A). They are the largest bones in the body and make up most of the appendicular skeleton. Long bones are basically tubular shaped with a shaft (diaphysis) and two bulbous ends (epiphysis). The wide part of the shaft nearest the epiphysis is called the **metaphysis** (see Fig. 2–3). The diaphysis consists of compact bone surrounding the marrow cavity. The metaphysis and epiphysis consist of cancellous bone covered by a thin layer of compact bone. Over the articular surfaces of the epiphysis is a thin layer of hyaline cartilage. Bone growth occurs at the epiphysis.

Short bones tend to have more equal dimensions of height, length, and width, giving them a cubical shape (Fig. 2–4B). They have a great deal of articular surface and, unlike long bones, usually articulate with more than one bone. Their composition is similar to long bones: they have a thin layer of compact bone covering cancellous bone, which has a marrow cavity in the middle. Examples include the bones of the wrist and ankle (carpals).

Flat bones have a very broad surface but are not very thick. They tend to have a curved surface rather than a flat one (Fig. 2–4C). They are made up of two layers of compact bone with cancellous bone and marrow in between. The ilium and scapula are good examples.

Irregular bones have a variety of mixed shapes, as their name implies (Fig. 2–4D). Examples are bones such as the vertebra and sacrum that do not fit into the other categories. They are also composed of cancellous bone and marrow encased in a thin layer of compact bone.

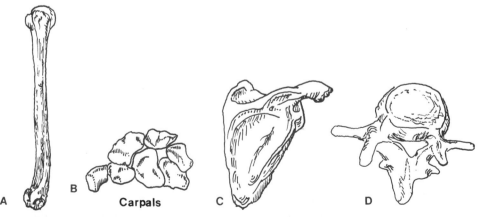

A   **B**   **Carpals**   **C**   **D**

FIGURE 2–4. Types of bones. (*A*) Long. (*B*) Short. (*C*) Flat. (*D*) Irregular.

Sesamoid bones, which resemble the shape of sesame seeds, are small bones located where tendons cross the ends of long bones in the extremities. They develop within the tendon and protect it from excessive wear. For example, the tendon of the flexor hallucis longus spans the foot and attaches on the great toe. If this tendon were not protected in some way at the ball of the foot, it would constantly be stepped on. Mother Nature is too clever to allow this to happen. Sesamoid bones are located on either side of the tendon near the head of the first metatarsal, providing a protective "groove" for the tendon to pass through this weight-bearing area.

Sesamoid bones also change the angle of attachment of a tendon. The patella can be considered a sesamoid bone because it is encased in the quadriceps tendon and improves the mechanical advantage of the quadriceps muscle. Sesamoid bones are also found in the flexor tendons that pass posteriorly into the foot on either side of the ankle. In the upper extremity they are found in the flexor tendons of the thumb near the metacarpophalangeal and interphalangeal joints. Occasionally, a sesamoid bone is located near the metacarpophalangeal joint of the index and little fingers. Table 2–2 summarizes the types of bones of the axial and appendicular skeletons. It should be noted that there are no long or short bones in the axial skeleton, and there are no irregular bones in the appendicular skeleton. Sesamoid bones are not included in Table 2–2 because they are considered accessory bones and their shape and number vary.

When looking at various bones, you will see holes, depressions, ridges, bumps, grooves, and various other kinds of markings. Each of these markings serves different purposes. Table 2–3 describes the different kinds of bone markings and their purposes.

TABLE 2–2	**TYPES OF BONES**		
Appendicular Skeleton	**Upper Extremity**	**Lower Extremity**	**Axial Skeleton**
Long bones	Clavicle	Femur	
	Humerus	Fibula	
	Radius	Tibia	
	Ulna	Metatarsals	
	Metacarpals	Phalanges	
	Phalanges		
Short bones	Carpals	Tarsals	None
Flat bones	Scapula	Ilium	Cranial bones (frontal, parietal)
		Patella	Ribs
			Sternum
Irregular bones	None	None	Vertebrae
			Cranial bones (sphenoid, ethmoid)
			Sacrum
			Coccyx
			Mandible, facial bones

TABLE 2–3	BONE MARKINGS	
Marking	**Description**	**Examples**
DEPRESSIONS AND OPENINGS		
1. Foramen	Hole through which blood vessels, nerves, and ligaments pass	Vertebral foramen of cervical vertebra
2. Fossa	Hollow or depression	Glenoid fossa of scapula
3. Groove	Ditchlike groove containing a tendon or blood vessel	Bicipital (intercondylar) groove of humerus
4. Meatus	Canal or tubelike opening in a bone	External auditory meatus
5. Sinus	Air-filled cavity within a bone	Frontal sinus in frontal bone
PROJECTIONS OR PROCESSES THAT FIT INTO JOINTS		
1. Condyle	Rounded knuckle-like projection	Medial condyle of femur
2. Eminence	Projecting, prominent part of bone	Intercondylar eminence, tibia
3. Facet	Flat or shallow articular surface	Articular facet of rib
4. Head	Rounded articular projection beyond a narrow necklike portion of bone	Femoral head
PROJECTIONS/PROCESSES THAT ATTACH TENDONS, LIGAMENTS, AND OTHER CONNECTIVE TISSUE		
1. Crest	Sharp ridge or border	Iliac crest of hip
2. Epicondyle	Prominence above or on a condyle	Medial epicondyle of humerus
3. Line	Less prominent ridge	Linea aspera of femur
4. Spine	Long, thin projection (spinous process)	Scapular spine
5. Trochanter	Very large prominence for muscle attachment	Greater trochanter of femur
6. Tubercle	Small, rounded projection	Greater tubercle of humerus
7. Tuberosity	Large, rounded projection	Ischial tuberosity

REVIEW QUESTIONS

1. What are the differences between the axial and appendicular skeletons?

2. Give an example of compact bone and one of cancellous bone.

3. Which is heavier, compact bone or cancellous bone?

4. What type of bone is mainly involved in an individual's growth in height? In what portion of the bone does this growth occur?

5. What is the purpose of sesamoid bone?

6. Identify the bone markings that can be classified as:
    a. Depressions and openings
    b. Projection or processes that fit into joints
    c. Projections or processes that attach connective tissue

Classify the following bone markings:

7. Bicipital groove

8. Humeral head

9. Acetabulum

10. Scapular spine

11. Supraspinous fossa

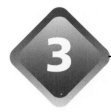

Articular System

A joint is a connection between two bones. Although joints have several functions, perhaps the most important is to allow motion. Joints also help to bear the weight of the body and to provide stability. This stability may be mostly due to the shape of the bones making up the joint, as with the hip joint, or due to soft-tissue features, as seen in the shoulder and knee. Joints also contain synovial fluid, which lubricates the joint and nourishes the cartilage.

Types of Joints

A joint may allow a great deal of motion, as in the shoulder, or very little motion as in the sternoclavicular joint. As with all differences, there are trade-offs. A joint that allows a great deal of motion will provide very little stability. Conversely, a joint that is quite stable tends to have little motion. There is often more than one term that can be used to describe the same joint. These terms tend to describe either the structure or amount of motion allowed.

A **fibrous joint** has a thin layer of fibrous periosteum between the two bones, as in the sutures of the skull. There are three types of fibrous joints: synarthrosis, syndesmosis, and gomphosis. A **synarthrosis,** or suture joint, has a thin layer of fibrous periosteum between the two bones, as in the sutures of the skull. The ends of the bones are shaped to allow them to interlock (Fig. 3–1A). With this type of joint there is essentially no motion between the bones. The purpose of this type of joint is to provide shape and strength. Another type of fibrous joint is a **syndesmosis,** or ligamentous joint. There is a great deal of fibrous tissue, such as ligaments and interosseous membranes, holding the joint together (Fig. 3–1B). A small amount of

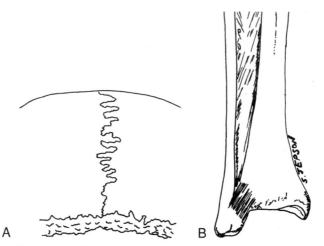

FIGURE 3–1.   Fibrous joint. (*A*) Synarthrosis (suture type). (*B*) Syndesmosis (ligamentous type).

twisting or stretching movement can occur in this type of joint. The distal tibiofibular joint at the ankle and the distal radioulnar joint are examples. The third type of fibrous joint is called *gomphosis,* which is Greek for "bolting together." This joint occurs between a tooth and the wall of its dental socket.

A **cartilaginous joint** (Fig. 3–2) has either hyaline cartilage or fibrocartilage between the two bones. The symphysis pubis is an example of a joint in which fibrocartilage directly connects the bones. The first sternocostal joint is an example of the direct connection made by hyaline cartilage. Cartilaginous joints are also called **amphiarthrodial joints** because they allow a small amount of motion, such as bending or twisting, and some compression. At the same time, these joints provide a great deal of stability.

A **synovial joint** (Fig. 3–3) has no direct union between the bone ends. Instead, there is a cavity filled with synovial fluid contained within a sleeve-like capsule. The outer layer of the capsule is made up of a strong fibrous tissue that holds the joint together. The inner layer is lined with a synovial membrane that secretes the synovial fluid. The articular surface is very smooth and covered with cartilage called *hyaline* or *articular cartilage.* The synovial joint is also called a **diarthrodial joint** because it allows free motion. It is not as stable as the other types of joints but does allow a great deal more motion. Table 3–1 provides a summary of the types of joints.

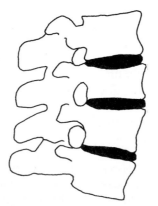

FIGURE 3–2.   Cartilaginous joint.

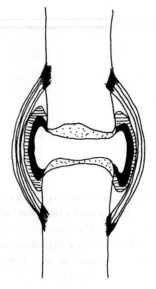

FIGURE 3–3. Synovial joint.

The number of axes, the shape of the joint, and the type of motion allowed by the joint (Table 3–2) could further classify synovial, or diarthrodial, joints.

In **a nonaxial joint,** movement tends to be linear instead of angular (Fig. 3–4). The joint surfaces arc relatively flat and glide over one another instead of one moving around the other. The motion that occurs between the carpal bones is an example of this type of motion. Unlike most other types of diarthrodial joint motion, nonaxial motion occurs secondarily to other motion. For example, you can flex and extend your elbow without moving other joints; however, you cannot move your carpal bones by themselves. Motion of the carpals occurs when the wrist joint moves in either flexion/extension or abduction/adduction.

A **uniaxial joint** has angular motion occurring in one plane around one axis, much like a hinge. The elbow, or humeroulnar joint, is a good example of the convex shape of the humerus fitting into the concave-shaped ulna. The only motions possible are flexion and extension, which occur in the sagittal plane around the frontal axis. There are no other motions possible at this joint. The interphalangeal joints of the hand and foot also have this hinge motion (Fig. 3–5). The knee is a hinge joint, but this example must be clarified. During the last few degrees of extension, the femur rotates medially on the tibia. This rotation is not an active motion but the result of certain mechanical features present. Therefore, the knee is best classified as a uniaxial joint because it has *active* motion only around one axis.

TABLE 3–1	JOINT CLASSIFICATION		
Type	**Motion**	**Structure**	**Example**
Synarthrosis	None	Fibrous—suture	Bones in the skull
Syndesmosis	Slight	Fibrous—ligamentous	Distal tibiofibular
Amphiarthrosis	Little	Cartilaginous	Symphysis pubis, vertebrae
Diarthrosis	Free	Synovial	Hip, elbow, knee

TABLE 3-2	CLASSIFICATION OF DIARTHROIDAL JOINTS		
Number of Axes	**Shape of Joint**	**Joint Motion**	**Example**
Nonaxial	Irregular (plane)	Gliding	Intercarpals
Uniaxial	Hinge	Flexion/extension	Elbow and knee
	Pivot	Rotation	Atlas/axis, radius/ulna
Biaxial	Condyloid	Flexion/extension, abduction/adduction	Wrist, MPs
	Saddle	Flexion/extension, abduction/adduction, rotation (accessory)	Thumb, CMC
Triaxial (multiaxial)	Ball and socket	Flexion/extension, abduction/adduction, rotation	Shoulder, hip

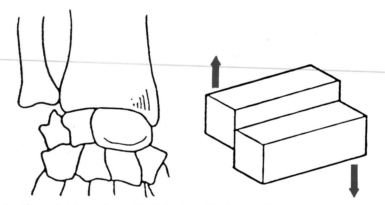

FIGURE 3–4.   Plane joint. (From Swan, B [ed]: Body on File. Facts on File, New York, 1983, p 05.006, with permission.)

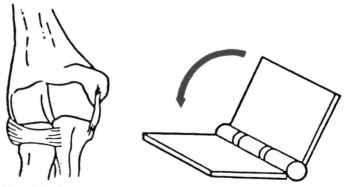

FIGURE 3–5.   Hinge joint. (From Swan, R [ed]: Body on File. Facts on File, New York, 1983, p 05.006, with permission.)

Also at the elbow is the radioulnar joint, which demonstrates another type of uniaxial motion. The head of the radius pivots around the stationary ulna during pronation and supination of the forearm. This pivot motion is in the transverse plane around the longitudinal axis. The motion of the atlantoaxial joint of C1 and C2 is also pivot motion (Fig. 3–6). The first cervical vertebra (*atlas*), on which the head rests, rotates around the odontoid process of the second cervical vertebra (*axis*). This allows the head to rotate.

Biaxial joint motion, such as that found at the wrist, occurs in two different directions (Fig. 3–7). Flexion and extension occur around the frontal axis, and radial and ulnar deviation occur around the sagittal axis. This bidirectional motion also occurs at the metaphalangeal (MP) joints, where they are referred to as **condyloid** or **ellipsoidal** joints because of their shape.

The carpometacarpal (CMC) joint of the thumb is biaxial but differs somewhat from the condyloid joint. In this joint, the articular surface of each bone is concave in one direction and convex in the other. The bones fit together like a horseback rider in a saddle, which is why this joint is also called a **saddle joint** (Fig. 3–8).

The CMC joint is unlike the condyloid joint in that it allows a slight amount of rotation. Like the motion within the carpal bones, this rotation cannot occur by itself. If you try to rotate your thumb without also flexing and abducting, you find that you cannot do it. Yet, rotation does occur. Look at the direction to which the pad of your thumb is pointing when it is adducted. Abduct and flex your thumb and notice that the direction to which the pad is pointing has changed by approximately 90 degrees. This rotation has not occurred actively; rotation has occurred because of the shape of the joint. Therefore, although the CMC joint of the thumb is not a true biaxial joint because of the rotation allowed, it fits into this category best because the *active* motion allowed is around two axes.

With a **triaxial joint,** sometimes referred to as a *multiaxial joint,* motion occurs actively in all three axes (Fig. 3–9). The hip and shoulder allow motion in the frontal axis (flexion and extension), in the sagittal axis (abduction and adduction), and in the vertical axis (rotation). Obviously, triaxial joints allow more motion than any other type of joint. The triaxial joint is also referred to as a **ball-and-socket joint** because in the hip, for example, the ball-shaped femoral head fits into the concave socket of the acetabulum.

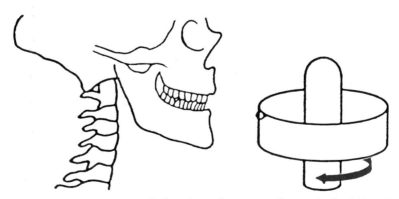

FIGURE 3–6.   Pivot joint. (From Swan, R [ed]: Body on File. Facts on File, New York, 1983, p 05.006, with permission.)

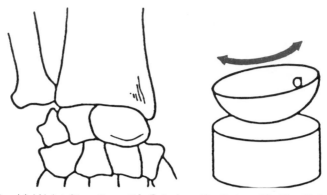

FIGURE 3–7.   Gondyloid joint. (From Swan, R [ed]: Body on File. Facts on File, New York, 1983, p 05.006, with permission.)

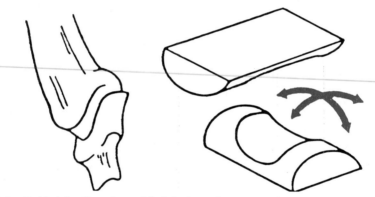

FIGURE 3–8.   Saddle joint. (From Swan, R [ed]: Body on File. Facts on File, New York, 1983, p 05.006, with permission.)

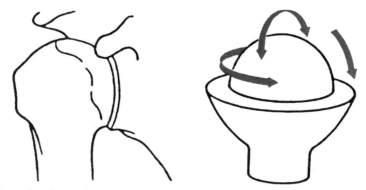

FIGURE 3–9.   Ball-and-socket joint. (From Swan, R [ed]: Body on File. Facts on File, New York, 1983, p 05.006, with permission.)

Joint Structure

There are many other structures associated with synovial joints (Fig. 3–10). First, there are **bones,** usually two, that articulate with each other. The amount of motion allowed at each joint and the direction of that motion are dictated by the shape of the bone ends and by the articular surface of each bone. For example, the shoulder joint has a smooth articular surface over most of the humeral head as well as over the *glenoid fossa* (shoulder socket). As a result, there is a great deal of shoulder motion, and that motion occurs in all directions. The knee, on the other hand, has a great deal of motion but in a specific direction. In examining the distal end of the femur, you will note that there are two ridges much like the rocker surfaces of a rocking chair. The proximal end of the tibia has two articular surfaces with a high area (intercondylar eminence) in between them. These articular surfaces allow a great deal of motion but, like the rocking chair, in only one direction.

The two bones of a joint are held together and supported by **ligaments,** which are bands of fibrous connective tissue. Ligaments also provide attachment for cartilage, fascia, or, in some cases, muscle. Ligaments are flexible but not elastic. This flexibility is needed to allow joint motion, but the nonelasticity is needed to keep the bones in close approximation to each other and to provide some protection to the joint. When ligaments surround a joint, they are called *capsular ligaments*.

In every synovial joint there is a joint **capsule** that surrounds and encases the joint and protects the articular surfaces of the bones (Fig. 3–11). In the shoulder joint, the capsule completely encases the joint, forming a partial vacuum that helps hold the head of the humerus against the glenoid fossa. In other joints, the capsule may not be as complete.

There are two layers to the capsule. There is the outer layer, which is made up of fibrous tissue and provides the support and protection to the joint. This fibrous layer is usually reinforced by ligaments. The inner layer is lined with a **synovial membrane,** which is a thick, vascular connective tissue that secretes synovial fluid.

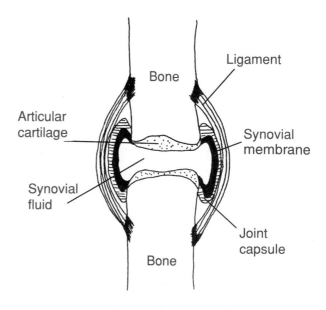

FIGURE 3–10. Synovial joint, longitudinal cross-section.

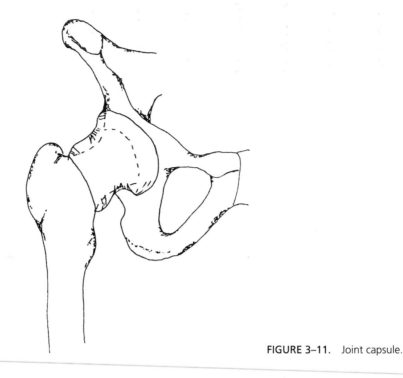

FIGURE 3–11.   Joint capsule.

Synovial fluid is a thick, clear fluid, much like the white of an egg that lubricates the articular cartilage. This substance reduces friction and helps to keep the joint moving freely. It provides some shock absorption and is the major source of nutrition for articular cartilage.

Cartilage is a dense fibrous connective tissue capable of withstanding a great amount of pressure and tension. There are basically three types of cartilage in the body: hyaline, fibrocartilage, and elastic. **Hyaline cartilage,** also called **articular cartilage,** covers the ends of opposing bones. With the help of synovial fluid, it provides a smooth articulating surface in all synovial joints. Hyaline cartilage has no blood or nerve supply of its own and must get its nutrition from the synovial fluid. Therefore, when it is damaged it is unable to repair itself.

Fibrocartilage acts as a shock absorber. This is especially important in weight-bearing joints such as the knee and vertebrae. At the knee, the semilunar-shaped cartilage called *menisci* build up the sides of the relatively flat articular surface of the tibia. Between the vertebral bones are the intervertebral **disks.** Because of their very dense structure, these disks are capable of absorbing an amazing amount of shock that is transmitted upward from weight-bearing forces.

In the upper extremity there is a fibrocartilaginous disk located between the clavicle and sternum. It is important for absorbing the shock transmitted along the clavicle to the sternum should you fall on your outstretched hand. This disk helps prevent dislocation of the sternoclavicular joint. It is also important in allowing motion. The disk, which is attached to the sternum at one end and the clavicle at the other, is much like a swinging door hinge that allows motion in both directions. This double-hung hinge allows the clavicle to move on the sternum as the acromial end is elevated and depressed. In effect, the fibrocartilage divides the joint into two cavities, allowing two sets of motion.

There are other functions of fibrocartilage in joints. The shoulder fibrocartilage, called **labrum,** deepens the shallow glenoid fossa, making it more of a socket to hold the humeral head (Fig. 3–12). Fibrocartilage also fills the gap between two bones. If you examine the wrist, you will notice that the ulna does not extend all the way to the carpal bones as does the radius. In this gap there is located a small triangular disk that acts as a space filler and allows force to be exerted on the ulna and carpals without causing damage.

The third type of cartilage, **elastic cartilage,** is designed to allow a certain amount of motion. It is found in the symphysis pubis and allows the motion necessary for childbirth. It is also found in the larynx, where its motion is important to speech.

Muscles provide the contractile force that causes joints to move. They must, therefore, span the joint to have an effect on that joint. Muscles are soft and cannot attach directly to the bone. A **tendon** must connect them. The tendon may be a cylindrical cord, like the long head of the biceps tendon, or a flattened band, like the rotator cuff. In certain locations tendons are encased in **tendon sheaths.** These fibrous sleeves surround the tendon when it is subject to pressure or friction, such as when it passes between muscles and bones or through a tunnel between bones. The tendons passing over the wrist all have tendon sheaths. These sheaths are lubricated by fluid secreted from their lining. An **aponeurosis** is a broad, flat tendinous sheet. Aponeuroses are found in several places where muscles attach to bones. The large, powerful latissimus dorsi muscle is attached at one end over a large area to several bones by means of an aponeurosis. In the anterior abdominal wall aponeuroses provide a base of muscular attachment where no bone is present but where great strength is needed. As the abdominal muscles approach the midline from both sides, they attach to an aponeurosis called the **linea alba.**

Found around most joints are small padlike sacs called **bursae.** Bursae are located in areas of excessive friction, such as under tendons and over bony prominences (Fig. 3–13). These sacs are lined with synovial membrane and filled with a clear fluid. Their purpose is to reduce friction between moving parts. For example, in the shoulder the deltoid muscle passes directly over the acromion process. Repeated motion would cause excessive wearing of the muscle tissue. However, the subdeltoid bursa, located between the muscle and acromion process, prevents excessive friction and reduces the likelihood of damage. The same arrangement occurs in the elbow where the triceps tendon attaches to the olecranon process. Some joints, such as the knee, have many bursae.

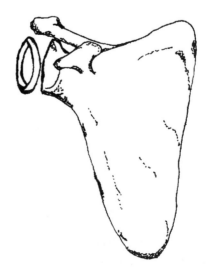

FIGURE 3–12. Labrum.

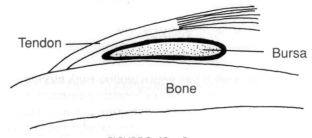

FIGURE 3–13.   Bursa.

There are two types of bursa: natural bursa, which has just been discussed, and acquired bursa. It is possible to develop a bursa in an area that normally does not have excessive friction if, for some reason, this area has become the site of excessive friction. These *acquired bursae* tend to occur in places other than joints. For example, a person may develop a bursa on the lateral side of the third finger of the writing hand. This is often called the "student's bursa" because students often do a lot of writing and note taking. These bursae disappear when the activity is stopped or greatly reduced.

Planes and Axes

Planes of action are fixed lines of reference along which the body is divided. There are three planes, and each plane is at right angles, or perpendicular, to the other two planes (Fig. 3–14).

The **sagittal plane** passes through the body from front to back and divides the body into right and left parts. Think of it as a vertical wall that the extremity moves along. Motions occurring in this plane are flexion and extension.

The **frontal plane** passes through the body from side to side and divides the body into front and back parts. It is also called the *coronal plane*. Motions occurring in this plane are abduction and adduction.

The **transverse plane** passes through the body horizontally and divides the body into top and bottom parts. It is also called the *horizontal plane*. Rotation occurs in this plane.

Whenever a plane passes through the midline of a part, whether it is the sagittal, frontal, or transverse plane, it is referred to as a cardinal plane because it divides the body into equal parts. The point where the three cardinal planes intersect each other is the **center of gravity.** In the human body that point is in the midline at about the level of, though slightly anterior to, the second sacral vertebra (Fig. 3–15).

Axes are points that run through the center of a joint around which a part rotates (Fig. 3–16). The **sagittal axis** is a point that runs through a joint from front to back. The **frontal axis** runs through a joint from side to side. The **vertical axis,** also called the *longitudinal axis,* runs through a joint from top to bottom.

Joint movement occurs around an axis that is always perpendicular to its plane. Another way of stating this is that joint movement occurs *in a plane* and *around an axis.* A particular motion will always occur in the same plane and around the same axis. For example, flexion/extension will always occur in the sagittal plane around the frontal axis. Abduction/adduction will always occur in the frontal plane around the sagittal axis. Similar motions, such as radial and ulnar deviation of the wrist, will also occur in the frontal plane around the sagittal axis. The thumb is the exception

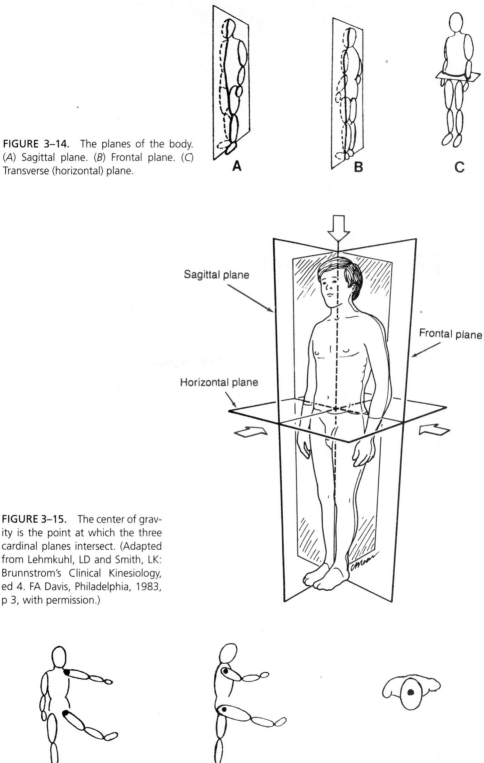

FIGURE 3–14. The planes of the body. (*A*) Sagittal plane. (*B*) Frontal plane. (*C*) Transverse (horizontal) plane.

Sagittal plane

Frontal plane

Horizontal plane

FIGURE 3–15. The center of gravity is the point at which the three cardinal planes intersect. (Adapted from Lehmkuhl, LD and Smith, LK: Brunnstrom's Clinical Kinesiology, ed 4. FA Davis, Philadelphia, 1983, p 3, with permission.)

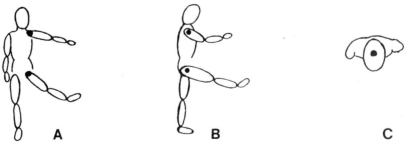

FIGURE 3–16. The axes of the body. (*A*) Sagittal axis. (*B*) Frontal axis. (*C*) Vertical axis.

TABLE 3–3	JOINT MOTIONS	
Plane	**Axis**	**Joint Motion**
Sagittal	Frontal	Flexion/extension
Frontal	Sagittal	Abduction/adduction
		Radial/ulnar deviation
		Eversion/inversion
Transverse	Vertical	Medial/lateral rotation
		Supination/pronation
		Right/left rotation
		Horizontal abduction/adduction

because flexion/extension and abduction/adduction do not occur in these traditional planes. These motions, and their planes and axes, will be discussed in Chapter 11. Table 3–3 summarizes joint motion in relation to planes and axes.

Degrees of Freedom

Joints can also be described by the **degrees of freedom,** or number of planes, in which they can move. For example, a uniaxial joint has motion around one axis and in one plane. Therefore, it has one degree of freedom. A biaxial joint would have two degrees of freedom, and a triaxial joint would have three, which is the maximum number of degrees of freedom that an individual joint can have.

This concept becomes significant when dealing with one or more distal joints. For example, the shoulder has three degrees of freedom, the elbow and radioulnar joints each have one, and together they have five degrees of freedom. The entire limb from the finger to the shoulder would have 11 degrees of freedom.

REVIEW QUESTIONS

1. There are three types of a joint that allows no motion. They are:

2. The two terms for a joint that allows a great deal of motion are:

3. Diarthrodial joints can be described in terms of three features.

   They are:

   a. _____

   b. _____

   c. _____

   Give an example of each feature and of a joint that has that feature.

4. What type of joint structure connects bone to muscle?

5. What type of joint structure pads and protects *areas* of great friction?

6. What are the five features of a synovial joint?

7. How does hyaline cartilage differ from fibrocartilage? Give an example of each type of cartilage.

8. When the anterior surface of the forearm moves toward the anterior surface of the humerus, what joint motion is involved? In what plane is the motion occurring? Around what axis?

9. What joint motion is involved in turning the palm of the hand? In what plane and around what axis does that joint motion occur?

10. What joint motion is involved in returning the fingers to anatomical position from the fully spread position? In what plane and around what axis does the joint motion occur?

11. Identify the 11 degrees of freedom of the upper limb.

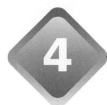

Muscular System

Muscle Attachments

When a muscle contracts, it knows no direction; it simply shortens. If a muscle were unattached at both ends and stimulated, the two ends would move toward the middle. However, muscles are attached to bones and cross at least one joint, so when a muscle contracts, one end of the joint moves toward the other bone (Fig. 4–1A). The more movable bone, often referred to as the **insertion,** moves toward the more stable bone, the **origin.** For example, when the biceps brachii muscle contracts, the forearm moves toward the humerus, as when bringing a glass toward your mouth. The humerus is more stable because it is attached to the axial skeleton at the shoulder joint. The forearm is more movable because it is attached to the hand, which is quite movable. Therefore, the insertion is moving toward the origin or, explained another way, the more movable end is moving toward the more stable end. Another point that can be made about muscle attachments is that origins tend to be closer to the trunk and insertions tend to be more toward the distal end.

This arrangement can be reversed if the more movable end becomes less movable. For example, what would happen if the hand were holding onto a thinning bar when the biceps contracted? The biceps would still flex the elbow, but now the humerus would move toward the forearm. In other words, the origin would move toward the insertion (Fig. 4–1B). Some sources refer to this as **reversal of muscle action.** However, you should realize that the same joint motion is occurring (in this

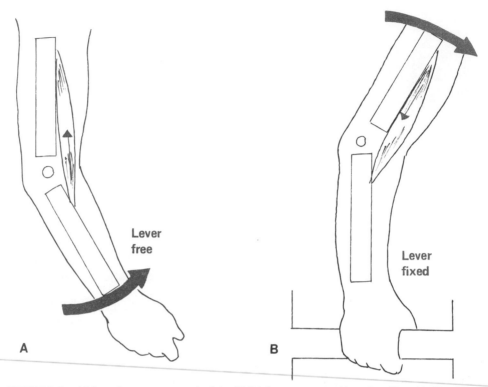

FIGURE 4–1.   (A) Insertion moves toward origin. (B) Origin moves toward insertion. (From Norkin, CN and Levangie, PK: Joint Structure and Function, ed 2. FA Davis, Philadelphia, 1992, p 107, with permission.)

case, elbow flexion). What has changed is that instead of the insertion moving toward the origin, the origin is now moving toward the insertion. The proximal bone, which is usually more stable, has become more movable.

Consider another example in a very simplistic form. Lying on your back, bring your knees up toward your chest. Using your hip flexors to flex your hip, you are moving the femur (more movable) toward your chest (more stable), or insertion toward origin. If someone holds your feet down, your femur would become the more stable end and your trunk, the more movable end. When your hip flexors contracted, the origin would move toward the insertion. Closed kinetic chain exercises are based on the distal segment being fixed, which is another way of applying reversal of muscle action. Open and closed kinetic chains will be discussed later in this chapter.

Muscle Names

The name of a muscle can often tell you a great deal about that muscle. Muscle names tend to fall into one or more of the following categories:

1. Location
2. Shape
3. Action
4. Number of heads or divisions
5. Attachments = origin/insertion
6. Direction of the fibers
7. Size of the muscle

The tibialis anterior, as its name indicates, is located on the anterior surface of the tibia. The rectus (straight) abdominis muscle is a vertical muscle located on the abdomen. The trapezius muscle has a trapezoid shape, and the serratus anterior muscle (Fig. 4–2) has a serrated or jagged-shaped attachment located anteriorly. The name of the extensor carpi ulnaris muscle tells you that its action is to extend the wrist (carpi) on the ulnar side. The triceps brachii muscle is a three-headed muscle on the arm, and the biceps femoris muscle is a two-headed muscle on the thigh. The sternocleidomastoid muscle (Fig. 4–3) attaches on the sternum, clavicle, and mastoid bones. The names of the external and internal oblique muscles describe the direction of the fibers and their location to one another. In the same way, the names pectoralis major and pectoralis minor indicate that although both of these muscles are in the same area, one is greater in size than the other.

Muscle Fiber Arrangement

Muscle fibers are arranged within the muscle in a direction that is either parallel or oblique to the long axis of the muscle. **Parallel muscle** fibers tend to be longer, thus having a greater range of motion potential. **Oblique muscle fibers** tend to be shorter but are more numerous per given area than parallel fibers, which means that oblique-fibered muscles tend to have a greater strength potential but a smaller range-of-motion potential than parallel-fibered muscles. There are many types of each muscle fiber arrangement in the body.

Parallel-fibered muscles can be strap, fusiform, rhomboidal (rectangular), or triangular in shape. **Strap muscles** are muscles that are long and thin with fibers running the entire length of the muscle (Fig. 4–4A). The sartorius muscle in the lower extremity, the rectus abdominis in the trunk, and the sternocleidomastoid in the neck are examples of strap muscles.

A **fusiform muscle** has a shape similar to that of a spindle (Fig. 4–4B). It is wider in the middle and tapers at both ends where it attaches to tendons. Most, but not all, fibers run the length of the muscle. The muscle may be any length or size,

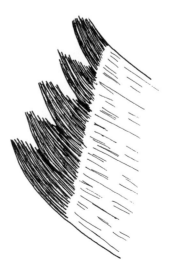

FIGURE 4–2. The serratus anterior muscle has a saw-toothed shape.

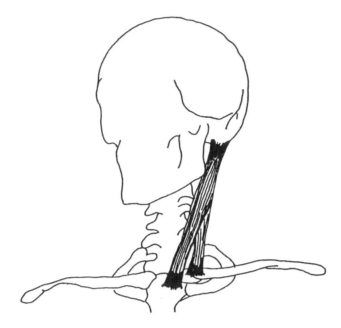

FIGURE 4–3. The sternocleido-mastoid muscle is named for its attachments on the sternum, clavicle, and mastoid bone.

from long to short or large to small. Examples of fusiform muscles can be found in the elbow flexors; that is, the biceps, brachialis, and brachioradialis.

A **rhomboidal muscle** is four-sided, usually flat, with broad attachments at each end (Fig. 4–4C). Examples of this muscle shape are the pronator quadratus in the forearm, the rhomboids in the shoulder girdle, and the gluteus maximus in the hip region.

Triangular muscles are flat and fan shaped with fibers radiating from a narrow attachment at one end to a broad attachment at the other (Fig. 4–4D). An example of this type of muscle is the pectoralis major in the chest.

Oblique-fibered muscles have a feather arrangement in which a muscle attaches at an oblique angle to its tendon, much like feather tendrils attach to the quill. The different types of oblique-fibered muscles are unipennate, bipennate, and multipennate.

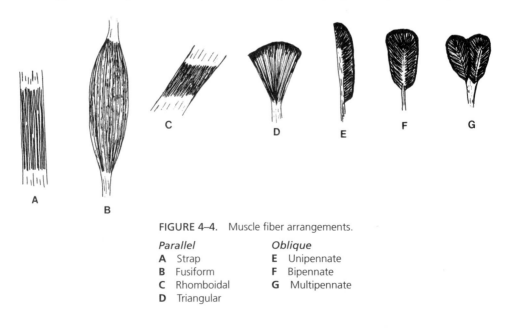

FIGURE 4–4. Muscle fiber arrangements.

Parallel	*Oblique*
A Strap	**E** Unipennate
B Fusiform	**F** Bipennate
C Rhomboidal	**G** Multipennate
D Triangular	

Unipennate muscles look like one side of a feather (Fig. 4–4E). There are a series of short fibers attaching diagonally along the length of a central tendon. Examples are the tibialis posterior muscle of the ankle, semimembranosus of the hip and knee, and the flexor pollicis longus muscle of the hand.

The **bipennate muscle** pattern looks like that of a common feather (Fig. 4–4F). Its fibers are obliquely attached to both sides of a central tendon. The rectus femoris muscle of the hip and the interossei muscles of the hand are examples of this pattern.

Multipennate muscles have many tendons with oblique fibers in between (Fig. 4–4G). The deltoid and subscapularis muscles at the shoulder demonstrate this pattern.

Functional Characteristics of Muscle Tissue

Muscle tissue has the properties of irritability, contractility, extensibility, and elasticity. No other tissue in the body has all of these characteristics. To better understand these properties, you might find it helpful to know that muscles have a normal resting length. This is defined as the length of a muscle when it is unstimulated, that is, when there are no forces or stresses placed upon it. **Irritability** is the ability to respond to a stimulus. A muscle contracts when stimulated. This can be a natural stimulus from a motor nerve or an artificial stimulus such as an electrical current. **Contractility** is the ability to shorten or contract, thus producing tension between its ends. This may result in the muscle shortening, staying the same, or lengthening. **Extensibility** is the ability of a muscle to stretch or lengthen when a force is applied. **Elasticity** is the ability to recoil or return to normal resting length when the stretching or shortening force is removed. Saltwater taffy has extensibility, but not elasticity. You can stretch it, but once the force is removed the taffy will remain stretched. A wire spring has both extensibility and elasticity. Stretch the wire, and it will lengthen. Remove the stretch, and the wire spring will return to its original length. The same can be said of a muscle. However, unlike the taffy or wire spring, a muscle is able to shorten from its normal resting length.

The properties of a muscle are summarized as follows: Stretch a muscle, and it will lengthen (extensibility). Remove the stretch, and it will return to its normal resting position (elasticity). Stimulate a muscle, and it will respond (irritability) by shortening (contractility); then remove the stimulus and it will return to its normal resting position (elasticity).

Length-Tension Relationship in Muscle Tissue

Tension refers to the force built up within the muscle, which is necessary for a muscle to contract or recoil. Stretching a muscle builds up tension within the muscle, and contracting that muscle releases tension.

A muscle is capable of being shortened to approximately one half of its normal resting length. For example, a muscle that is approximately 6 inches long can shorten to approximately 3 inches. Also, a muscle can be stretched twice as far as it can be shortened. Therefore, this same muscle can be stretched 3 inches beyond its resting length to an overall length of 9 inches; in other words, the muscle can be stretched 3 inches beyond its resting length. The **excursion** of a muscle is that distance from maximum elongation to maximum shortening. In this example, the excursion would be 6 inches (Fig. 4–5). The excursion ratio from maximum elongation to maximum shortening in most muscles is approximately 2:1.

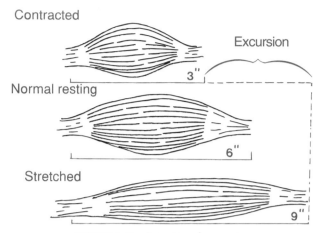

FIGURE 4–5. Excursion of a muscle.

Usually a muscle has sufficient excursion to allow the joint to move through the joint's entire range. This is certainly true of muscles that span only one joint. However, a muscle that spans two or more joints may not have sufficient excursion to allow the joint to move through its full range.

It has been demonstrated that a muscle is strongest if put on a slight stretch prior to contracting. Many examples of this concept can be cited. Think of what you do when kicking a ball. First you hyperextend your hip and then flex it forcefully. In other words, you put the hip flexors on a stretch before contracting them. There is an optimum range of a muscle where it contracts effectively. As with a rubber band, a muscle contraction is strongest when it is on a stretch, and it loses power quickly as it becomes shortened. Therefore, two-joint muscles have the advantage over one-joint muscles of maintaining maximum contractile force through a greater range. They do so by contracting over one joint while being elongated over another. Consider your hamstring muscles as you climb up stairs. Remember that they extend the hip and flex the knee. When you go up stairs, your hip goes into extension while your knee also goes into extension. In other words, the hamstring muscles are being shortened over the hip while they are being elongated over the knee. So instead of them becoming actively insufficient, they maintain an optimum length-tension relationship throughout the range.

ACTIVE AND PASSIVE INSUFFICIENCY

In a one-joint muscle, the excursion of the muscle will be greater than the range allowed by the joint. However, with a two-joint or a multijoint muscle, the muscle's excursion is less than the combined range allowed by the joints. The tension within the muscle becomes insufficient at both extremes. Brunnstrom uses the terms "active" and "passive insufficiency" to describe these conditions. When a muscle reaches a point where it cannot shorten any farther, it is called **active insufficiency.** Active insufficiency occurs to the agonist (the muscle that is contracting). When a muscle cannot be elongated any farther without damage to the fibers, it is called **passive insufficiency.** Passive insufficiency occurs to the antagonist (the muscle that is relaxed and is on the opposite side of the joint from the agonist).

Consider the example given for active insufficiency. The hamstring muscles are two-joint muscles located on the posterior thigh. They extend the hip and flex the knee. There is sufficient tension to perform either one of these motions but not both simultaneously. If you flex your knee while your hip is slightly flexed, you complete the full range of motion. However, if you flex your knee while your hip is extended, you will notice that you cannot complete the full range because the muscles do not have enough power (Fig. 4–6). They have become actively insufficient. Be careful when trying this exercise that you do not get a muscle cramp. In other words, in this two-joint muscle contracting over both joints at the same time, the muscle (hamstring) will run out of the ability to contract before the joints (hip and knee) run out of range of motion.

For an example of passive insufficiency, consider the hamstring muscle as an antagonist. This muscle is long enough to be stretched over each joint individually, but not both. If you flex your hip with your knee flexed, you can complete the range (Fig. 4–7). You can also extend your knee fully when the hip is extended. However, in a sitting position, put your foot on the ground with the knee fully extended. Now flex your hip by leaning forward. Note that well before you reach full hip flexion, you are experiencing pain in the posterior thigh. Your hamstring muscles are telling you to stop. They have become passively insufficient, and they cannot be stretched farther.

Stretching

Generally speaking, an agonist usually becomes actively insufficient (cannot contract any farther) before the antagonist becomes passively insufficient (cannot be stretched farther). In physical therapy, we will purposely stretch a muscle to either maintain or regain its normal resting length. Some activities require a great deal of flexibility, so stretching is done to lengthen the resting length of a muscle. In all of these situations, stretching is performed on *relaxed* muscles. A person is put in a position that

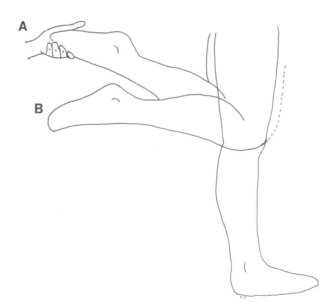

FIGURE 4–6.   Active insufficiency of the hamstring muscle. (*A*) Passive range of motion. (*B*) Active range of motion. (Adapted from Backhouse, KM and Hutchings, RT: Color Atlas of Surface Anatomy: Clinical and Applied. Williams & Wilkins, Baltimore, 1986, p 16.)

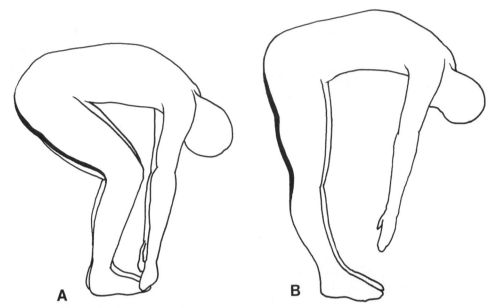

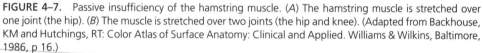

FIGURE 4–7. Passive insufficiency of the hamstring muscle. (*A*) The hamstring muscle is stretched over one joint (the hip). (*B*) The muscle is stretched over two joints (the hip and knee). (Adapted from Backhouse, KM and Hutchings, RT: Color Atlas of Surface Anatomy: Clinical and Applied. Williams & Wilkins, Baltimore, 1986, p 16.)

will stretch a muscle, usually a two-joint muscle, over all joints simultaneously within the pain limits of that muscle. So if you wanted to stretch your hamstring muscles, you would put the knee in extension and slowly flex the hip to the point where you feel discomfort but not beyond to the point of extreme pain. To stretch a one-joint muscle, it is necessary to put any two-joint muscles on a slack over the joint not spanned by the one joint-muscle. In other words, to stretch the soleus muscle, which spans the ankle only, the gastrocnemius muscle, which spans the ankle and knee, must be put on a slack over the knee. This can be accomplished by flexing the knee while dorsiflexing the ankle. Otherwise, if you attempt to dorsiflex the ankle and the knee is extended, you may be stretching the gastrocnemius more than the soleus.

There are various methods of stretching used for different situations and sometimes for different results. These different methods are important, but beyond the scope of this discussion.

Tendon Action of a Muscle (Tenodesis)

Some degree of opening and closing the hand can be accomplished by using this principle of passive insufficiency. The finger flexors and extensors are multijoint muscles. They span the wrist, the metaphalangeal (MP) joints, and the interphalangeal (IP) joints. We have already noticed that a two-joint or a multijoint muscle does not have sufficient length to be stretched over all joints simultaneously. Therefore, something has to give. If you rest your elbow on the table and flex your wrist, you will notice that your fingers have a tendency to open (Fig. 4–8). Conversely, if you hyperextend your wrist, your fingers have a tendency to close. If these tendons were a little tight, this opening and closing would be more pronounced. This is called *tenodesis* or tendon action of a muscle. A person who has quadriplegic movement

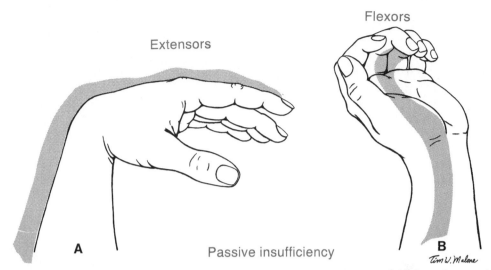

Extensors

Flexors

A   Passive insufficiency   **B**

Tim W. Malone

FIGURE 4–8.   An example of tenodesis, the functional use of passive insufficiency of the finger flexor and extensor muscles. (*A*) Passive insufficiency of the finger extensor muscles. These muscles cannot be stretched over the wrist and the MP and IP joints at the same time; therefore, when the wrist is flexed, the fingers extend. (*B*) Passive insufficiency of the finger flexor muscles. These muscles cannot be stretched over the wrist and the MP and IP joints at the same time; therefore, when the wrist is extended, the fingers flex. (From Norkin, CN and Levangie, PK: Joint Structure and Function, ed 2. FA Davis, Philadelphia, 1992, p 117, with permission.)

and has no voluntary ability to open and close the fingers can use this principle to grasp and release some objects. By supinating the forearm, gravity causes the wrist to fall into hyperextension, thus closing the fingers. Pronating the forearm causes the wrist to fall into flexion, thus opening the fingers.

Types of Muscle Contraction

There are three basic types of muscle contraction: isometric, isotonic, and isokinetic. An **isometric contraction** occurs when muscle contracts, producing force without changing the length of muscle (Fig. 4–9A). To demonstrate this action, in the sitting position place your right hand under your thigh and place your left hand on your right biceps muscle. Now, pull up with your right hand or, in other words, attempt to flex your right elbow. Note that there was no real motion at the elbow joint, but you did feel the muscle contract. This is an isometric contraction of your right biceps muscle. The muscle contracted, but no joint motion occurred.

Next, hold a weight in your hand while flexing your elbow to bring the weight up toward your shoulder (Fig. 4–9B). You will feel the biceps muscle contract, but this time there is joint motion. This is an **isotonic contraction.** An isotonic contraction occurs when a muscle contracts, the muscle length changes, and the joint angle changes.

Occasionally you will read a text that describes an isometric contraction as a *static,* or *tonic, contraction* and an isotonic contraction as *phasic.* Although these terms mean essentially the same thing, they have fallen into disuse, and specific differences between these terms no longer seem relevant.

An isotonic contraction can be subdivided into concentric and eccentric con-

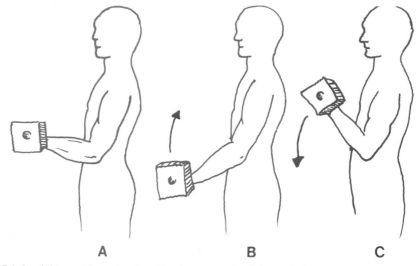

FIGURE 4–9. (*A*) Isometric contraction. Muscle *contracts* but joint angle does not change. (*B*) Isotonic contraction—concentric. Muscle contracts and joint angle increases. (*C*) Isotonic contraction—eccentric. Muscle contracts and joint angle decreases.

tractions. A **concentric contraction** occurs when there is joint movement, the muscles shorten, and the muscle attachments (O and I) move toward each other (Fig. 4–9B). Picking up the weight, as described earlier, is an example of a concentric contraction of the biceps muscle.

If you continue to palpate the biceps muscle while setting the weight back down on the table, you will feel that the biceps muscle (not the triceps muscle) continues to contract, even though the joint motion is elbow extension. What is occurring is an eccentric contraction of the biceps muscle.

An **eccentric contraction** occurs when there is joint motion but the muscle appears to lengthen; that is, the muscle attachments separate (Fig. 4–9C). Realize that after bringing the weight up to shoulder level, if you relaxed your biceps muscle, your hand and weight would drop to the table. If you used your triceps muscle, (which would extend the elbow concentrically), your hand and weight would fall onto the tabletop with some force and speed. However, what you did by slowly returning the weight to the tabletop was to slow down the pull of gravity.

Eccentric contractions are sometimes referred to as *lengthening contractions*. This is somewhat misleading because, although the muscle is lengthening at a gross level, it is shortening microscopically. What the muscle is actually doing is returning to its normal resting position from a shortened position. This type of contraction can produce much greater forces than a concentric contraction can.

In physical therapy, we frequently use these different types of muscle contractions in various exercises. Quadriceps "setting" exercises are isometric contractions of the quadriceps muscle. Flexing and extending the knee are isotonic contractions. Sitting on a table and straightening the knee is a concentric contraction of the quadriceps muscle, whereas bending the knee would be an eccentric contraction of the quadriceps muscle. If you were lying on the floor in a prone position and flexed your knee, it would be a concentric contraction of the hamstring muscles. Straightening your knee would be an eccentric contraction of the same muscles. What is happening? Straightening the knee while sitting, and bending the knee while prone involve moving the part *against gravity*. Bending the knee while sitting, and straightening the knee while prone involve moving the part *with gravity* and actually slowing down gravity. Generally speaking, eccentric contractions are used in deceleration activities and concentric contractions are used in acceleration activities.

Changing this example slightly will illustrate another feature of concentric contractions. In the sitting position, have someone give resistance while you flex your leg. What type of contraction is it, and what muscle group is contracting? The answer is a concentric contraction of the hamstring muscles. In this case, gravity is not being slowed down, but a force greater than the pull of gravity is being overcome. Therefore, it can be summarized that isotonic contractions have the following features.

CONCENTRIC CONTRACTIONS
1. Muscle attachments move closer together.
2. Movement is occurring against gravity (a "raising" motion).
3. If movement is occurring with gravity, the muscle is overcoming a force greater than the pull of gravity.
4. The contraction is used with an acceleration activity.

ECCENTRIC CONTRACTIONS
1. Muscle attachments move farther apart.
2. Movement occurs with gravity (a "lowering" motion).
3. The contraction is used with a deceleration activity.
4. The contraction produces greater forces.

Another, less common type of muscle contraction is an **isokinetic contraction.** It is a fairly new concept and relatively speaking can be done only with special equipment. The *Cybex* and *Orthotron* were the first machines to introduce such contractions. With an isokinetic contraction, the resistance to the part varies, but the velocity, or speed, stays the same. This differs from an isotonic contraction in which the resistance remains constant but the velocity varies.

Consider the example of the person with the 5-pound weight attached to the leg. While that person straightens and flexes the knee (isotonic contraction), the amount of resistance stays the same. That 5-pound weight remained 5 pounds throughout the range. Because of other factors, such as angle of pull, it is easier to move the leg in the middle and at the end of the range than at the beginning. In other words, the speed at which the person is able to move the leg varies throughout the range.

In an isokinetic contraction, the speed is preset and will stay the same no matter how hard a person pushes. However, the resistance will vary. If the person pushes harder, the machine will give more resistance, and if the person does not push as hard, there will be less resistance.

Why are isokinetic muscle contractions significant? A complete discussion of the merits of isokinetic exercise in comparison to other forms of exercise is best covered in a more detailed discussion of therapeutic exercise, which is beyond the scope of this book. However, there are two significant advantages. Isokinetic exercises can alter or adjust the amount of resistance given through the range of motion, whereas an isotonic contraction cannot. This is important because a muscle is not as strong at the beginning or end of its range as it is in the middle. Because the muscle is strongest in the midrange, more resistance should be given there, and less resistance at the beginning and end. An isotonic contraction cannot do this; therefore, there may be too much resistance in the weaker parts of the range and not enough resistance in the stronger parts.

Accommodating resistance is important because of the pain factor. If pain suddenly develops during the exercise, the person's response is to stop exercising, or to not work as hard. With an isotonic contraction, this response cannot happen quickly or even safely. With an isokinetic exercise, if the person stops working, the machine also stops. If the person does not contract as hard, the machine does not give as much resistance.

Hopefully, this will give you some idea of the value of isokinetic exercise. There are, however, some drawbacks. For example, isokinetic exercise requires special equipment, and that equipment is expensive. There is a time and place for all of these types of muscle contractions. It is important that you recognize the differences among them. Table 4–1 summarizes the major differences among these three types of muscle contractions.

Roles of Muscles

Muscles assume different roles during joint motion, depending on such variables as the motion being performed, the direction of the motion, and the amount of resistance the muscle must overcome. If any of these variables change, the muscle's role may also change. The roles a muscle can assume are those of an agonist, antagonist, stabilizer, or neutralizer. An **agonist** is a muscle or muscle group that causes the motion. It is sometimes referred to as the **prime mover.** A muscle that is not as effective but does assist in providing that motion is called an **assisting mover.** Factors that determine whether a muscle is a prime mover or an assisting mover are such factors as size, angle of pull, leverage, and contractile potential. During elbow flexion, the biceps muscle is an agonist, and the pronator teres muscle, because of its size and angle of pull, is an assisting mover.

An **antagonist** is a muscle that performs the opposite motion of the agonist. In the case of elbow flexion, the antagonist is the triceps muscle. Keep in mind that the role of a muscle is specific to a particular joint action. In the case of elbow extension, the triceps muscle is the agonist and the biceps muscle is the antagonist. In elbow flexion, the biceps muscle is the agonist and the triceps muscle is the antagonist.

The antagonist has the potential to oppose the agonist, but it is usually relaxed while the agonist is working. When the agonist does contract at the same time as the antagonist, a **cocontraction** has occurred. A cocontraction occurs when there is a need for accuracy. Some experts feel that cocontractions are common when a person learns a task, especially a difficult one; thus, as the task is learned, cocontraction activity tends to disappear.

TABLE 4–1	**TYPES OF MUSCLE CONTRACTION**		
	Speed	**Resistance**	**Joint Motion**
Isometric	Fixed	Fixed (0 degrees/sec)	No
Isotonic	Variable	Fixed	Yes
Isokinetic	Fixed	Variable (accommodating)	Yes

A **stabilizer** is a muscle or muscle group that supports, or makes firm, a part and allows the agonist to work more efficiently. For example, when you do a push-up, the agonists are the elbow extensor muscles. The abdominal muscles (trunk flexor muscles) act as stabilizers to keep the trunk straight, while the arms move the trunk up and down. A stabilizer is sometimes referred to as a fixator.

A **neutralizer** prevents unwanted motion because a muscle knows no direction when it contracts. What action it performs depends mostly on the angle of pull. A neutralizer may also allow a muscle to do more than one motion. For example, the biceps muscle can flex the elbow and supinate the forearm. If only elbow flexion is wanted, the supination component must be ruled out. Therefore, the pronator teres muscle, which pronates the forearm, would contract to counteract the supination component of the biceps muscle, and only elbow flexion would occur. Another example is wrist ulnar deviation. The flexor carpi ulnaris muscle causes flexion and ulnar deviation of the wrist. The extensor carpi ulnaris muscle causes extension and ulnar deviation. In ulnar deviation, these muscles contract, doing two things: They neutralize each other's flexion/extension component and act as agonists in wrist ulnar deviation.

A **synergist** is a term used by some authors to encompass the role of agonists assisting movers, stabilizers, and neutralizers. It is a muscle that works with another muscle to enhance a particular motion. The disadvantage of this term is that although it indicates that the muscle is working, it does not indicate how.

Angle of Pull

Several factors determine the role that a muscle will play in a particular joint motion. Determining whether a muscle has a major role (prime mover), a minor role (assisting mover), or no role at all will depend on such factors as its size, angle of pull, the joint motions possible, and the location of the muscle in relation to the joint axis. Visualizing the muscle, particularly in relation to other muscles performing the same action will give you an idea about size as a factor. For example, compare the size of the triceps with that of the anconeus (see Figs. 9–17 and 9–18). It is easy to see that the anconeus will have little effect on joint motion compared to the triceps. Next, you know the motions allowed that a particular joint allows. In the case of the elbow, the motions possible are flexion and extension. The triceps and anconeus cross the joint posterior to the joint axis. Because the triceps is much larger than the anconeus, it crosses the elbow posteriorly, and extensors must cross the elbow posteriorly, it is logical that the triceps is a prime mover in elbow extension.

Not all muscles are so obvious in their action. Angle of pull is usually a major factor. Most muscles pull at a diagonal. As will be discussed in Chapter 6 regarding torque, most muscles have a diagonal line of pull. That diagonal line of pull is the resultant force of a vertical force and a horizontal force. In the case of the shoulder girdle, muscles with a greater vertical angle of pull will be effective in pulling the scapula up or down (elevating or depressing the scapula). Muscles with a greater horizontal pull will be more effective in pulling the scapula in or out (protracting or retracting). Muscles with a more equal horizontal and vertical pull will have a role in both motions. Figure 4–10 gives an example of each. The levator scapula has a stronger vertical component, the middle trapezius has a stronger horizontal component, and the rhomboids have a more equal pull in both directions. As you will see

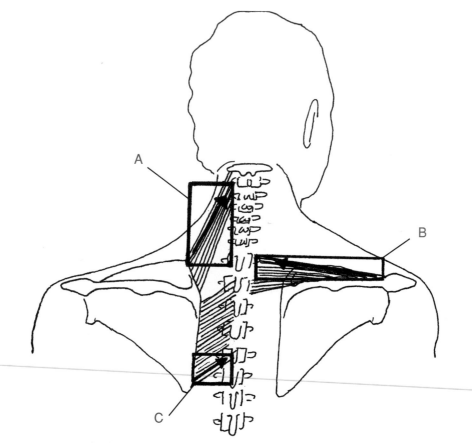

FIGURE 4–10.   Angle of pull as a determinant of muscle action. (*A*) Vertical pull will be effective in elevating or depressing the scapula. (*B*) Horizontal pull will retract or protract the scapula. (*C*) Diagonal pull, which is nearly equal amounts of vertical and horizontal pull, will cause motion in both planes.

when these muscles are described later in Chapter 7, the levator scapula is a prime mover in scapular elevation, the middle trapezius is a prime mover in retraction, and the rhomboids are prime movers in both elevation and retraction.

Kinetic Chains

In recent years, the concept of open versus closed kinetic chain exercises has evolved into physical therapy. In engineering terms, a kinetic chain consists of a series of rigid links connected in such a way as to allow motion. Because these links are connected, movement of one link causes motion at other links in a predictable way. Applying this to the human body, a **closed kinetic chain** requires that the distal segment be fixed (closed) and the proximal segment(s) move (Fig. 4–11). For example, when you rise from a sitting position, your knees extend, causing your hips and ankles to move as well. With your foot fixed on the ground, there is no way you can move your knee without causing movement at the hip and knee.

However, if you were to remain seated and extend your knee, your hip and ankle would not move. This is an **open kinetic chain** activity. The distal segment is

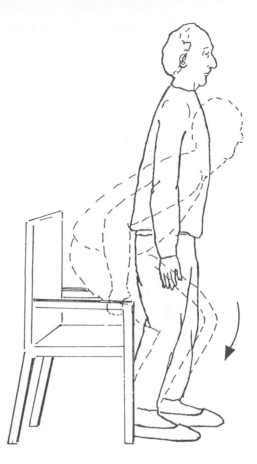

FIGURE 4–11. Closed kinetic chain (distal segment fixed, proximal segment(s) move).

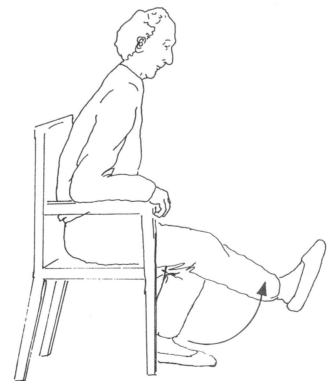

FIGURE 4–12. Open kinetic chain (distal segment moves, proximal segment(s) fixed).

free to move while the proximal segment(s) can remain stationary (Fig. 4–12). With open chain activities, the limb segments are free to move in many directions. For example, if you are lying on a bed with your arm in the air, you can move your shoulder, elbow, wrist, and hand in many directions, either together or individually. This is open chain activity. The distal segment is not fixed but is free to move.

However, if you took hold of an overhead trapeze, your hand, the distal segment, would be fixed or closed. As you flexed your elbow, your shoulder would have to go into some extension. As your elbow extended, your shoulder would have to go into some flexion. With closed chain activities, the limb segments move in limited and predictable directions. Other examples of upper extremity closed chain activities occur during crutch walking and pushing a wheelchair.

Closed chain exercise equipment includes such things as the bench press, rowing machine, stationary bicycle, and StairMaster. Examples of open chain exercise equipment would be the Cybex, treadmill, and the StairMaster in which full-sized stairs revolve around the treadmill. Manual muscle testing is all open chain movement.

REVIEW QUESTIONS

1. Usually, when a muscle contracts, the distal attachment moves toward the proximal attachment. Another name for the distal attachment is
_____. Another name for the proximal attachment is
_____.

2. What is the term for a muscle contraction in which the proximal end moves toward the distal end?

For questions 3 and 4, answer the following questions:

   a. What is the joint motion involved?
   b. Is the muscle action an isometric or isotonic contraction?
   c. If the contraction is isotonic, is it concentric or eccentric?

3. Sitting with a weight in your hand, forearm pronated, elbow extended, and shoulder medially rotated, slowly abduct your shoulder.

At the shoulder

a.

b.

c.

At the elbow

a.

b.

c.

4. Lying supine with a weight in your hand (starting in an anatomical position) raise the weight up and over your shoulder.

a.

b.

c.

5. The flexor carpi radialis muscle performs wrist flexion and radial deviation. The flexor carpi ulnaris muscle performs wrist flexion and ulnar deviation. In what wrist action do the two muscles act as agonists? In what wrist action do they act as antagonists?

6. The gluteus maximus muscle is a hip extensor and lateral rotator. The semitendinosus muscle is a hip extensor. The gluteus minimus muscle is a hip medial rotator. Which of these three muscles must act as a neutralizer for hip extension to occur?

7. What is the term for the situation in which a muscle contracts until it can contract no farther even though more joint range of motion is possible?

8. Walking downhill, do you tend to use your quadriceps muscle in a concentric or eccentric contraction?

9. Identify following activities in terms of open or closed kinetic chain activities:
   a. Wheelchair push-ups
   b. Exercises with weight cuffs
   c. Overhead wall pulleys

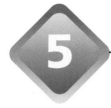

The Nervous System

The nervous system is the highly complex mechanism in our bodies that controls, stimulates, and coordinates all other body systems. As outlined in Figure 5–1, it can be anatomically divided into the central nervous system (CNS), the peripheral nervous system (PNS), and the autonomic nervous system (ANS). The CNS includes the brain and spinal cord, and the PNS includes nerves outside the spinal cord. The ANS controls mostly visceral structures. The subdivisions of the ANS are the sympathetic nervous system and the parasympathetic nervous system. These operate as a check-and-balance system for each other. The sympathetic system deals with stress and stimulation whereas the parasympathetic system deals with conserving energy.

Specific description of the various parts of each system and their functions is beyond the scope of this text. A fairly brief anatomical and functional description of the CNS and PNS as they affect muscle movement will be made. This description will be focused at the gross, not the cellular, level.

Nervous Tissue (Neurons)

The fundamental unit of nervous tissue is the neuron (Fig. 5–2). It contains a **cell body** and fiber branches coming into and going away from it. The term "nerve cell" is synonymous with *neuron,* including all of its processes (dendrites and axons).

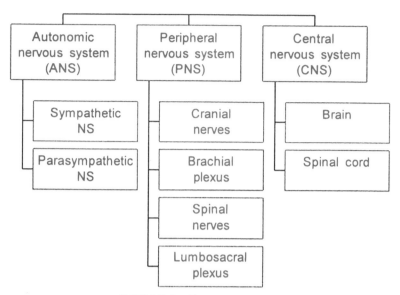

FIGURE 5–1.   The nervous system.

Dendrites are fiber branches that receive impulses from other parts of the nervous system and bring them toward the cell body. **Axons** transmit impulses away from the cell body, are located on the side opposite the dendrites, and usually consist of a single branch. The inner part of the axon is often surrounded by a fatty sheath called the **myelin,** which in turn is surrounded by a transparent **neurilemma.** The myelin is interrupted approximately every half millimeter. Such a break in the myelin is referred to as the **node of Ranvier.**

Myelin is a white, fatty substance found in the CNS and PNS. One of its functions is to increase the speed of impulse conduction in the myelinated fiber. Myelin does not cover cell bodies or certain nerve fibers. Areas that contain mostly unmyelinated fibers are referred to as **gray matter,** whereas areas that contain mostly myelinated fibers are called **white matter** (Fig. 5–3). Areas of gray matter include the cerebral cortex and the central portion of the spinal cord. White matter includes the major tracts within the spinal cord and fiber systems, such as the internal capsule within the brain.

A **nerve fiber** is the conductor of impulses for the neuron. Transmission of impulses from one neuron to another occurs at a **synapse,** which is a minute gap between neurons involving very complex physiologic actions.

A **tract** is a group of myelinated nerve fibers within the CNS that carries a specific type of information from one area to another. Depending on location within the CNS, the group of fibers may be referred to as a *fasciculus, peduncle, brachium, column,* or *lemniscus.* A group of fibers within the PNS may be called a *spinal nerve, nerve root, plexus,* or *peripheral nerve,* depending on location. An example of the pathway tract can be seen in Fig. 5–18.

There are two major types of nerve fibers in peripheral nerves. A **motor (efferent) neuron** has a large, multipolar cell body with multibranched dendrites and a long axon (Fig. 5–2b). The cell body and dendrites are located within the anterior horn of the spinal cord (Fig. 5–4). Depending upon authors use of terms, ventral and anterior are synonomous as are dorsal and posterior. The axon leaves the anterior horn through the white matter and is organized with other similar axons in the **an-**

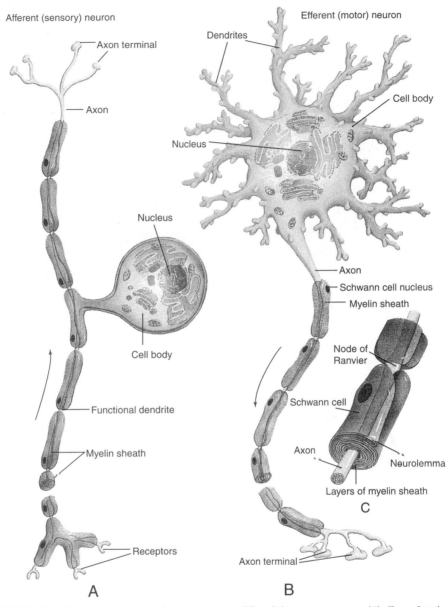

FIGURE 5–2. Neuron structure are the motor neuron (*B*) and the sensory neuron (*A*). (From Scanlon, VC and Sandrus, T. Essentials of Anatomy and Physiology, Ed 3, FA Davis, Philadelphia 1999, p 155, with permission.)

terior (ventral) root, located just outside the spinal cord in the area of the intervertebral foramen. The axon continues down the peripheral nerve to its termination in a **motor endplate (axon terminal)** of a muscle fiber. A motor neuron conducts **efferent** impulses from the spinal cord to the periphery.

The **sensory afferent neuron** has a dendrite, which arises in the skin and runs all the way to its cell body in the dorsal root ganglion (see Fig. 5–2a), located in the intervertebral foramen. The axon travels through the posterior (dorsal) root of the

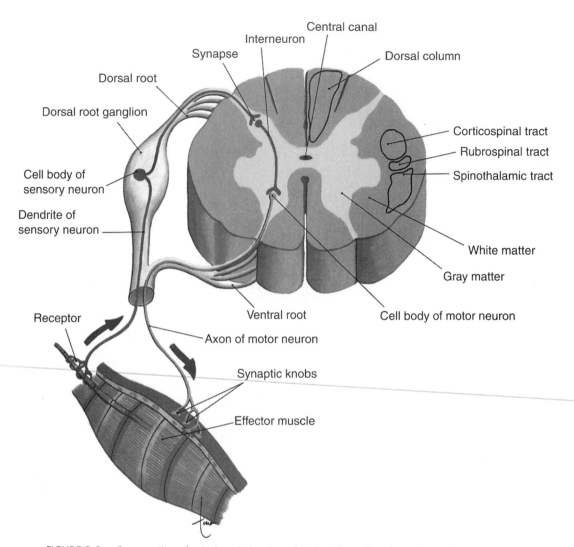

FIGURE 5–3. Cross section of spinal cord, showing white (myelinated) and gray (unmyelinated) matter.

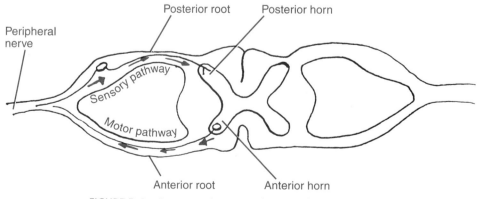

FIGURE 5–4. Sensory and motor pathways within the spinal cord.

spinal nerve and into the spinal cord through the posterior horn. The axon may end at this point, or it may enter the white matter and ascend to a different level of the spinal cord or to the brain stem. Therefore, a sensory neuron sends **afferent** impulses from the periphery to the spinal cord. Both sensory and motor impulses travel along nerve fibers located outside the spinal cord, within peripheral nerves.

A third type of neuron is an **interneuron** (Fig. 5–3). It is found within the CNS. It transmits only sensory or motor impulses, or integrates these impulses.

The Central Nervous System

The main components of the CNS are the brain and the spinal cord. The brain is made up of the cerebrum, brain stem, and cerebellum. (Trivia fans will note that the brain weighs about 3 pounds.)

BRAIN

Cerebrum

The **cerebrum** is the largest and main portion of the brain (Fig. 5–5), and it is responsible for the highest mental functions. It occupies the anterior and superior area of the cranium above the brain stem and cerebellum. The cerebrum is made up of right and left **cerebral hemispheres** joined in the center by the **corpus callosum.**

Each cerebral hemisphere has a **cortex,** or outer coating, that is many cell layers deep, and each hemisphere is divided into four **lobes** (Fig. 5–6). The **frontal lobe** occupies the anterior portion of the skull, and the **occipital lobe** takes up the posterior portion. The **parietal lobe** lies between the frontal and occipital lobe, and the **temporal lobe** lies under the frontal and parietal lobes, just above the ear.

Each lobe has many known functions; the locations of some functions have yet to be discovered. The area of brain activity that has to do with such characteristics as personality is located in the frontal lobe. The frontal lobe also controls motor movement and expressive speech. The occipital lobe is responsible for vision and recognition of size, shape, and color. The parietal lobe controls gross sensation, such as touch and pressure, and fine sensation, such as the determination of texture, weight, size, and shape. The center of brain activity associated with reading skills is also located in the parietal lobe. The temporal lobes are the centers for behavior, hearing, and language reception and understanding. The interested student can find detailed maps of the brain functions in most anatomy and neurology texts.

Deep within the cerebral hemispheres, beneath the cortex, is the **thalamus** (see Fig. 5–5). This mass of nerve cells serves as a relay station for body sensations; it is here where pain is perceived. Also deep inside the brain is the **hypothalamus,** which is important to hormone function and behavior. The **basal ganglia,** also in this area, are important in coordination of motor movement.

Brain stem

Lying below the cerebrum is the brain stem, which can be divided into three parts: the midbrain, pons, and medulla (see Fig. 5–5). The upper portion of the brain stem is the **midbrain,** located somewhat below the cerebrum. The midbrain is the center for visual reflexes. *Pons* is Latin for "bridge"; the pons is located between the mid-

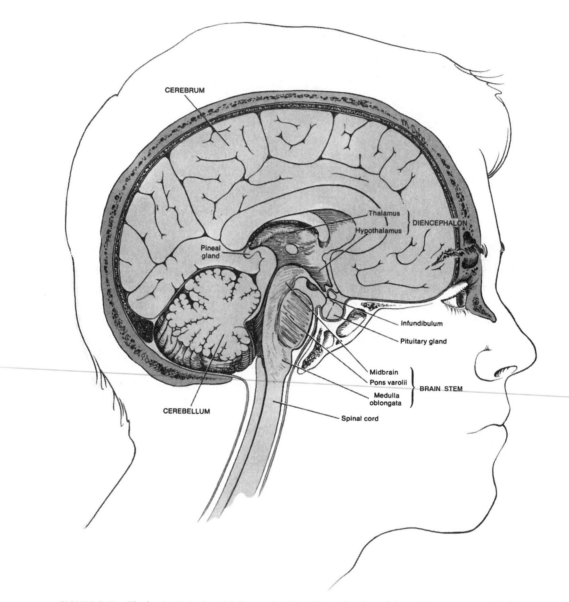

FIGURE 5–5. The brain. Note that this illustration identifies only a few of the major structures of the brain. (From Tortora, GJ and Anagnostakos, NP: Principles of Anatomy and Physiology, ed 3. Harper & Row, New York, 1981, p 327, with permission.)

brain and medulla. The **medulla oblongata** is the most caudal or inferior portion of the brain stem. It is usually referred to simply as the *medulla,* meaning "middle" or "inner." The medulla is continuous with the spinal cord, with the transition being at the base of the skull where it passes through foramen magnum. The medulla is the center for automatic control of respiration and heart rate.

Most of the cranial nerves come from the brain stem area, and all fiber tracts from the spinal cord and peripheral nerves to and from higher centers of the brain go through this area.

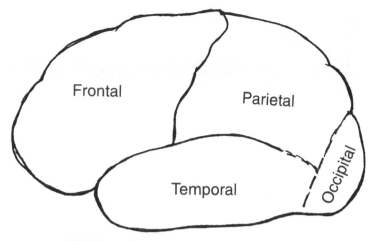

FIGURE 5–6. Each cerebral hemisphere has four lobes.

Cerebellum

In Latin, *cerebellum* means "little brain"; it is located in the posterior portion of the cranium behind the pons and medulla (see Fig. 5–5). It is covered superiorly by the posterior portion of the cerebrum. The main functions of the cerebellum are control of muscle coordination, tone, and posture.

Brain Protection

The brain has basically three levels of protection: bony, membranous, and fluid. Surrounding the brain is the **skull,** made up of several bones with joints fused together for greater strength (Fig. 5–7).

Within the skull are three layers of membrane, called *meninges* (Fig. 5–8), that cover the brain and provide support and protection. The thickest, most fibrous, tough outer layer is called the *dura mater,* which means "hard mother" in Latin. The middle, thinner layer is called **arachnoid** or, less commonly, *arachnoid mater. (Arachnoid,* from Greek for "spider," means "spider-like.") The inner, delicate layer is called the *pia mater* (Latin for "tender mother"), which carries blood vessels to the brain. These cranial meninges are continuous with the spinal meninges that surround the spinal cord.

Between the layers of the arachnoid and pia mater is the **subarachnoid space** through which circulates **cerebrospinal fluid** (Fig. 5–9). This fluid surrounds the brain and fills the four **ventricles** (small cavities) within the brain. The main function of the cerebrospinal fluid is shock absorption.

Brain Blood Supply

The blood supply to the brain comes from branches of the internal carotid and vertebral arteries (Fig. 5–10). The common carotid arteries (right and left) arise from the aortic arch and run the length of the neck in an anterior lateral position. At about the level of the jaw, each divides into the external and internal carotid arteries. The **external carotid arteries** supply the scalp, dura, and skull. The **internal carotid arteries** enter the middle cranial fossa through the carotid canal in the temporal

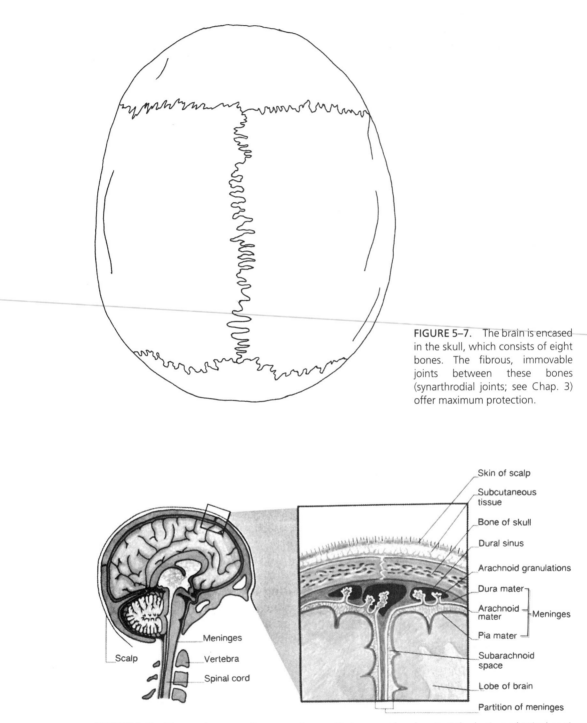

FIGURE 5–7. The brain is encased in the skull, which consists of eight bones. The fibrous, immovable joints between these bones (synarthrodial joints; see Chap. 3) offer maximum protection.

Skin of scalp
Subcutaneous tissue
Bone of skull
Dural sinus
Arachnoid granulations
Dura mater
Arachnoid mater — Meninges
Pia mater
Subarachnoid space
Lobe of brain
Partition of meninges

Meninges
Scalp
Vertebra
Spinal cord

FIGURE 5–8. The meninges are three membranes that surround and protect the brain and spinal cord. (From Hole, JW Jr: Human Anatomy and Physiology, ed 2. Wm C Brown, Dubuque, Iowa, 1978, p 338, with permission.)

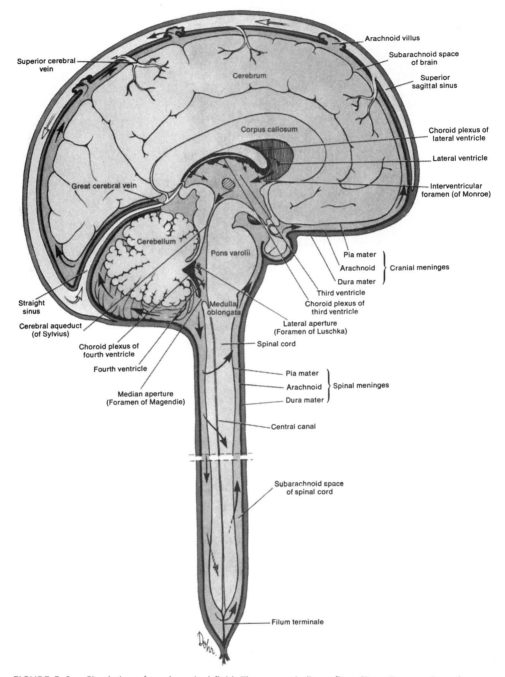

FIGURE 5–9.   Circulation of cerebrospinal fluid. The arrows indicate flow. (From Tortora, GJ and Anagnostakos, NP: Principles of Anatomy and Physiology, ed 3. Harper & Row, New York, 1981, p 328, with permission.)

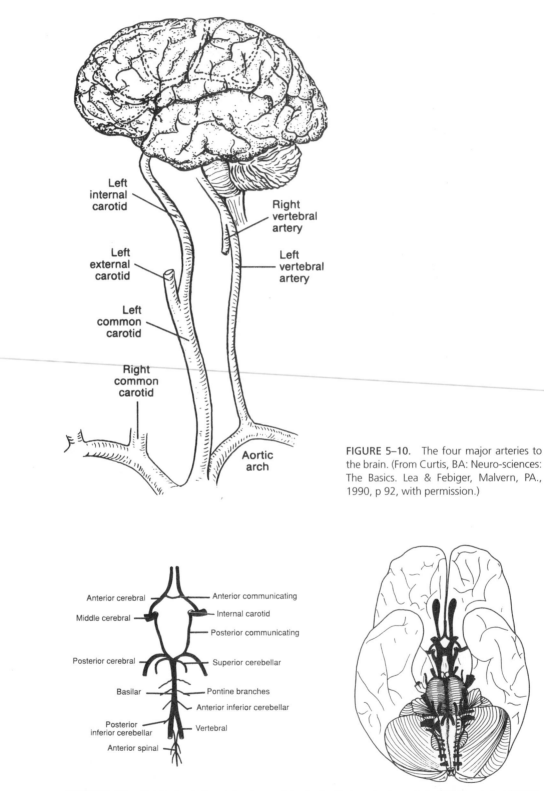

FIGURE 5–10. The four major arteries to the brain. (From Curtis, BA: Neuro-sciences: The Basics. Lea & Febiger, Malvern, PA., 1990, p 92, with permission.)

FIGURE 5–11. Cerebral arteries at the base of the brain, their major branches, and the circle of Willis. (From Curtis, BA: Neurosciences: The Basics. Lea & Febiger, Malvern, PA, 1990, p 93, with permission.

bone to supply primarily the anterior portion of the brain. Immediately upon entering the cranial cavity, the internal carotid artery branches into the middle and anterior cerebral arteries (Fig. 5–11). The middle cerebral artery is actually a continuation of the internal carotid and supplies the lateral cerebral hemispheres. The anterior cerebral arteries supply the medial surface of the brain.

The right and left vertebral arteries also branch off the aortic arch (see Fig. 5–10). They ascend the neck through the transverse foramens of the cervical vertebrae and enter the base of the brain through the foramen magnum to supply primarily the posterior portion of the brain. The vertebral arteries give off branches to the medulla and cerebellum and join together to form the **basilar artery** (see Fig. 5–11), which also supplies parts of the cerebellum, as well as the pons and midbrain. The basilar artery branches to form the **posterior cerebral arteries,** which supply the occipital lobes and part of the temporal lobes.

The anterior and posterior cerebral arteries are connected at the base of the brain and form a cerebral arterial circle, often referred to as the **circle of Willis** (see Fig. 5–11) after the English physician, Thomas Willis, who first described this interconnection. The anterior and posterior cerebral arteries are joined by the **posterior communicating artery.** The right and left anterior cerebral arteries are joined by the **anterior communicating artery.** The significance of this circle is that failure of one of these major arteries usually does not seriously decrease blood flow to the region supplied by that artery.

SPINAL CORD

A continuation of the medulla, the spinal cord runs within the vertebral canal from the foramen magnum to the cone-shaped **conus medullaris** at approximately the level of the second lumbar vertebra (Fig. 5–12). Below this level is a collection of nerve roots running down from the spinal cord much like a horse's tail, hence the name **cauda equina.** The cauda equina is made up of the nerve roots for L2 through S5. A threadlike, nonneural filament running from the conus medullaris is the **filium terminale.**

The spinal cord is approximately 17 inches in length. It is enclosed in the same three protective layers as the brain: the outer dura mater, the arachnoid membrane, and the inner pia mater (Fig. 5–13). As with the brain, cerebrospinal fluid flows in the space between the arachnoid layer and pia mater.

The **vertebral foramen** is the passageway for the spinal cord and is surrounded and protected by the bony structures of each individual vertebra (Fig. 5–14). Each vertebra is made up of a **body,** the anterior weight-bearing portion, and the posterior **neural arch** consisting of pedicles, transverse processes, lamina, and a spinous process (Fig. 5–15). The opening formed between these two parts is the vertebral foramen. This opening is not to be confused with the **intervertebral foramen** located on the sides of the vertebral column. The intervertebral foramen is the opening formed by the superior vertebral notch of the vertebra below and the inferior vertebral notch of the vertebra above (Fig. 5–16). Through this opening, the spinal nerve root exits the vertebral canal.

A cross-sectional view of the spinal cord reveals peripheral white matter and central gray matter. The **gray matter** is in the middle of the cord in an **H** or "butterfly" shape (Fig. 5–17). It contains neuronal cell bodies and synapses. The top portion of the **H** is the **posterior horn,** which transmits sensory impulses. The lower portion, the **anterior horn,** transmits motor impulses.

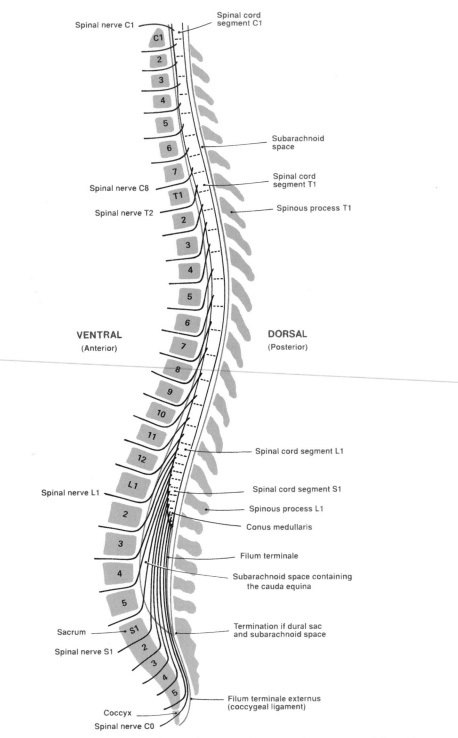

FIGURE 5–12. The spine and spinal cord. (From Gilman, S and Newman, SW: Manter and Gatz's Essentials of Clinical Neuroanatomy and Neurophysiology, ed 8. FA Davis, Philadelphia, 1992, p 11, with permission.)

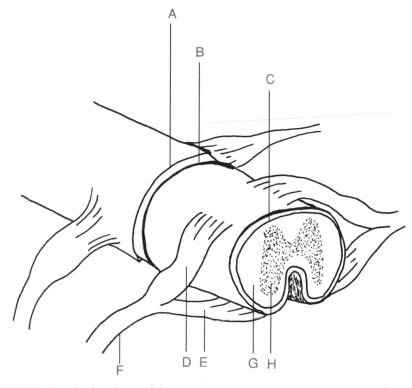

FIGURE 5–13. The three layers of the meninges surround the spinal cord as well as the brain.

A	Dura mater	**E**	Anterior root
B	Archnoid	**F**	Spinal nerve
C	Pia mater	**G**	White matter
D	Posterior root	**H**	Gray matter

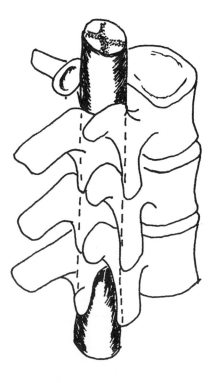

FIGURE 5–14. The spinal cord runs through the vertebral foramen.

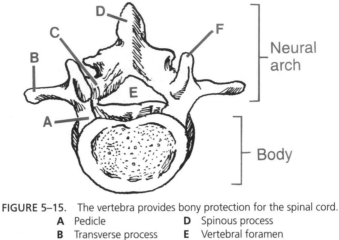

FIGURE 5–15. The vertebra provides bony protection for the spinal cord.
A Pedicle   **D** Spinous process
B Transverse process   **E** Vertebral foramen
C Lamina   **F** Articular process

The **posterior columns,** also called the *dorsal columns,* are located in the posterior medial portions of the spinal cord. These columns transmit the sensations of proprioception pressure and vibration (see Fig. 5–17).

White matter contains ascending (sensory) and descending (motor) fiber pathways. Each pathway carries a particular type of impulse, such as touch, from and to a specific area. These various pathways cross over from one side of the body to the other at different levels. It is this crossover phenomenon that results, for example, in a stroke on the left side of the brain affecting the right side of the body.

The pathway of particular significance to muscle control is the **corticospinal tract** (Fig. 5–18). It is located lateral to the posterior column and horn. As its name implies, it runs from the motor area of the cerebral cortex to the spinal cord crossing over at about the level of the lower part of the brain stem. Corticospinal pathways synapse in the anterior horn just prior to leaving the spinal cord.

Motor neurons that synapse above this level are called **upper motor neurons.** Those that synapse at or below the anterior horn are called **lower motor neurons.**

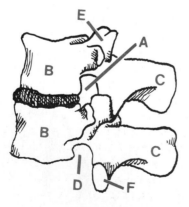

FIGURE 5–16. Two vertebrae combine to form openings (intervertebral foramen) on each side. A Spinal nerve roots pass through this opening.
A Invertebral foramen   **D** Inferior vertebral notch
B Body of vertebra   **E** Superior articular
process
C Spinous process   **F** Inferior articular process

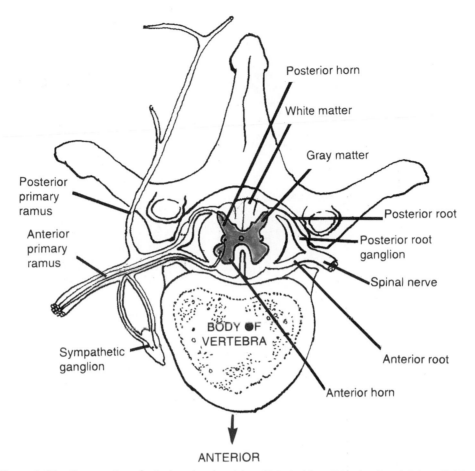

Posterior horn

White matter

Gray matter

Posterior root

Posterior root ganglion

Spinal nerve

Posterior primary ramus

Anterior primary ramus

Sympathetic ganglion

BODY OF VERTEBRA

Anterior root

Anterior horn

ANTERIOR

Figure 5–17. Cross section of spinal cord and vertebra. (Adapted from Tyldesley, B and Grieve. JI: Muscles, Nerves and Movement: Kinesiology in Daily Living. Blackwell Scientific, Boston, 1989, p 75, with permission.)

Injury to these two types of neurons results in quite different clinical signs. In other words, if a lesion occurs between the brain and the spinal cord proximal to the anterior horn, it will be considered an upper motor neuron lesion. If the lesion occurs between the anterior horn of the spinal cord and the periphery, it will be a lower motor neuron lesion. Paralysis will usually result in either case; however, clinical signs differ greatly (these are contrasted in Table 5–1).

Examples of diagnoses involving upper motor neuron lesions include spinal cord injuries, multiple sclerosis, parkinsonism, cerebral vascular accident, and various types of head injuries. Examples of diagnoses involving lower motor neuron lesions are muscular dystrophy, poliomyelitis, myasthenia gravis, and peripheral nerve injuries.

To summarize, motor impulses travel from the brain down the spinal cord through the anterior horn and out to the periphery via spinal nerves. Sensory impulses from the periphery travel up the nerves into the spinal cord via the posterior, or dorsal, horn, then up the spinal cord to the brain.

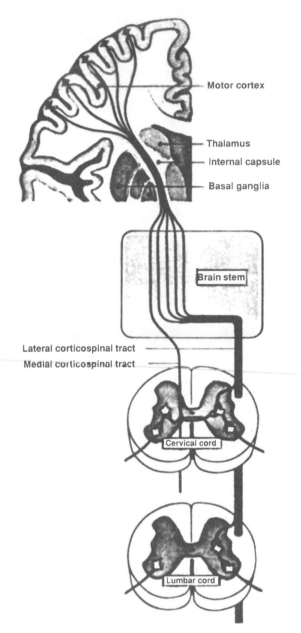

FIGURE 5–18.   Schematic diagram of the course of the corticospinal tract from the brain's motor cortex to the spinal cord. (From Lehmkuhl, LD and Smith, LK: Brunnstrom's Clinical Kinesiology, ed 4. FA Davis, Philadelphia, 1983, p 105, with permission.)

TABLE 5–1	CLINICAL DIFFERENCES BETWEEN UPPER AND LOWER MOTOR NEURON LESIONS	
Sign	**Upper Motor Neuron Lesion**	**Lower Motor Neuron Lesion**
Paralysis	Spasticity present	Flaccid
Muscle atrophy	Not significant	Marked
Fasciculations and fibrillations	Not present	Present
Reflexes	Hyperreflexia	Hyporeflexia
Babinski reflex	Reflex	Not present
Clonus	Present	Not present

The Peripheral Nervous System

The PNS is, for the most part, made up of all the nervous tissue outside the vertebral canal. It actually begins at the anterior horn of the spinal cord, sending motor impulses out to the muscles and receiving sensory impulses from the skin.

CRANIAL NERVES

There are 12 pairs of cranial nerves that are both numbered and named. They have their origins in the brain and can best be seen at their origins on the inferior surface of the brain (Fig. 5–19). They are sensory and/or motor nerves, as summarized in Table 5–2.

Of the 12 cranial nerves, the trigeminal (V), facial (VII), and spinal accessory (XI) (often shortened to accessory) nerves are the ones of most concern in physical therapy because of their control over certain muscles. In the following chapters, innervation of muscles will be given along with the summary description of each muscle.

SPINAL NERVES

There are 31 pairs of spinal nerves. The spinal nerves are made up of 8 cervical, 12 thoracic, 5 lumbar, 5 sacral, and 1 coccygeal nerves (Fig. 5–20). The first seven cervical nerves (C1 to C7) exit the vertebral column over the corresponding vertebra. For example, C3 nerve exits over C3 vertebra. Because there is one more cervical nerve than vertebra, this arrangement changes with the eighth cervical nerve (C8). It exits over the T1 vertebra. T1 nerve exits *under* the T1 vertebra, and so on down the vertebral column.

Branches of Spinal Nerves

Once outside the spinal cord the anterior (motor) and posterior (sensory) roots join together to form the spinal nerve (Fig. 5–21), which passes through the intervertebral foramen. Almost immediately, the nerve sends a branch called the **posterior (dorsal) ramus.** This branch on all spinal nerves innervates the deep muscles of the

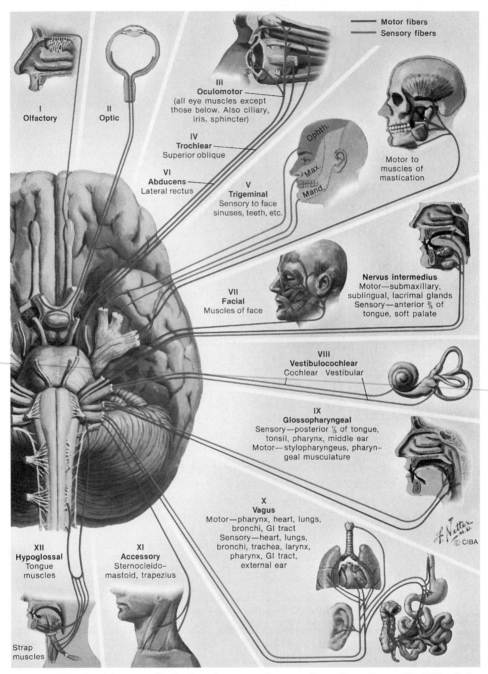

FIGURE 5–19. Cranial nerves: distribution of motor and sensory fibers. (From Netter, FH: ©Ciba Collection of Medical Illustrations: Nervous System, Part I, Anatomy and Physiology. Ciba Pharmaceutical, West Caldwell, NJ, 1983, p 93, with permission.)

TABLE 5–2	**CRANIAL NERVES**		
Number	**Name**	**Type**	**Function**
I	Olfactory	Sensory	Smell
II	Optic	Sensory	Vision
III	Oculomotor	Motor	Muscles of eye
IV	Trochlear	Motor	Muscles of eye
V	Trigeminal	Mixed (sensory and motor)	Sensory: Face area Motor: Chewing muscles
VI	Abducens	Motor	Muscles of eye
VII	Facial	Mixed	Sensory: Tongue area Motor: Muscles of face
VIII	Vestibulocochlear (auditory)	Sensory	Hearing
IX	Glossopharyngeal	Mixed	Sensory: Tongue, pharynx, middle ear Motor: Muscles of pharynx
X	Vagus	Mixed	Sensory: Heart, lungs, GI tract, ear Motor: Heart, lungs, GI tract
XI	Spinal accessory	Motor	Sternocleidomastoid and trapezius muscles
XII	Hypoglossal	Motor	Muscles of tongue

back as well as the skin covering these muscles. The spinal nerve continues as the **anterior (ventral) ramus.** These rami (plural of ramus) innervate all muscles and skin areas not innervated by the posterior rami. Located just peripheral to the posterior ramus is a branch to the ANS. It is involved with such functions as blood pressure regulation. Although these functions are vital, they will not be discussed here. Instead, emphasis will be on the motor functions that occur mostly via the anterior ramus.

Dermatomes

The area of skin supplied with the **sensory fibers** of a spinal nerve is called the **dermatome** (Fig. 5–22). There is often much overlap of contiguous dermatomes; therefore, anesthesia will not occur unless more than two spinal nerves have lost function. If an injury involves only one spinal nerve, sensation will be decreased or altered, but it will not be absent.

Thoracic Nerves

There are 12 pairs of thoracic nerves. With the exception of T1, which is part of the brachial plexus, they maintain their segmental relationship and do not join with the other nerves. Each nerve branches into a posterior and anterior ramus (see Fig. 5–20). The posterior rami innervate the muscles of the back and the overlying skin. The anterior rami become **intercostal nerves,** innervating the anterior trunk and intercostal muscles as well as the skin of the anterior and lateral trunk.

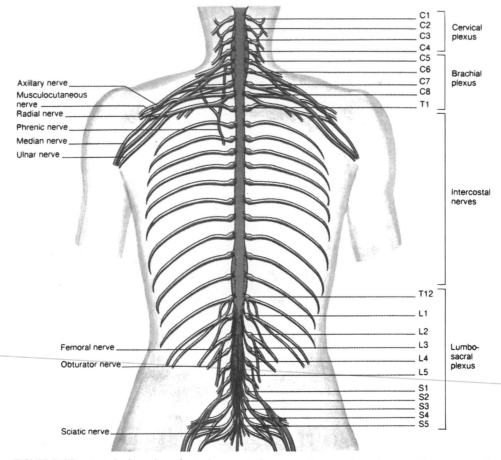

FIGURE 5–20. Anterior branches of spinal nerves in thoracic region give rise to intercostal nerves. Spinal nerves in other regions combine to form complex networks called plexuses. (From Hole, JW Jr: Human Anatomy and Physiology, ed 2. Wm C Brown, Dubuque, Iowa, 1978, p 372, with permission.)

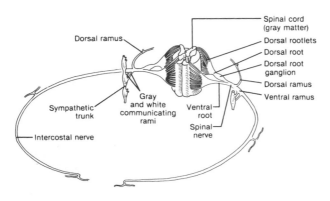

FIGURE 5–21. Anterolateral view of a thoracic spinal cord segment and the formation and branches of its spinal nerves. (From Pratt, NE: Clinical Musculoskeletal Anatomy. JB Lippincott, Philadelphia, 1991, p 44, with permission.)

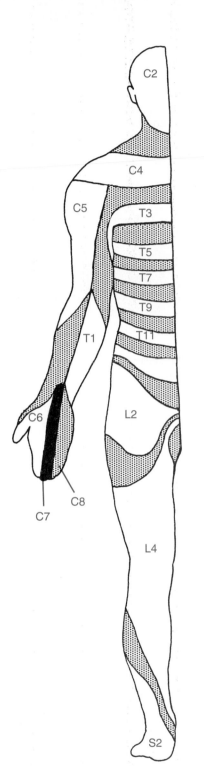
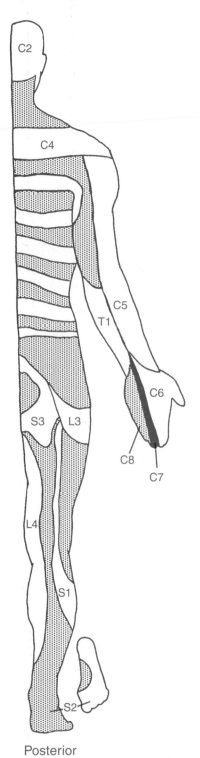

Anterior   Posterior

FIGURE 5–22. Dermatomes: segmental areas of innervation of the skin. (Modified from Manter, JT and Gatz, AJ: Essentials of Clinical Neuroanatomy and Neurophysiology, ed 2. FA Davis, Philadelphia, 1961, p 24.)

PLEXUS FORMATION

Except for the thoracic nerves, the anterior rami of the spinal nerves will join together and/or branch forming a network known as a **plexus.** There are three major plexuses (see Fig. 5–20):

1. The cervical plexus, made up of C1 through C4 spinal nerves, innervates the muscles of the neck.
2. The brachial plexus, made up of C5 through T1, innervates muscles of the upper limb.
3. The lumbosacral plexus, made up of L1 through S5, innervates muscles of the lower limb.
   a. Lumbar portion, L1 through L4, supplies mostly muscles of the thigh.
   b. Sacral portion, L5 through S5, supplies mostly muscles of the leg and foot.

Cervical Plexus

The anterior rami of the first four cervical nerves (C1 to C4) join together in various ways to form the **cervical plexus** (see Fig. 5–20). This plexus will not be described in detail because only a few muscles covered in this text receive their innervation from the cervical plexus.

There is a branch from C2 going to the sternocleidomastoid, and branches from C3 and C4 supply the trapezius. The levator scapulae receive innervation from C3 through C5. The anterior scalene gets some innervation from C4, and the middle scalene from C3 and C4. Perhaps one of the most significant nerves of the cervical plexus is the *phrenic nerve,* which is formed from branches of C3 through C5 and innervates the diaphragm.

Brachial Plexus

The **brachial plexus** is formed by the anterior rami of C5 through T1 spinal nerves. It splits and joins several times before ending in five main peripheral nerves. Its network arrangement consists of roots, trunks, divisions, cords, and finally peripheral (terminal) nerves, as shown in Figure 5–23.

There are five roots made up of the anterior rami of C5, C6, C7, C8, and T1. These roots join together forming three **trunks.** The three trunks, named for their position relative to each other, are:

1. The superior trunk coming from C5 and C6
2. The middle from C7
3. The inferior trunk coming from C8 and T1

Each trunk splits into an anterior and posterior **division,** named for their position relative to each other.

Next are the three **cords,** named according to their relationship to the axillary artery. They are formed by the joining of various trunk divisions. The lateral cord comes from the anterior division of the superior and middle trunks. The posterior cord arises from the posterior divisions of all three trunks, and the medial cord comes from the anterior division of the inferior trunk. The five **peripheral nerves,** which are branches of the cords, form the terminal nerves of the plexus as follows:

1. *Musculocutaneous:* From the lateral cord
2. *Axillary:* A branch of the posterior cord
3. *Radial:* A branch of the posterior cord

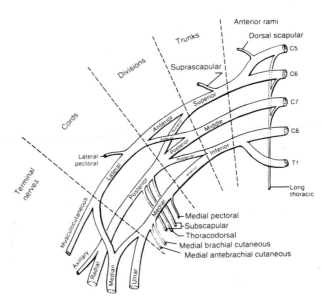

FIGURE 5–23. The organization of the brachial plexus. (From Pratt, NE: Clinical Musculoskeletal Anatomy. JB Lippincott, Philadelphia, 1991, p 65, with permission.)

4. *Median:* From the lateral and medial cords

5. *Ulnar:* From the medial cord

This network arrangement is not a plot to make learning more difficult; rather, it provides muscles with innervation from more than one level. In the event of trauma or disease, perhaps not all levels of innervation will be involved. Therefore, a muscle may be weakened but not completely paralyzed.

For the most part, these five nerves innervate the muscles of the upper limb; however, some muscles receive innervation from nerves that have branched off the plexus earlier. These branches are noted in Figure 5–23. The medial pectoral nerve branches off the medial cord to innervate the pectoralis major and minor muscles. The subscapular nerve, a branch of the posterior cord, innervates the subscapularis muscle, and the thoracodorsal nerve also branches off the posterior cord to innervate the latissimus dorsi muscle.

Terminal Nerves of the Brachial Plexus

The five terminal nerves of the brachial plexus have been summarized below according to (1) the segment, or root, of the spinal cord from which they came, (2) the major muscles they innervate, (3) the major sensory distribution, and (4) the main motor impairments that would be seen following severance of the nerve.

Axillary Nerve (Fig. 5–24)	
Spinal cord segment	C5, C6
Muscle innervation	Deltoid
	Teres minor
Sensory distribution	Lateral arm over lower portion of deltoid
Clinical motor features of paralysis	Loss of shoulder abduction
	Weakened shoulder external rotation

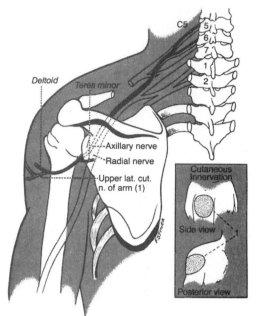

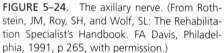

FIGURE 5–24. The axillary nerve. (From Rothstein, JM, Roy, SH, and Wolf, SL: The Rehabilitation Specialist's Handbook. FA Davis, Philadelphia, 1991, p 265, with permission.)

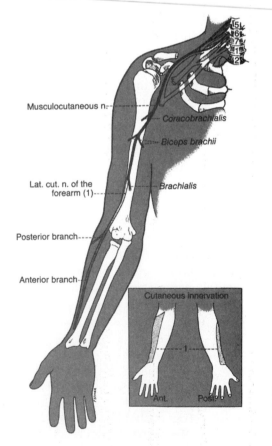

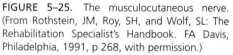

FIGURE 5–25. The musculocutaneous nerve. (From Rothstein, JM, Roy, SH, and Wolf, SL: The Rehabilitation Specialist's Handbook. FA Davis, Philadelphia, 1991, p 268, with permission.)

Musculocutaneous Nerve (Fig. 5–25)

Spinal cord segment	C5, C6
Muscle innervation	Coracobrachialis
	Biceps
	Brachialis
Sensory distribution	Anterolateral surface of forearm
Clinical motor features of paralysis	Loss of forearm flexion when supinated
	Weakened supination

Radial Nerve (Fig. 5–26)

Spinal segment	C6, C7, C8, T1
Muscle innervation	Triceps
	Anconeus
	Brachioradialis
	Supinator
	Wrist, finger, and thumb extensors
Sensory distribution	Posterior arm, posterior forearm, and radial side of posterior hand
Clinical motor features of paralysis	Loss of elbow, wrist, finger, and thumb extension: "wrist drop"

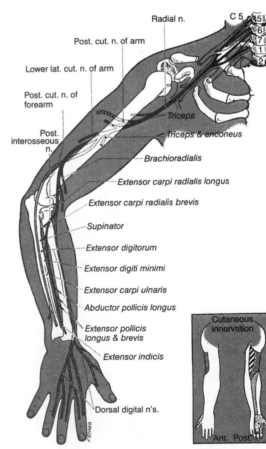

FIGURE 5–26. The radial nerve. (From Rothstein, JM, Roy, SH, and Wolf, SL: The Rehabilitation Specialist's Handbook. FA Davis, Philadelphia, 1991, p 286, with permission.)

Median Nerve (Fig. 5–27)

Spinal cord segment	C6, C7, C8, T1
Muscle innervation	Pronators
	Wrist and finger flexors on radial side
	Most thumb muscles
Sensory distribution	Palmar aspect of thumb, second, third, and fourth (radial half) fingers
Clinical motor features of paralysis	Loss of forearm pronation
	Loss of thumb opposition, flexion, and abduction ("ape hand")

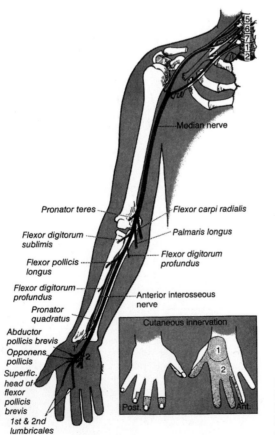

FIGURE 5–27.   The median nerve. (From Rothstein, JM, Roy, SH, and Wolf, SL: The Rehabilitation Specialist's Handbook. FA Davis, Philadelphia, 1991, p 272, with permission.)

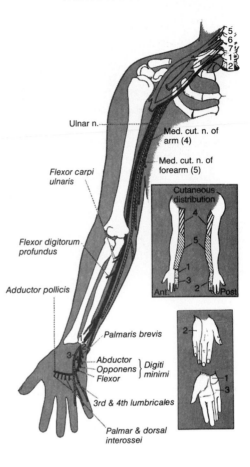

Ulnar n.

Med. cut. n. of arm (4)

Med. cut. n. of forearm (5)

Flexor carpi ulnaris

Cutaneous distribution

Flexor digitorum profundus

Adductor pollicis

Palmaris brevis

Abductor
Opponens } Digiti
Flexor } minimi

3rd & 4th lumbricales

Palmar & dorsal interossei

FIGURE 5–28. The ulnar nerve. (From Rothstein, JM, Roy, SH, and Wolf, SL: The Rehabilitation Specialist's Handbook. FA Davis, Philadelphia, 1991, p 280, with permission.)

Ulnar Nerve (Fig. 5–28)

Spinal cord segment	C8, T1
Muscle innervation	Flexor carpi ulnaris
	Flexor digitorum profundus (medial half)
	Interossei
	Fourth and fifth lumbricales
Sensory distribution	Fourth finger (medial portion), fifth finger
Clinical motor features of paralysis	Loss of wrist ulnar deviation
	Weakened wrist, finger flexion
	Weakened fourth and fifth finger flexion ("pope's blessing")
	Loss of thumb adduction
	Loss of most intrinsics ("claw hand")

Lumbosacral Plexus

The lumbosacral plexus is formed by the anterior rami of L1 through S3 (Fig. 5–29). Some sources will separate this into a **lumbar plexus** (L1 through L4), which innervates most muscles of the thigh, and a **sacral plexus** (L5 through S3), which innervates

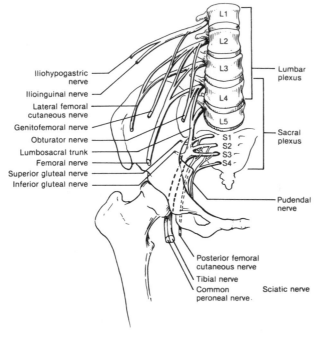

Iliohypogastric nerve
Ilioinguinal nerve
Lateral femoral cutaneous nerve
Genitofemoral nerve
Obturator nerve
Lumbosacral trunk
Femoral nerve
Superior gluteal nerve
Inferior gluteal nerve

L1
L2
L3
L4
L5
S1
S2
S3
S4

Lumbar plexus

Sacral plexus

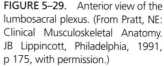

Pudendal nerve

Posterior femoral cutaneous nerve
Tibial nerve
Common peroneal nerve.

Sciatic nerve

FIGURE 5–29. Anterior view of the lumbosacral plexus. (From Pratt, NE: Clinical Musculoskeletal Anatomy. JB Lippincott, Philadelphia, 1991, p 175, with permission.)

mostly muscles of the leg and foot. Because there are several muscles of the lower limb that receive innervation from both plexuses, they will be discussed here as one plexus.

The lumbosacral plexus does not have as much dividing and joining of nerves as does the brachial plexus. It has eight roots that each divide into an upper and lower branch. L3 is the only root that does not divide. Most of these branches divide into an anterior and posterior division. These divisions join in various ways to form the six main peripheral nerves.

The upper branch of L1 divides into the iliohypogastric and ilioinguinal nerves. The lower branch of L1 and the upper branch of L2 form the genitofemoral nerve. These three nerves are primarily sensory in nature and will not be discussed in detail.

The anterior divisions of L2, L3, and L4 form the **obturator nerve,** and the posterior divisions of the same roots form the **femoral nerve.** The posterior divisions of L4 through S1 form the **superior gluteal nerve,** and the posterior divisions of L4 through S2 make up the **inferior gluteal nerve** and **common peroneal nerve.** The **tibial nerve** is made up of anterior divisions of L4 through S2. The **sciatic nerve** is actually the tibial and common peroneal nerves joined by a common sheath—it separates into the two nerves just above the knee.

If all of this is confusing, perhaps the illustrations in Figures 5–29 and 5–30 plus the summary that follows will provide some clarity. This summary is similar to the one provided for the brachial plexus.

Terminal Nerves of the Lumbosacral Plexus

Like the nerves of the upper extremity, the nerves of the lower extremity have been summarized according to (1) the segment, or root, of the spinal cord from which they came, (2) the major muscles they innervate, (3) the major sensory distribution, and (4) the main motor impairments that would be seen following severance of the nerve.

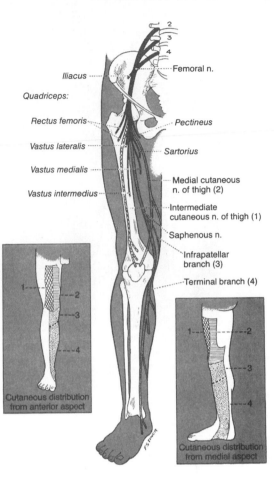

Iliacus

Quadriceps:

Rectus femoris

Vastus lateralis

Vastus medialis

Vastus intermedius

Femoral n.

Pectineus

Sartorius

Medial cutaneous n. of thigh (2)

Intermediate cutaneous n. of thigh (1)

Saphenous n.

Infrapatellar branch (3)

Terminal branch (4)

Cutaneous distribution from anterior aspect

Cutaneous distribution from medial aspect

FIGURE 5–30. The femoral nerve. (From Rothstein, JM, Roy, SH, and Wolf, SL: The Rehabilitation Specialist's Handbook, FA Davis, Philadelphia, 1991, p 300, with permission.)

Femoral Nerve (See Fig. 5–30)

Spinal cord segment	L2, L3, L4
Muscle innervation	Iliopsoas
	Sartorius
	Pectineus
	Quadriceps femoris
Sensory distribution	Anterior and medial thigh, medial leg, and foot
Clinical motor features of paralysis	Weakened hip flexion
	Loss of knee extension

Obturator Nerve (Fig. 5–31)

Spinal cord segment	L2, L3, L4
Muscle innervation	Hip adductors
	Obturator externus
Sensory distribution	Middle medial thigh
Clinical motor features of paralysis	Loss of hip adduction
	Weakened hip lateral rotation

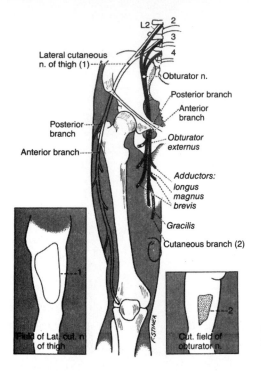

FIGURE 5–31. The obturator nerve. (From Rothstein, JM, Roy, SH, and Wolf, SL: The Rehabilitation Specialist's Handbook. FA Davis, Philadelphia, 1991, p 297, with permission.)

Sciatic Nerve (Fig. 5–32)

Spinal segment	L4, L5, S1, S2, S3
Muscle innervation	Hamstring muscles
Sensory distribution	None
Clinical motor features of paralysis	Weakened hip extension
	Loss of knee flexion

Tibial Nerve (divides into the medial and lateral plantar nerves) (See Fig. 5–32)

Spinal cord segment	L4, L5, S1, S2, S3
Muscle innervation	Popliteus
	Ankle plantar flexors
	Tibialis posterior
	Foot intrinsics (medial and lateral plantar)
Sensory distribution	Posterior lateral leg, lateral foot
Clinical motor features of paralysis	Loss of ankle plantar flexion
	Weakened ankle inversion
	Loss of toe flexion

Common Peroneal Nerve (divides into superficial and deep peroneal nerves (Figs. 5–33 and 5–34)

Spinal segment	L4, L5, S1, S2
Muscle innervation	Peroneals (mostly superficial peroneal)
	Tibialis anterior (deep peroneal)
	Toe extensors (deep peroneal)
Sensory distribution	Anterior lateral aspect of leg and foot
Clinical motor features of paralysis	Loss of ankle dorsiflexion ("foot drop")
	Loss of toe extension
	Loss of ankle eversion

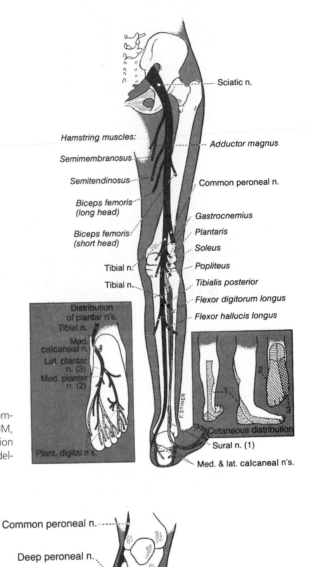

FIGURE 5–32. The sciatic, tibial, and common peroneal nerves. (From Rothstein, JM, Roy, SH, and Wolf, SL: The Rehabilitation Specialist's Handbook. FA Davis, Philadelphia, 1991, p 307, with permission.)

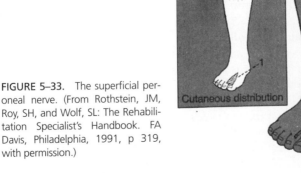

FIGURE 5–33. The superficial peroneal nerve. (From Rothstein, JM, Roy, SH, and Wolf, SL: The Rehabilitation Specialist's Handbook. FA Davis, Philadelphia, 1991, p 319, with permission.)

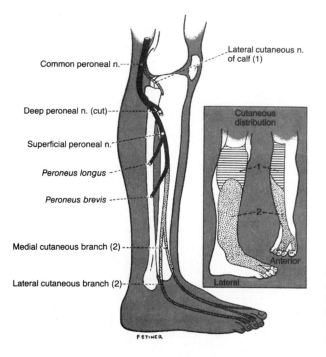

FIGURE 5–34. The deep peroneal nerve. (From Rothstein, JM, Roy, SH, and Wolf, SL: The Rehabilitation Specialist's Handbook. FA Davis, Philadelphia, 1991, p 322, with permission.)

Functional Significance of Spinal Cord Level

It should be remembered that in the cervical region, the spinal nerves come out above the vertebra. For example, the C7 spinal nerve comes out above the C7 vertebra, and the C8 spinal nerve comes out below. Starting with the T1 spinal nerve, all spinal nerves at and below T1 come out below the vertebra. For example, the T5 spinal nerve comes out between the T5 and T6 vertebra. This is illustrated in Figure 5–35.

In this same illustration, one can gain an appreciation for the general innervation level of major muscles. It should be noted that most muscles take innervation from more than one spinal level. Therefore, an injury at one level may weaken a muscle, but some function will remain. For example, the elbow flexors receive innervation from C5 and C6; therefore, an injury at C5 vertebral level will weaken elbow flexion but function will not be completely absent.

Although there is slight variation among individuals, some general statements can be made about level of function at various levels of the spinal cord. A person with a spinal cord injury at C3 or above would not have the function of the diaphragm and would be unable to breathe without assistance. Below that level, although breathing would be compromised, a person would probably be able to breathe without assistance. With C5 spinal cord involvement, the shoulder abductors and elbow flexors remain intact allowing increased function of the upper extremities. The wrist extensors receive innervation from C6 to C8 whereas the triceps are innervated at C7 to C8. The intrinsic muscles of the hand are the last to be innervated in the upper extremity at C8 to T1.

In the thoracic level, muscles receive innervation at each spinal level. Because the intercostals and erector spinae muscles received innervation throughout the thoracic region, the lower the level, the more muscles remain intact. The abdominal muscles receive innervation from the lower thoracic levels.

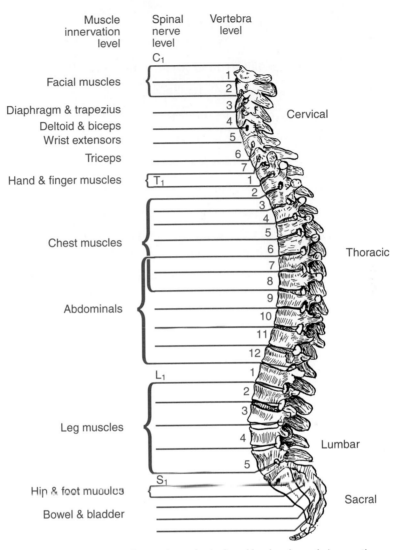

Muscle innervation level	Spinal nerve level	Vertebra level	
	C_1		
Facial muscles		1	Cervical
		2	
Diaphragm & trapezius		3	
Deltoid & biceps		4	
Wrist extensors		5	
Triceps		6	
		7	
Hand & finger muscles	T_1	1	
		2	
		3	
		4	
Chest muscles		5	
		6	Thoracic
		7	
		8	
		9	
Abdominals		10	
		11	
		12	
	L_1	1	
		2	
		3	
Leg muscles		4	Lumbar
		5	
	S_1		
Hip & foot muscles			Sacral
Bowel & bladder			

FIGURE 5–35. Comparison of spinal cord level and muscle innervation.

The lumbar and sacral region is controlled by plexus innervation, so once again, level of injury will be important in knowing which muscles are functioning. The hip flexors and knee extensors are innervated between L2 and L4. Next come the hip adductors at L2 to L3 and the hip abductors at L4 to L5. The hip extensors and knee flexors are innervated at L5 through S2. The ankle motions are innervated between L4 and S2. Last to receive innervation is bowel and bladder control at S4 to S5.

Sensation changes as one proceeds down the spinal cord. Figure 5–22 shows the sensory innervation (dermatomes) at various levels. A person with a C3 spinal cord injury will have sensation only from the top of the head to the neck. At T3, the entire upper extremity and the chest level with the axilla are innervated. An injury at L3 would show innervation in an irregular pattern to approximately the midthigh level.

REVIEW QUESTIONS

1. The spinal cord extends to about what vertebral level?

2. What makes up gray matter? White matter?

3. What protects the brain from trauma?

4. What is the circle of Willis? Why is the circle of Willis significant?

5. What are the differences between upper and lower motor neurons?

6. How do thoracic nerves differ from cervical or lumbar nerves?

7. What is the difference between an afferent and an efferent nerve fiber?

8. In an individual who has lost the ability to oppose his or her thumb, what nerve is involved? What is a common term for this condition?

9. In an individual who has lost the ability to pick up his or her toes (ankle dorsiflexion), what nerve is involved? What is a common term for this condition?

10. Claw hand involves the loss of what muscle group? What nerve is primarily involved?

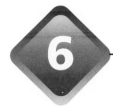

Basic Biomechanics

Introduction

The human body, in many respects, can be referred to as a living machine. It is important, when learning about how the body moves (kinesiology), to also learn about the forces that are placed on the body causing movement. As illustrated in Figure 6–1, **mechanics** is the branch of physics dealing with the study of forces and the motion produced by their actions. **Biomechanics** involves taking the principles and methods of mechanics and applying them to the structure and function of the human body. As mentioned in Chapter 1, mechanics can be divided into two main areas: statics and dynamics. **Statics** deals with factors associated with nonmoving, or nearly nonmoving systems. **Dynamics** involves factors associated with moving systems and can be divided into kinetics and kinematics. **Kinetics** deals with forces causing movement in a system, whereas kinematics involves the time, space, and mass aspects of a moving system. **Kinematics** can be divided into osteokinematics and arthrokinematics. **Osteokinematics** deals with the manner in which bones move in space without regard to the movement of joint surfaces, such as shoulder flexion/extension. **Arthrokinematics** deals with the manner in which adjoining joint surfaces move in relation to each other, that is, in the same or opposite direction.

Various mechanical terms must be defined before we begin a discussion of these topics. **Force** is any action or influence that moves an object. A **vector** is a quantity having both magnitude and direction. Force is a vector. For example, if you were to

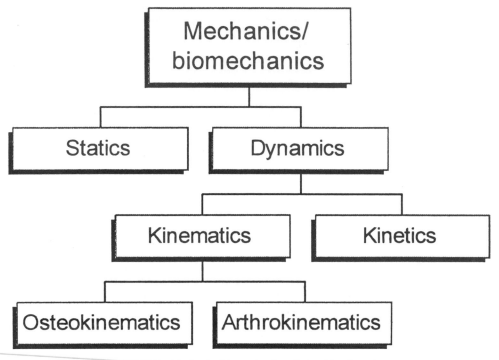

FIGURE 6–1.   Mechanics/biomechanics relationships flow chart.

throw a ball, you would throw it in a certain direction and with certain speed. **Mass** refers to the amount of matter that a body contains. In this example, the amount of matter within and making up the ball is the mass. **Inertia** is the property of matter that causes it to resist any change of its motion in either speed or direction. Mass is a measure of inertia; that is, its resistance to a change in motion.

Kinetics is a description of motion with regard to what causes motion. **Torque** is the tendency of force to produce rotation about an axis. **Friction** is a force developed by two surfaces, which tends to prevent motion of one surface across another. For example, there is a great deal of friction between the bottom of a foot covered by a sock and the carpeted floor making sliding difficult; however, there is relatively little friction between the sock and a highly polished hardwood floor. **Velocity** is a vector that describes displacement and is measured in units such as feet per second or miles per hour.

Laws of Motion

Motion is happening all around you—people walking, cars traveling on highways, airplanes flying in the air, water flowing in rivers, balls being thrown, and so on. Isaac Newton's three laws explain all types of motion. Newton's first law of motion states that an object at rest tends to stay at rest, and an object in motion tends to stay in motion. This is sometimes referred to as the **law of inertia,** because inertia is the tendency of an object to stay at rest or in motion. To demonstrate this law, consider riding in a car. If the car moves forward quickly from a starting position, your body pushes against the back of the seat and your neck probably hyperextends. Your body was at rest before the car moved, and it tended to stay at rest as the car started to move. Once moving, if the car were to stop suddenly, your body would be thrown forward and your neck would go into extreme flexion because your body was in motion and tended to stay in motion when the car stopped. Many of the people with neck injuries seen in physical therapy have, unfortunately, demonstrated this law.

A force is needed to overcome the inertia of an object and cause the object to move, stop, or change direction. The speed of the object depends on the strength of the force applied and the mass of the object. For example, kick a soccer ball and it will roll along the grass. If no forces act on it, the ball will roll forever. However, the force of friction acting on the ball causes the ball to stop. There is friction between any two surfaces. In this case, it is the friction of the grass on the surface of the ball that causes the ball to stop rolling.

A soccer ball can be used to demonstrate Newton's second law. First, mildly kick the ball and notice how far it travels. Next, kick the ball again about twice as hard as the first kick. Notice that the ball will travel approximately twice as far. **Acceleration** is any change in the speed of an object. The soccer ball is accelerating when it starts moving. If you were to kick the ball again even harder, it would travel proportionately farther. This is Newton's second **law of acceleration:** the amount of acceleration depends on the strength of the force applied to an object. Acceleration can also deal with a change in direction. Force is needed to change direction and, according to the law, the change in direction of an object depends on the force applied to it.

Another part of Newton's second law deals with the mass of an object. **Mass** is the amount of matter in an object. Acceleration is inversely proportional to the mass of an object. Thus, if you apply the same amount of force to two objects of differing mass, the object with greater mass will accelerate less than the object with less mass. You can demonstrate this by first kicking a soccer ball, then kicking a medicine ball with the same amount of force. The heavier medicine ball will not travel nearly as far.

Newton's third **law of action-reaction** states that for every action there is an equal and opposite reaction. The strength of the reaction is always equal to the strength of the action, and it occurs in the opposite direction. This can be demonstrated by jumping on a trampoline. The action is you jumping down on the trampoline. The reaction is the trampoline pushing back with the same amount of force. This causes you to rebound up in the opposite direction that you jumped. The harder you jump, the higher you rebound.

As stated, no motion can occur without a force. There are basically two types of force that will cause the body to move. Forces can be internal, such as muscular contraction, ligamentous restraint, or boney support or external, which could be gravity or any externally applied resistance such as weight, friction, and so on.

Force

Force is one of those concepts that everyone understands, but is difficult to define. To create a force, one object must act on another. Force can either be a push, which creates compression, or pull, which creates tension. Movement occurs if one side pushes (or pulls) harder than the other.

There are two quantities that describe forces: scalar and vector. A **scalar** quantity describes only magnitude. Common scalar terms are length, area, volume, and weight. Everyday examples would be such things as 5 feet, 2 acres, 12 fluid ounces, and 150 pounds. A **vector** quantity describes both magnitude and direction. A person pulling a heavy load with a rope would be an example of a vector. The tension in the rope represents the magnitude of the vector, and the direction of the rope represents the direction of the vector.

A vector force can be shown graphically by a straight line of appropriate length and direction. Figure 6–2 represents the diagram of two people (forces) pulling on a box, but at right angles to each other. The characteristics of force include (1) magnitude (which is equal, in this case), (2) direction (shown by the arrow), and (3) point of application (tail of arrow).

Forces can be described by the effect they produce. A **linear force** results when two or more forces are acting along the same line or plane. Figure 6–3*A* shows two people pulling a boat with the same rope in the same direction. Figure 6–3*B* shows two people pushing the hospital bed in the same direction with the same force. In both cases, movement occurs in the direction of force. Figure 6–3*C* shows two people pushing on opposite sides of the bed with equal force, but in the same plane. Although this is an example of linear force because the two people are pushing in the same plane, no motion occurs because they are pushing with equal force in opposite directions.

Parallel forces occur in the same plane and direction with a counter force in the middle but in the opposite direction. An example, as shown in Figure 6–4, is two children sitting on a seesaw. The forces are the two children, and the counter force is the support bar in the middle. Because of this counter force, a rotary movement occurs when one force is greater than the other is. Another example of parallel forces would be the three-point pressure of bracing (Fig. 6–5). Two forces, in this case the *X* and *Y*, are parallel to each other and pushing in the same direction, while a third

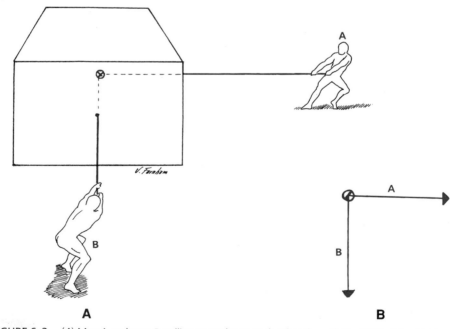

FIGURE 6–2. (*A*) Man A and man B pulling at angles to each other through the COG of the block represent a concurrent force system. (*B*) Illustration of the forces. (Adapted from Norkin, CC and Levangie, PK: Joint Structure and Function, ed 2. FA Davis, Philadelphia, 1992, p 29.)

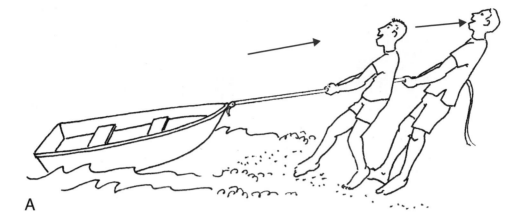

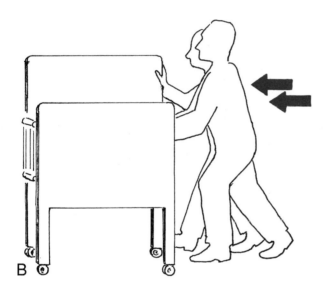

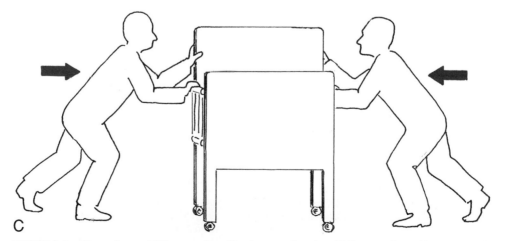

FIGURE 6–3.   Linear forces. (*A*) Two people pulling in same direction. (*B*) Two people pushing in same direction with same force. (*C*) Two people pushing with same force in opposite directions.

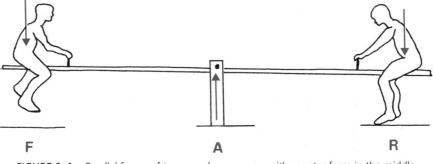

FIGURE 6–4. Parallel forces of two people on seesaw with counter force in the middle.

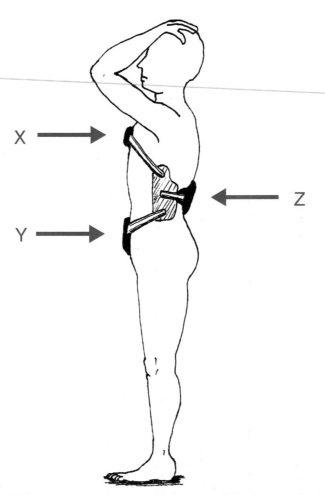

FIGURE 6–5. Parallel forces of body brace. Force *x* and *y* are parallel in the same direction while force *z* is parallel, but in the opposite direction. Force *z* must be in between forces *x* and *y* to provide stability. If force *z* were at either end, instead of the middle, motion would occur.

parallel force, the back brace is pushing against them. This third force must always be located between the two parallel forces. To be effective, it must be of sufficient strength to counter the two forces.

To produce **concurrent forces,** two or more forces act from a common point but pull in different (divergent) directions, such as the two people pulling on the box in Figure 6–6. The net effect of these two divergent forces is called the **resultant force,** and lies somewhere in between.

Because forces are vectors, they can be shown graphically using what is called the **parallelogram method.** Using Figure 6–6 as an example, first draw in vectors for the two forces (solid lines). Secondly, complete the parallelogram using dotted lines. Lastly, draw in the diagonal of the parallelogram (middle line and arrow). This diagonal line represents the resultant force.

An example of resultant force in the body is the anterior and posterior parts of the deltoid muscle (Fig. 6–7). Both parts have a common attachment (the insertion) but they pull in different directions. When both parallel forces are equal, the resultant force causes the shoulder to abduct. If the pull of the two forces were not equal, that is, if the pull of the anterior deltoid were stronger than that of the posterior, the resultant force would show that the motion would be more in the direction of the anterior deltoid (Fig. 6–8). The shoulder would flex and abduct in a forward, diagonal direction.

A **force couple** occurs when two forces act in an equal but opposite direction resulting in a turning effect. An example would be the fingers (force *a*) and the thumb (force *b*) unscrewing a jar lid (Fig. 6–9). With the jar lid in the right hand, the fingers move to the left while the thumb moves to the right; together they move the jar lid counterclockwise.

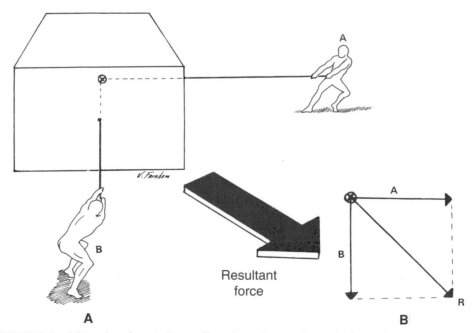

Resultant force

A   **B**

FIGURE 6–6.   (*A*) Resultant force is the net effect of two divergent forces. (*B*) Forces shown graphically using the parallelogram method. (Adapted from Norkin, CC and Levangie, PK: Joint Structure and Function, ed 2. FA Davis, Philadelphia, 1992, p 29.)

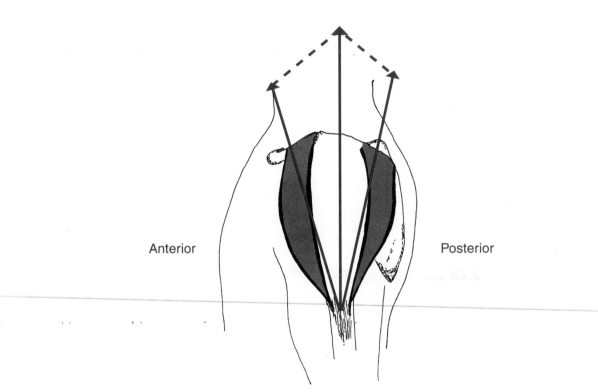

Anterior

Posterior

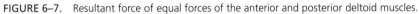

FIGURE 6–7.   Resultant force of equal forces of the anterior and posterior deltoid muscles.

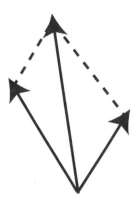

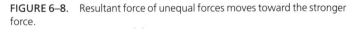

FIGURE 6–8.   Resultant force of unequal forces moves toward the stronger force.

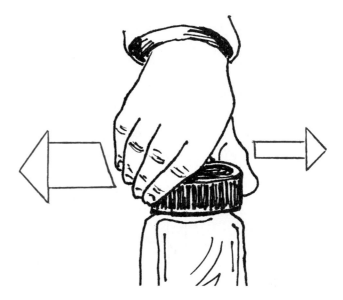

FIGURE 6–9.   Force couple.

Torque

Torque, also known as **moment of force,** is the ability of force to produce rotation about an axis. It can be thought of as rotary force. The amount of torque a lever has depends on the amount of force exerted and the distance it is from the axis. Use of a wrench demonstrates torque. The twisting force (torque) exerted by the wrench can be increased either by (1) increasing the force applied to the handle or (2) by increasing the length of the handle. Torque is also the amount of force needed by a muscle contraction to cause rotary joint motion.

Torque about any point (axis) equals the product of the force magnitude (how strong the force is) and its perpendicular distance from the axis of rotation to the line of force. The perpendicular distance is called the **moment arm** or **torque arm** (Fig. 6–10). Therefore, the moment arm of a muscle is the perpendicular distance between the muscle's line of force (line of pull) and the center of the joint (joint axis). Torque is greatest when the angle of pull is at 90 degrees, and decreases as the angle of pull either increases or decreases from that perpendicular position (Fig. 6–11). No torque would be produced if the force were directed exactly through the axis of rotation. Although this is not quite possible for a muscle, it comes very close. For example, if the biceps were to contract when the elbow was completely extended, there would be very little torque produced (Fig. 6–11B). The perpendicular distance between the joint axis and the angle of pull is very small. Therefore, the force generated by the muscle would be primarily a **stabilizing force,** in that nearly all of the force generated by the muscle is directed back into the joint, pulling the two bones together. Contrary to that, when the angle of pull is at 90 degrees (Fig. 6–11A), the perpendicular distance between the joint axis and the angle of pull is much larger. Therefore, the force generated by the muscle would be primarily an **angular force,** in that most of the force generated by the muscle is directed at moving the joint.

As a muscle contracts through its range of motion (ROM), the amount of angu-

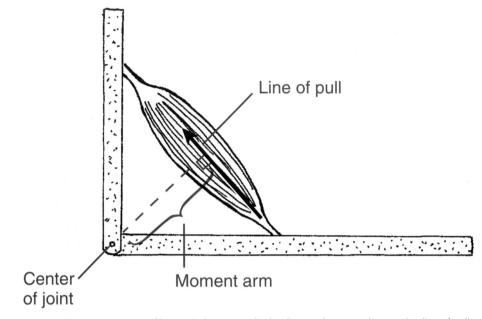

FIGURE 6–10. Moment arm of biceps is the perpendicular distance between the muscle's line of pull and the center of the joint.

lar or stabilizing force will change. As the muscle increases its angular force, it decreases its stabilizing force and vice versa. At 90 degrees, or half way through its range, the muscle has its greatest angular force. Past 90 degrees, the stabilizing force becomes a **dislocating force** because the force is directed away from the joint (Fig. 6–11*C*).

Some muscles that have a much greater stabilizing force than angular force throughout the range, and therefore, are more effective at stabilizing the joint than moving it. The coracobrachialis of the shoulder joint is a good example (see Fig. 8–17). Its line of pull is mostly vertical and quite close to the axis of the shoulder joint. Therefore, it has a very short moment arm, which makes this muscle more effective at stabilizing than at flexing the shoulder joint.

The angular force of the quadriceps muscle is increased by the presence of the patella. The patella, a sesamoid bone encapsulated in the tendon, increases the moment arm of the quadriceps muscle, allowing the muscle to have a greater angular force (Fig. 6–12). Without a patella, the moment arm is smaller and much of the force of the quadriceps is directed back into the joint (Fig. 6–13). Although this is good for stability, it is not effective for motion. To have an effective knee, it is vital that the quadriceps provide a strong angular force.

In summary, the greater the moment arm, the greater the angular force (torque). Moment arm is determined by measuring the perpendicular distance between the axis of rotation (joint axis) and the line of force (muscle's line of pull). Moment arm, size of the muscle, and contractile strength of the muscle all determine how effective a muscle is in causing joint motion.

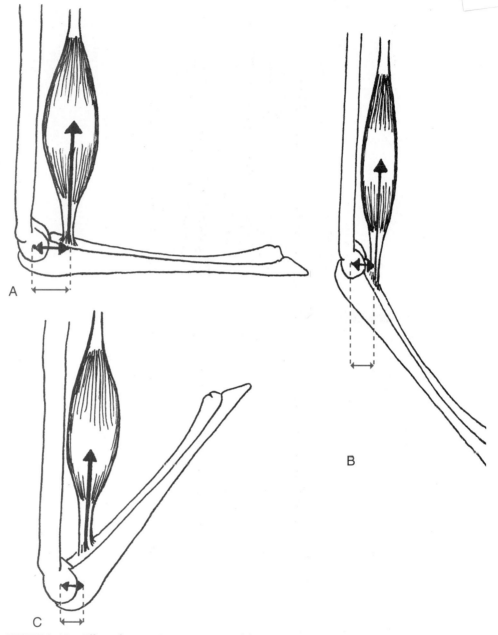

FIGURE 6–11. Effect of moment arm on torque. (*A*) Moment arm and angular force are greatest at 90 degrees. (*B*) Moment arm decreases as joint moves toward 0 degrees and stabilizing force increases. (*C*) Moment arm decreases as joint moves beyond 90 degrees toward 180 degrees and dislocating force increases. In both cases, when the stabilizing and dislocating forces are increasing, the angular force is decreasing. Stated another way, a muscle is most efficient at moving a joint when the joint is at 90 degrees. It becomes less efficient at moving when the joint angle either increasing or decreasing.

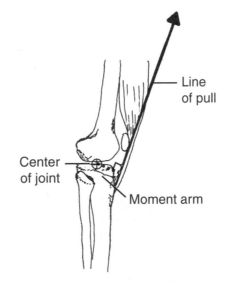

FIGURE 6–12. Moment arm of quadriceps muscle with a patella has larger moment arm and is thus more efficient at causing joint motion.

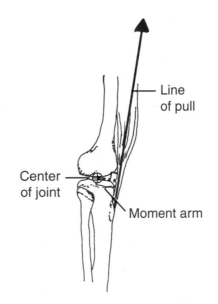

FIGURE 6–13. Moment arm of quadriceps muscle without a patella has smaller moment arm and is thus less efficient at causing joint motion.

Stability

When an object is balanced, all forces acting on it are even, and it is in a **state of equilibrium.** How secure or precarious this state of equilibrium is depends primarily on the relationship between the object's center of gravity and base of support. To understand the principles of stability, certain terms must be defined. **Gravity** is the mutual attraction between the earth and an object. **Gravitational force** is always directed vertically downward toward the center of the earth. Practically speaking, gravitational force is always directed toward the ground. **Center of gravity (COG)** is the balance point of an object at which weight on all sides is equal. It is also the point at which the planes of the body intersect, as shown in Figure 6–14.

In the human body, the COG is located in the midline at about the level of, though slightly anterior to, the second sacral vertebra of an adult. Because body proportions change with age, the COG of a child is higher than of an adult. To demonstrate this, move your right arm up over your head and touch your left ear. Now, ask a 3-year-old child to do the same. You will notice that while you can easily touch your ear, the child's hand reaches only to about the top of the head (Fig. 6–15). The child's head is much larger in proportion to the arms and rest of the body.

Base of support (BOS) is that part of a body that is in contact with the supporting surface. If you were to outline the surface of the body in contact with the ground, you would have identified the BOS. **Line of gravity (LOG)** is an imaginary

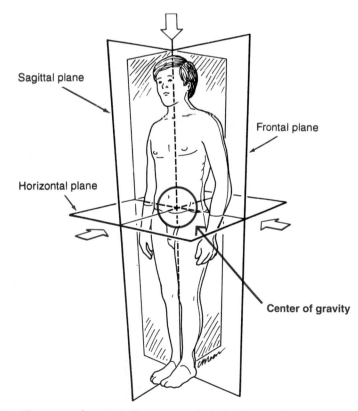

FIGURE 6–14. The center of gravity is the point at which the three cardinal planes intersect. (Adapted from Lehmkuhl, LD and Smith, LK: Brunnstrom's Clinical Kinesiology, ed 4. FA Davis, Philadelphia, 1983, p 3, with permission.)

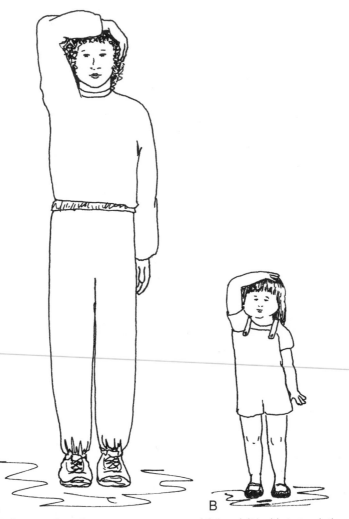

FIGURE 6–15. Body proportions change as a person grows. (*A*) An adult is able to touch the ear with opposite hand. (*B*) The child's head is larger proportionately to rest of body; thus, a child is unable to touch the opposite ear.

vertical line passing through the COG toward the center of the earth. These are shown in Figure 6–16.

There are basically three states of equilibrium (Fig. 6–17). **Stable equilibrium** occurs when an object is in a position that to disturb it would require its COG to be raised. A simple example is that of a brick. When the widest part of the brick is in contact with the surface (BOS), it is quite stable (Fig. 6–17A). To disturb it, the brick would have to be tipped up in any direction, thus raising its COG. **Unstable equilibrium** occurs when only a slight force is needed to disturb an object. Balancing a pencil by the pointed end is a good example. Once balanced, it takes very little force to knock the pencil over (Fig. 6–17B). **Neutral equilibrium** exists when an object's COG is neither raised nor lowered when it is disturbed. A good example would be a ball. As the ball rolls across the floor, its COG remains the same (Fig. 6–17C).

The following principles demonstrate the relationships between balance, stability, and motion.

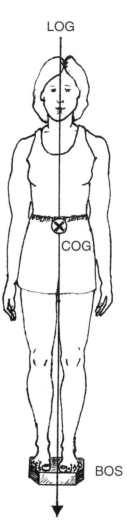

FIGURE 6–16. Center of gravity (COG), line of gravity (LOG), and base of support (BOS).

1. The lower the COG, the more stable the object. In Figure 6–18, both triangles have the same base of support. However, the triangle on the left is taller, has a higher COG, and thus is more unstable than the triangle on the right. It would take less force to disturb the taller triangle.
2. The COG and LOG must remain within the BOS for an object to remain stable. (Keep in mind that the LOG passes through the COG. Therefore what can be said of one can be said of the other. For the purpose of clarity, from this point forward, the term COG will be used.) The wider the BOS, the more stable the object. In the example in Figure 6–19, the book, resting entirely on its BOS (tabletop), is quite stable. As you push it off the edge, it becomes less stable. When its COG is no longer over the BOS, the book will fall.

   Another example would be a woman standing upright on both feet (Fig. 6–20). Her COG lies at or near the center of the base of support. As she leans to the side, her COG moves toward the border of her BOS. As soon as her COG passes beyond the BOS, she becomes unstable, and if her posture is not corrected or her BOS widened, she will fall. To lean further without los-

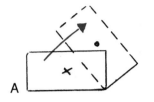

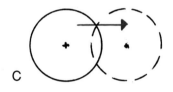

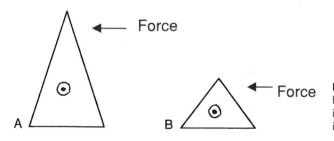

FIGURE 6–17. Three states of equilibrium. (*A*) Stable. (*B*) Unstable. (*C*) Neutral.

FIGURE 6–18. Relationship of height of center of gravity to stability. Triangle A is less stable because it has a higher COG.

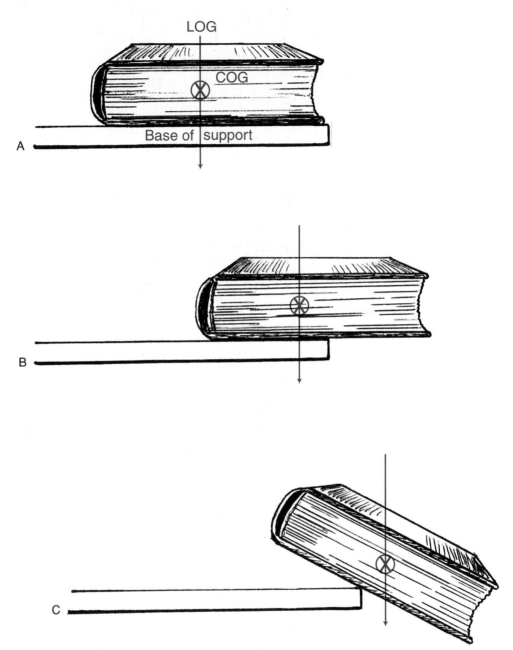

FIGURE 6–19. Relationship of COG to BOS. (*A*) The book is very stable because its COG is in the middle of its BOS. (*B*) The book is less stable because its COG is near the edge of its BOS. (*C*) The book is unstable and will fall because its COG is beyond its BOS.

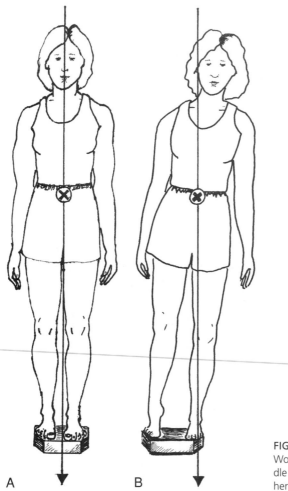

A   B

FIGURE 6–20. Relationship of COG to BOS. Woman in (*A*) is stable—her COG is in the middle of her BOS. In (*B*) she is less stable because her COG is near the edge of her BOS.

ing her balance she could either extend her opposite arm or widen her stance. In either case, her COG would move back over her BOS.

3. Stability increases as the BOS is widened in the direction of the force. A person standing at a bus stop on a very windy day would be more stable when facing into the wind and placing one foot behind the other, thus widening the BOS in the direction of the wind (Fig. 6–21).

4. The greater the mass of an object, the greater its stability. This concept is observed by looking at the size of players on a football team. Linebackers are traditionally heavier, and thus harder to push over. Halfbacks, whose job is to run with the ball, are much lighter. It can be said that what is gained in stability is lost in speed and vice versa.

5. The greater the friction between the supporting surface and the BOS, the more stable the body will be. Walking on an icy sidewalk is a slippery experience. Sanding the sidewalk increases the friction of the icy surface, thus improving traction. Having a surface with a great deal of friction is not always desirable. Pushing a wheelchair across a hardwood floor is much easier than pushing one across a carpeted floor. The carpet creates more friction, making it harder to push the wheelchair.

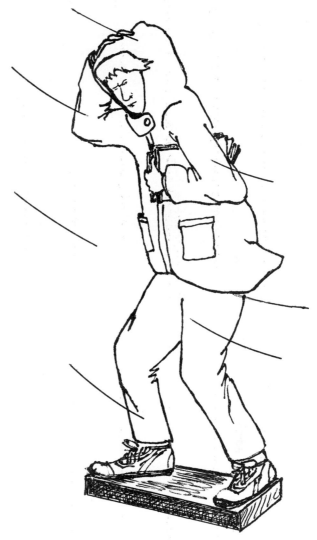

FIGURE 6–21. Wider base of support in direction of force increases stability.

6. People have better balance while moving if they focus on a stationary object rather than on a moving object. Therefore, people learning to walk with crutches would be more stable by focusing on an object down the hall than looking down at their moving feet or crutches.

Simple Machines

In engineering, various machines are used to change the magnitude or direction of a force. The four simple machines are the lever, the pulley, the wheel and axle, and the inclined plane. Examples of each of these machines, except for the inclined plane, can be found in the human body. The lever, the wheel and axle, and the inclined plane allow a person to exert a force greater than could be exerted by using muscle power alone; the pulley allows force to be applied more efficiently. This increase in force is usually at the expense of speed and can be expressed in terms of mechanical advantage, which will be described later.

LEVERS

There are three classes of levers, each with a different purpose and a different mechanical advantage. We use levers daily to help us accomplish various activities. The wheelbarrow, crowbar, manual can opener, scissors, golf club, tennis racket, and the playground seesaw are but a few examples. Different types of levers can also be found in the human body. To understand the structure and function of levers, you should be familiar with certain terms.

A **lever** is a rigid bar that can rotate about a fixed point when a force is applied to overcome resistance. The fixed point about which the lever rotates is the **axis (A),** sometimes referred to as the **fulcrum.** In the human body, the **force (F)** that causes the lever to move is usually muscular. The **resistance (R)** that must be overcome for motion to occur can include the weight of the part being moved, gravity, or an external weight. The **force arm (FA)** is the distance between the force and the axis and the **resistance arm (RA)** is the distance between the resistance and the axis (Fig. 6–22). The arrangement of the axis *A* in relation to the force *F* and the resistance *R* determines the type of lever.

Classes of Levers

In a **first-class lever,** the axis is located between the force and the resistance:

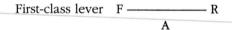

First-class lever   F ——————— R
                         A

A good example of this would be a playground seesaw (Fig. 6–23). The seesaw (lever arm) rotates on a crossbar (axis), which is located somewhere between a child sitting on one end of the board and pushing down against the ground (force) and the weight of the child sitting at the other end (resistance).

A **second-class lever** has the axis at one end, the resistance in the middle, and the force at the other end:

$$\text{Second-class lever} \quad \frac{\quad R \quad\quad F \quad}{A}$$

The wheelbarrow is a second-class lever (Fig. 6–24). The wheel at the front end is the axis, the contents of the wheelbarrow are the resistance, and the person pushing the wheelbarrow is the force.

A **third-class lever** has the axis at one end with the force in the middle and resistance at the opposite end:

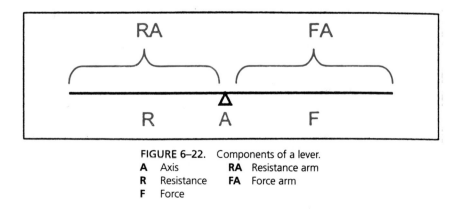

FIGURE 6–22.   Components of a lever.
A   Axis   **RA**   Resistance arm
R   Resistance   **FA**   Force arm
F   Force

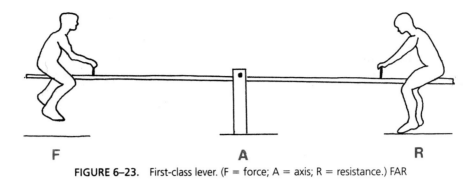

FIGURE 6–23. First-class lever. (F = force; A = axis; R = resistance.) FAR

$$\text{Third-class lever} \quad \frac{\text{F} \quad \text{R}}{\text{A}}$$

An example of this type of lever would be a screen door that has a spring attachment (Fig. 6–25). The axis is the door hinges, the force is the spring closing, and the resistance is the door itself.

As mentioned, each of these levers has a different purpose or mechanical advantage. The first-class lever is best designed for balance. An example in the human body would be the head sitting on the first cervical vertebra, moving up and down (Fig. 6–26). The vertebra would be the axis, the weight of one side of the head would be the resistance, and the muscles, pulling down on the opposite side of the head, would be the force. If, for example, you lowered your head to your chest, your head would rotate about the vertebra (axis). To return to the upright position, your posterior neck muscles (force) must contract to pull the weight of your head up against gravity (resistance). If you look up to the sky, your head would rock back, and you would need to use your anterior neck muscles to pull your head back to the upright position. Although force and resistance may change places, depending on the motion, the axis is always in the middle.

The second-class lever is best used for power, and there are surprisingly few, if any, examples in the body. Most authorities feel that there are no pure second-class levers in the body, in which the force is a muscle contracting concentrically. Some will give the example of the action of the ankle plantar flexor muscles when a per-

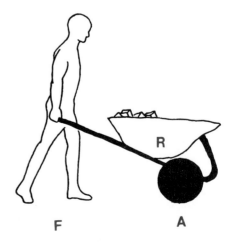

FIGURE 6–24. Second-class lever. (F = force; R = resistance; A = axis.) FRA

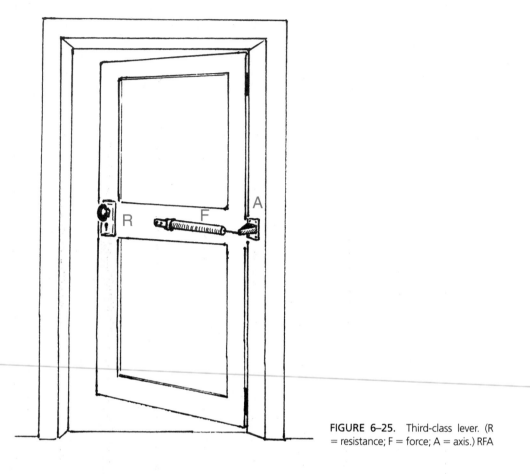

FIGURE 6–25. Third-class lever. (R = resistance; F = force; A = axis.) RFA

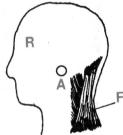

FIGURE 6–26. First-class lever. (R = resistance; A = axis; F = force.) RAF

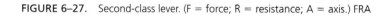

FIGURE 6–27. Second-class lever. (F = force; R = resistance; A = axis.) FRA

son stands on tiptoes (Fig. 6–27). In this case, the axis is the MP (metatarsal pha-langeal) joints in the foot, the resistance is the tibia and the rest of the body weight above it, and the force is provided by the ankle plantar flexors. As you can see, the plantar flexors do not have to move the joint very far, but they do have a great deal of weight or resistance to overcome.

The advantage of the third-class lever is ROM. This is, by far, the most common lever in the body. An example would be the biceps muscle during elbow flexion (Fig. 6–28). The axis is the elbow joint, the force is that exerted by the biceps mus-cle attached to the proximal radius, and the resistance is the weight of the forearm and hand. For the hand to be truly functional, it must be able to move through a wide ROM. The resistance will vary depending on what, if anything, is in the hand.

Why are there so many third-class levers, which favor ROM, and so few second-class levers, which favor power, in the body? Probably because the advantage gained from increased ROM is more important than the advantage gained from increased power. Examine the roles of the biceps and brachioradialis muscles in elbow flexion (Fig. 6–29). They both span the elbow but attach on the radius at very different places. The biceps muscle attaches to the proximal end of the radius, and the brachioradialis muscle attaches to the distal end. The biceps muscle acts as the force in a third-class lever because it attaches between the axis (elbow) and the resistance (forearm). The brachioradialis muscle is the force in a second-class lever because it attaches at the end of the lever arm, putting the resistance (forearm) in the middle. For example, say that each muscle is capable of contracting approximately four inches. Remember that a muscle is capable of being shortened one-half of its resting length. Therefore, the brachioradialis muscle will be able to move the distal end of the forearm and, subse-quently, the hand approximately four inches because its attachment is near the distal end. The biceps muscle will move the proximal end of the forearm approximately 4 inches, which will move the hand at the distal end much farther. Because the main function of the upper extremity is to allow the hand to move through a wide range, it makes sense that most of these muscles act as third-class levers.

Factors That Change Class

Under certain conditions a muscle may change from a second-class to a third-class lever, and vice versa. For example, the brachioradialis has been described as a second-class lever with the weight of the forearm being the main resistance. The weight of the forearm is located between the axis (elbow) and the force (distal muscle attachment)

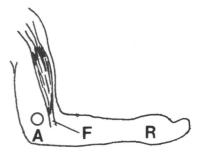

FIGURE 6–28.   Third-class lever. (A = axis; F = force; R = re-sistance.)

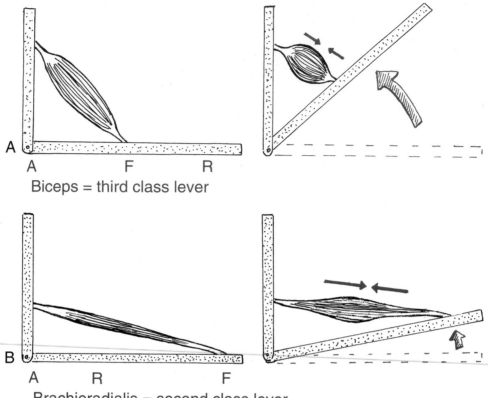

Biceps = third class lever

Brachioradialis = second class lever

FIGURE 6–29. (*A*) Third-class levers favor distance. The biceps moves a joint farther but requires more force. (*B*) Second-class levers favor force. The brachioradialis needs less force to move the joint, but the distance is much shorter.

as shown in Figure 6–29*B*. However, if you put a weight in the hand, that weight now becomes the resistance and is located farther from the axis than the force (muscle) (Fig. 6–30). Therefore, the brachioradialis is now working as a third-class lever.

The direction of the movement in relation to gravity is another factor that will effect lever class. For example, the biceps illustrated in Figure 6–31a is a third-class lever because it contracts concentrically to flex the elbow. The muscle is the force and the forearm is the resistance. The force is between the axis and resistance; therefore, it is a third-class lever. If you put a weight in the hand, it would still be a third-class lever. However, if the muscle contracted eccentrically, it would become a second-class lever. What has changed? As the elbow extends, moving the same direction as the pull of gravity, the biceps must contract eccentrically to slow the pull of gravity. Gravity and its pull on the forearm becomes the force. The biceps becomes the resistance, slowing elbow extension (Fig. 6–31). With the resistance now in the middle between the force and the axis, the biceps becomes a second-class lever.

MECHANICAL ADVANTAGE

Another important feature of levers and other machines, is **mechanical advantage,** which is defined as the ratio between the force arm and the resistance arm. The me-

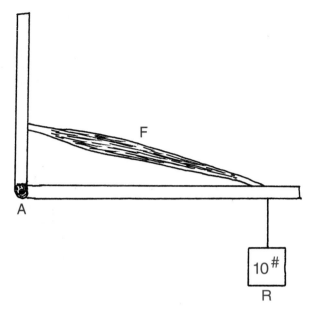

FIGURE 6–30. The brachioradialis becomes a third-class lever when a weight is placed in the hand.

chanical advantage (MA) of a lever is determined by dividing the length of the force arm by the length of the resistance arm

$$\left(MA = \frac{FA}{RA} \right)$$

When the force arm (*FA*) is greater than the resistance arm (*RA*), as with a second class lever, the mechanical advantage (*MA*) is greater than one. For example, if a force arm was 2 feet and the resistance arm was 1 foot, the mechanical advantage would be:

$$MA = \frac{FA}{RA} \qquad MA = \frac{2}{1} \qquad MA = 2$$

This means that the force arm has twice the force as the resistance arm. If, however, the force arm was shorter (1 foot) and the resistance arm was longer (2 feet) as with a third-class lever, the mechanical advantage would be:

$$MA = \frac{FA}{RA} \qquad MA = \frac{1}{2} \qquad MA = \frac{1}{2}$$

In other words, the force arm has half the force of the resistance arm.

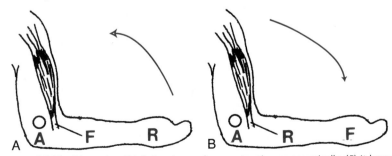

FIGURE 6–31. (*A*) The biceps is a third-class lever when contracting concentrically. (*B*) It becomes a second-class lever when contracting eccentrically.

What is always true of simple machines is that what is gained in force is lost in distance, and vice versa. In other words, to move an object using less force (mechanical advantage greater than 1) will also require that the force arm move a greater distance. Conversely, by using more force (mechanical advantage less than 1), the force arm will need to move a shorter distance. If the mechanical advantage equaled 1, the force arm and resistance arm would be equal and the system would be balanced, as in a first-class lever.

An example in physical therapy is the application of force to a patient's lower leg while the patient tries to keep the knee extended. It takes less force on your part if you place your hand distally versus proximally (Fig. 6–32). In this case the axis (A) is the knee joint, the resistance (R) is the insertion of the quadriceps muscle and the force (F) is your hand on the lower leg. In Figure 6–32A, the resistance arm is two inches and the force arm is 4 inches. The mechanical advantage can be calculated as follows:

$$MA = \frac{FA}{RA} \qquad\qquad MA = \frac{4}{2} \qquad\qquad MA = 2$$

In Figure 6–32B, the RA remains at 2 inches and the FA is 10 inches. Its mechanical advantage is calculated as follows:

$$MA = \frac{FA}{RA} \qquad\qquad MA = \frac{10}{2} \qquad\qquad MA = 5$$

Simply stated, the greater the mechanical advantage, the less force is needed to cause motion.

If the force arm and resistance arm are the same length, and the amount of force and resistance are equal, then the system is balanced and no motion will occur. In other words, if child A and child B each weigh 40 pounds, and are both sitting 5 feet from the crossbar, the seesaw will be balanced. If child A moved one foot closer to

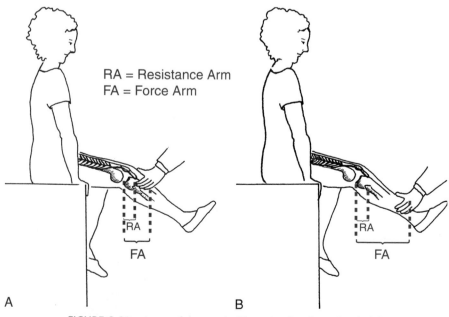

RA = Resistance Arm
FA = Force Arm

A

B

FIGURE 6–32.   Longer force arm in (*B*) requires less force than in (*A*).

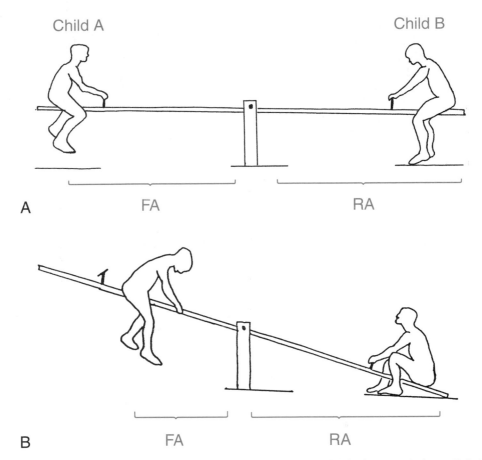

FIGURE 6–33. (*A*) When lever arms are equal, the system is balanced. (*B*) The force arm is shorter. To balance the system, the force arm needs to be lengthened or more weight (force) needs to be added to the force arm.

the crossbar, the system would no longer be balanced. Child A would go up, and child B would go down (Fig. 6–33). Child A would need either to add weight (more force) or move back (lengthen *FA*) to balance the seesaw again. Remember, with a longer force arm and a shorter resistance arm, less force is needed to cause motion.

Apply this concept to the wheelbarrow (Fig. 6–34). What is the difference between placing a load of bricks closer to the wheel axis (1 foot) or farther away (2 feet)? Although the force arm (where you place your hands on the handles) remains the same (3 feet), the length of the resistance arm changes. It becomes shorter as the bricks are placed closer to the wheel (Fig. 6–34*A*) and longer if the bricks are placed farther from the wheel (Fig. 6–34*B*). When there is a longer resistance arm, more force is needed; conversely, when there is a shorter resistance arm, less force is needed.

Another example involves lifting or carrying (Fig. 6–35). Which is going to take less energy, holding a box 2 inches from your body or 10 inches from your body? The answer is 2 inches. When the box is held 10 inches away from your body, the resistance arm is longer; therefore, more force is required to overcome its resistance.

There are many applications of the mechanical advantage of levers in physical therapy. The importance of levers can be seen in such things as saving energy or making tasks possible when strength is limited. To summarize, less force is required

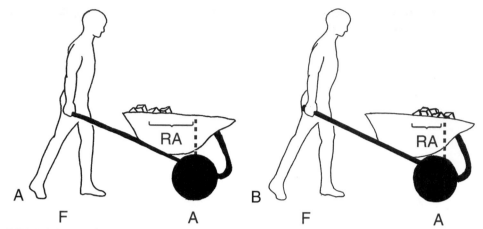

FIGURE 6–34. A shorter resistance requires less force. Loading bricks in front closer to axis (*B*) shortens the resistance arm.

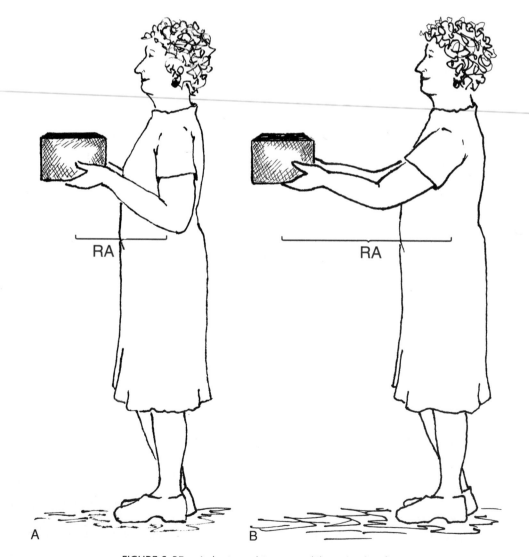

FIGURE 6–35. A shorter resistance arm (*A*) requires less force.

if you put the resistance as close to the axis as possible, and apply the force as far from the axis as possible.

PULLEYS

A **pulley** consists of a grooved wheel that turns on an axle with a rope or cable riding in the groove (Fig. 6–36). Its purpose is to either change the direction of a force, or to increase or decrease the magnitude of a force. A **fixed pulley** is a simple pulley attached to a beam. It acts as a first-class lever with *F* on one side of the pulley (axis) and *R* on the other. It is used only to change direction. Clinical examples of this can be found in both overhead and wall pulleys (Fig. 6–37) and home cervical traction units. In the body, the lateral malleolus of the fibula acts as a pulley for the tendon of the peroneus longus and changing its direction of pull (Fig. 6–38).

A **movable pulley** has one end of the rope attached to a beam then runs through the pulley to the other end where the force is applied. The load (resistance)

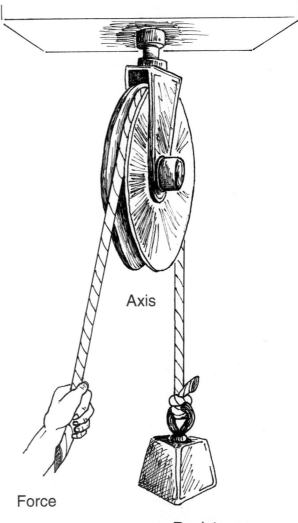

Axis

Force

Resistance

FIGURE 6–36. Pulley system.

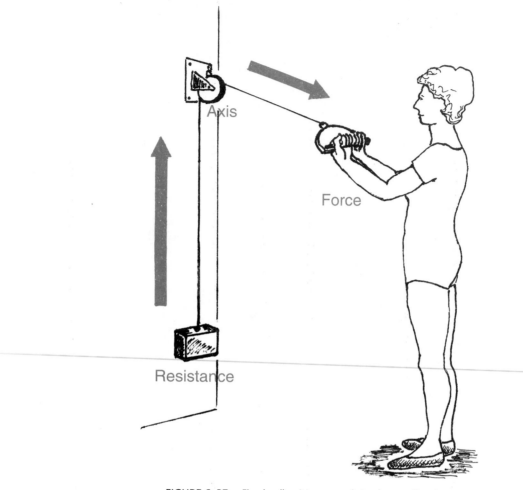

FIGURE 6–37.   Fixed pulley. Its purpose is to change direction.

is suspended from the movable pulley (Fig. 6–39). A single movable pulley acts as a second-class lever and increases the force of one of the levers (effort). The load is supported by both segments of the rope on either side of the pulley so it has a mechanical advantage of 2. It will require only half as much force to lift the load because the amount of force gained has doubled. Although only half of the force is needed to lift the load, the rope must be pulled twice as far. In other words, what is gained in force, is lost in distance. Examples of a movable pulley are not found in the human body.

WHEEL AND AXLE

The **wheel and axle** is another, though less common, type of simple machine found in the body. It is actually a lever in disguise. The wheel and axle consists of a wheel, or crank, attached to and turning together with an axle. It is typically used to increase the force exerted. Turning about a large radius (wheel) requires less force, whereas turning about a small radius (axle) requires a greater force. An example of a wheel

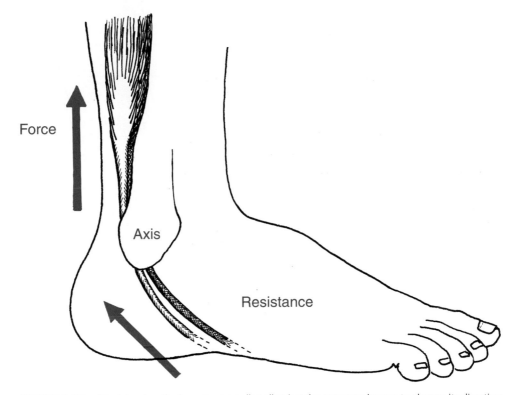

FIGURE 6–38. The lateral malleolus acts as a pulley allowing the peroneus longus to change its direction of pull.

and axle would be a faucet handle (Fig. 6–40). The handle(s) is the wheel and the stem is the axle. Turning the faucet requires a certain amount of force. However, take off the handle and you are left with only the axle (Fig. 6–41*B*). Try turning it and you will realize that a great deal more strength is needed to turn it. Simply stated, the larger the wheel in relation to the axle, the easier it is to turn the object. This is referred to as **mechanical advantage** (MA).

Calculation of the mechanical advantage of a wheel and axle is essentially the same as for a lever, only some of the terms are different. Wheel-and-axle mechanical advantage is calculated by dividing the radius of the wheel by the radius of the axle (Fig. 6–41).

$$MA = \frac{\text{radius of wheel}}{\text{radius of the axle}}$$

Therefore, calculating the mechanical advantage between the faucet *with* the handle and the faucet *without* the handle would be as follows:

$$MA \text{ (with handle)} = \frac{\text{radius of wheel}}{\text{radius of axle}}$$

$$MA = \frac{2 \text{ inches}}{1/8 \text{ inch}} = 16$$

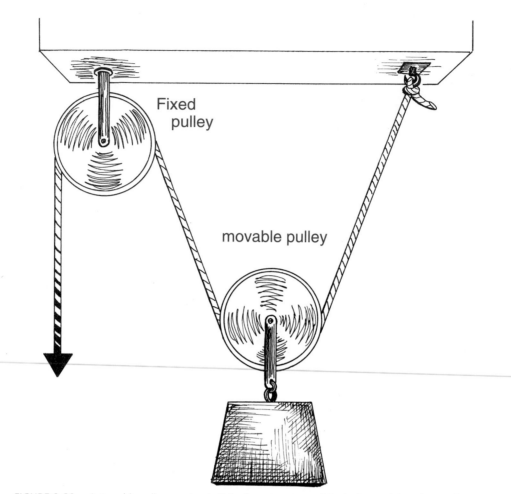

Fixed pulley

movable pulley

FIGURE 6–39. A movable pulley requires half the force to move weight (resistance), but the rope must be pulled twice as far.

The MA (without handle) is when the radius of the wheel and axle are the same, so the calculation would be as follows:

$$MA = \frac{1/8 \text{ inch}}{1/8 \text{ inch}} = 1$$

Hence, the larger the mechanical advantage, the easier it is to turn the handle, but the further the handle must be turned. Assume that you are treating a person with severe arthritis in the hands who is unable to turn the faucet handles easily. If you replace the handle with a long, lever-type handle (Fig. 6–42), you still have a wheel and axle. Visualize the 3-inch handle as one spoke of the wheel with the rest of the wheel missing. Its mechanical advantage would be calculated as follows:

$$MA = \frac{3 \text{ inches}}{1/8 \text{ inch}} = 24$$

The faucet handle will be much easier to turn because of greater mechanical advantage. The longer the handle of the faucet, the easier it is to turn. Keep in mind that although it is easier to turn the handle, the handle must be turned a greater distance.

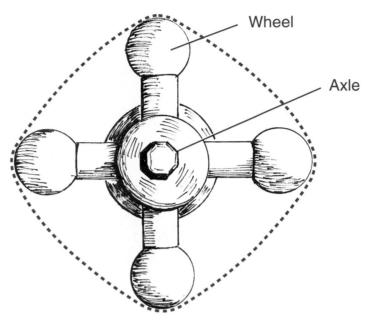

FIGURE 6–40.   A faucet handle is a wheel and axle.

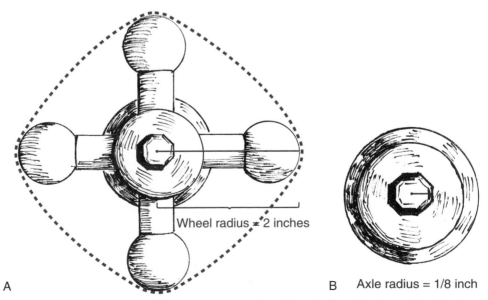

Wheel radius = 2 inches

A

B   Axle radius = 1/8 inch

FIGURE 6–41.   The radius of a wheel divided by the radius of the axle determines the mechanical advantage.

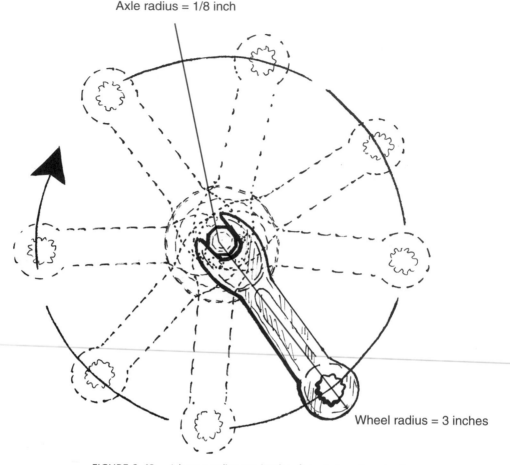

Axle radius = 1/8 inch

Wheel radius = 3 inches

FIGURE 6–42. A longer radius requires less force to turn the wheel.

To give an example of a wheel and axle in the human body, think of performing passive shoulder rotation on a patient. It can best be visualized by looking down on the shoulder from a superior view (Fig. 6–43). The shoulder joint serves as the axle and the forearm serves as the wheel. With the elbow flexed, the wheel is much longer than the axle, thus, much easier to turn.

INCLINED PLANE

Although there are no examples of an inclined plane in the human body, the concept of wheelchair accessibility often depends on this type of simple machine. An **inclined plane** is a flat surface that slants. It exchanges increased distance for less effort. The longer the length of a wheelchair ramp, the greater distance the wheelchair must travel, but the less effort required to propel the chair up the ramp. For example, if a porch is 2 feet from the ground and the ramp is 24 feet long, it would be fairly easy to propel the wheelchair up this fairly long ramp (Fig. 6–44A). If the ramp is only 12 feet long, it would be much steeper. The person would not have to propel the wheelchair as far, but would have to use more force to do so (Fig. 6–44B). Repeating the basic rule of simple machines: what is gained in force is lost in distance.

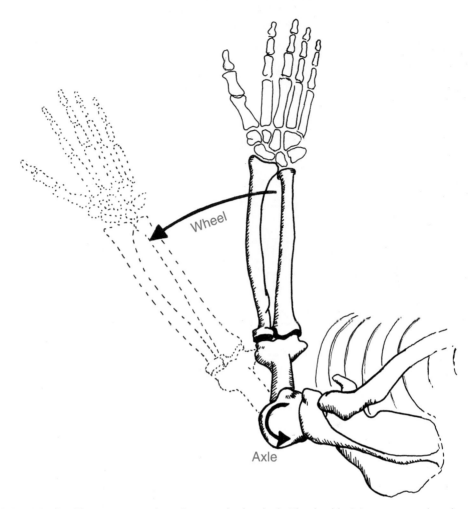

FIGURE 6–43. The upper extremity acting as a wheel and axle. The shoulder joint represents the axle and the flexed forearm is the wheel.

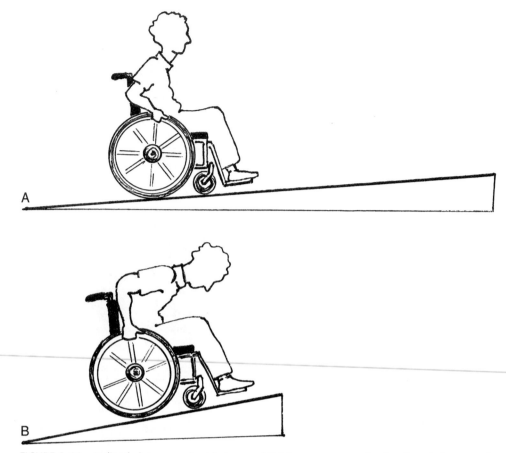

FIGURE 6–44. Inclined plane as a wheelchair ramp. (*A*) A longer ramp requires less force but greater distance. (*B*) A shorter ramp requires more force but shorter distance.

REVIEW QUESTIONS

1. Which weight cuff would provide more resistance to a patient, one placed around the wrist or around the elbow? Why?

2. Two people have the same weight and BOS, but one is on stilts. Which would be the most stable? Why?

3. What is the resultant force of the following muscles:

   a. Two heads of the gastrocnemius

   b. Sternal and clavicular portions of the pectoralis major

4. You are given two different sets of instructions. The first one tells you to run 5 miles, and the second one tells you to walk 30 feet to the north. Which instructions are vector and which are scalar?

5. Look at Figure 6–23, which illustrates a first-class lever. What would happen to the person on the left end of the seesaw (F) if another person got on behind the person on the right end of the seesaw (R)? Why?

6. Assuming it were possible, what would the person on the left end of the seesaw have to do to restore the balance?

7. Look at the illustration of a second-class lever (see Fig. 6–24). If the contents of the wheelbarrow shifted forward, would the load feel heavier or lighter?

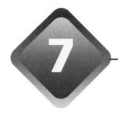

Shoulder Girdle

Clarification of Terms

The purpose of the shoulder and the entire upper extremity is to allow the hand to be placed in various positions to accomplish the multitude of tasks it is capable of performing. The shoulder, or glenohumeral joint, is the most mobile joint in the body and is capable of a great deal of motion. However, note that in talking about the shoulder motion, we must recognize that motion also occurs at three other joints or areas. The **shoulder complex** is a term that is sometimes used to include all of the structures involved with motion of the shoulder. The shoulder complex consists of the scapula, clavicle, sternum, humerus, and rib cage and includes the sternoclavicular joint, acromioclavicular joint, glenohumeral joint, and "scapulothoracic articulation" (Fig. 7–1). In other words, it includes the shoulder girdle (scapula and clavicle) and the shoulder joint (scapula and humerus). Note that the scapulothoracic articulation is not a joint in the pure sense of the word. Although the scapula and thorax do not have a point of fixation, the scapula does move over the rib cage of the thorax. The scapula and thorax are not directly attached but are connected indirectly via the clavicle and several muscles. The scapulothoracic articulation does provide motion and flexibility to the body.

Shoulder girdle is a term often used to discuss the activities of the scapula and

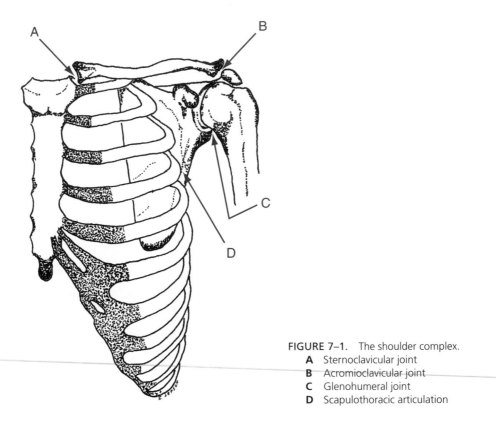

FIGURE 7–1. The shoulder complex.
A Sternoclavicular joint
B Acromioclavicular joint
C Glenohumeral joint
D Scapulothoracic articulation

clavicle and, to a lesser degree, the sternum. The sternoclavicular and acromioclavicular joints allow shoulder girdle motions; these motions are elevation and depression, protraction and retraction, and upward and downward rotation. There are five muscles that attach to the scapula, the clavicle, or both, providing motion of the shoulder girdle.

The **shoulder joint,** also called the glenohumeral joint, consists of the scapula and humerus. The motions of the shoulder joint are flexion, extension and hyperextension, abduction and adduction, medial and lateral rotation, and horizontal abduction and adduction. Because the shoulder joint is such a mobile joint, there are few ligaments. There are nine muscles that span the shoulder joint and are the prime movers.

Now that the various terms connected with the shoulder complex have been defined, the shoulder girdle will be discussed in more detail. The shoulder joint will be addressed in the Chapter 8.

Bones and Landmarks

The scapula is a triangular-shaped bone located superficially on the posterior side of the thorax that, along with the clavicle, makes up the shoulder girdle. The scapula attaches to the trunk indirectly through its ligamentous attachment to the clavicle. The scapula is slightly concave and glides over the convex rib cage posteriorly. Many muscles also connect the scapula to the trunk.

In the resting position, the scapula is located between the second and seventh ribs, with the vertebral border approximately 2 to 3 inches lateral from the spinous processes of the vertebra. The spine of the scapula is approximately level with the spinous process of the third and fourth thoracic vertebrae (Fig. 7–2).

The important bony landmarks of the scapula (Fig. 7–3) in terms of shoulder girdle function are the following.

Superior angle	Superior medial aspect, providing attachment for the levator scapula muscle.
Inferior angle	Most inferior point and where vertebral and axillary border meet. This point determines scapular rotation.
Vertebral border	Between superior and inferior angle medially, and attachment of the rhomboid muscles and the serratus anterior muscle.
Axillary border	The lateral side between glenoid fossa and inferior angle.
Spine	Projection on posterior surface running from medial border laterally to the acromion process. It provides attachment for the middle and lower trapezius muscles.
Coracoid process	Projection on anterior surface, providing attachment for the pectoralis minor muscles.
Acromion process	Broad, flat area on superior lateral aspect, providing attachment for the upper trapezius muscle.
Glenoid fossa	Slightly concave surface that articulates with humerus on superior lateral side above the axillary border and below acromion process.

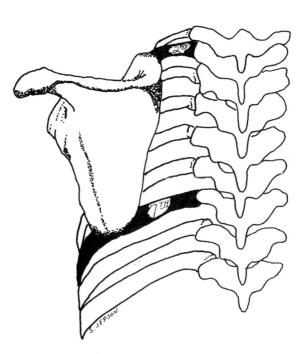

FIGURE 7–2. Resting position of the scapula on the thorax.

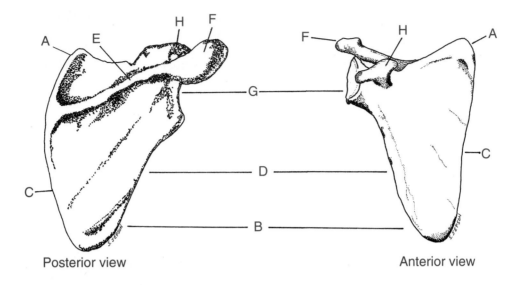

Posterior view

Anterior view

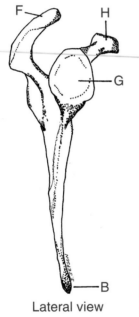

Lateral view

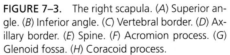

FIGURE 7–3. The right scapula. (*A*) Superior angle. (*B*) Inferior angle. (*C*) Vertebral border. (*D*) Axillary border. (*E*) Spine. (*F*) Acromion process. (*G*) Glenoid fossa. (*H*) Coracoid process.

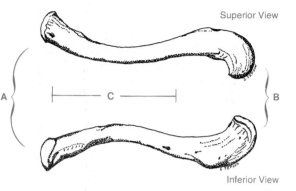

Superior View

Inferior View

FIGURE 7–4. The left clavicle. (*A*) Sternal end. (*B*) Acromial end. (C) Body.

The **clavicle** is an S-shaped bone that connects the upper extremity to the axial skeleton at the sternoclavicular joint. It also attaches to the scapula at the acromioclavicular joint. The important bony landmarks of the clavicle (Fig. 7–4) for shoulder girdle function are as follows:

Sternal end	Attaches medially to sternum
Acromial end	Attaches laterally to scapula, and provides attachment for the upper trapezius muscle
Body	Area between the two ends

The **sternum** is a flat bone located in the midline of the anterior thorax (Fig. 7–5). At its superior end it provides attachment for the clavicle, followed beneath by attachments for the costal cartilages of the ribs. It is divided into three parts:

Manubrium	The superior end, providing attachment for the clavicle and the first rib
Body	The middle two thirds of the sternum, providing attachment for the remaining ribs
Xiphoid process	Meaning "sword-shaped"; the inferior tip

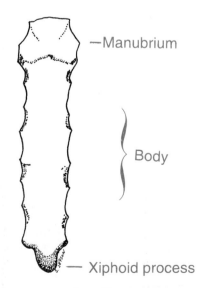

—Manubrium

Body

— Xiphoid process

FIGURE 7–5. The sternum (anterior view).

Joints and Ligaments

The **sternoclavicular joint** (Fig. 7–6) provides the shoulder girdle with its only direct attachment to the trunk. It is a synovial joint that is plane shaped and has a double gliding motion. Motions occur in three planes and accompany the motions of the shoulder girdle. Although these motions are more subtle than those at most other joints, they are nonetheless important. Basically, the clavicle moves while the sternum remains stationary.

The sternoclavicular joint, being a synovial joint, has a joint capsule. It also has three major ligaments and a joint disk. The joint capsule surrounds the joint and is reinforced by the anterior and posterior sternoclavicular ligaments. The articular disk serves as a shock absorber, especially from forces generated by falls on the outstretched hand. The disk and its ligamentous support are so effective that dislocation at the sternoclavicular joint is rare. This disk has a unique attachment that contributes to the motion of this joint: It has a double attachment much like that of a double-hung hinge found on doors that can swing in both directions. During shoulder girdle elevation and depression, motion occurs between the clavicle and the disk. During protraction and retraction motion occurs between the disk and the sternum.

The three major ligaments supporting this joint are the sternoclavicular, costoclavicular, and interclavicular ligaments. The sternoclavicular ligament connects the clavicle to the sternum on both the anterior and posterior surfaces and is therefore divided into the anterior and posterior sternoclavicular ligaments. As mentioned, it provides reinforcement to the joint capsule. The **costoclavicular ligament** is a short, flat, rhomboid-shaped ligament that connects the inferior surface of the clavicle to the superior surface of the costal cartilage of the first rib. The primary purpose of this ligament is to limit the amount of clavicular elevation. The **interclavicular ligament** is located on top of the manubrium, connecting the superior sternal ends of the clavicles. Its purpose is to limit the amount of clavicular depression.

The **acromioclavicular joint** (Fig. 7–7) connects the acromion process of the scapula with the lateral end of the clavicle. It is a plane-shaped synovial joint with three planes of motion. The motions are minimal but important to normal shoulder motion. The joint capsule surrounds the articular borders; it is quite weak and is reinforced above and below by the superior and inferior acromioclavicular ligaments. These ligaments also give support to the joint by holding the acromion process to the clavicle, thus preventing dislocation of the clavicle.

The coracoclavicular ligament and coracoacromial ligaments are two accessory ligaments of the acromioclavicular joint. Although the **coracoclavicular ligament**

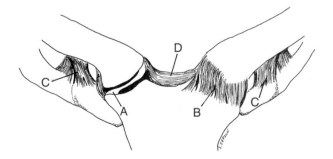

FIGURE 7–6. The sternoclavicular joint (left side cut away). (*A*) Articular disk. (*B*) Sternoclavicular ligament. (*C*) Costoclavicular ligament. (*D*) Interclavicular ligament.

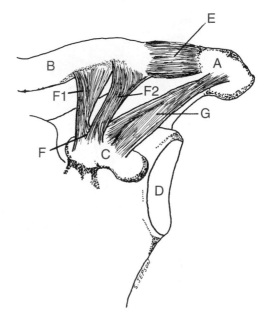

FIGURE 7–7. The acromioclavicular joint. (*A*) Acromion. (*B*) Clavicle. (*C*) Coracoid process. (*D*) Glenoid fossa. (*E*) Acromioclavicular ligament. (*F*) Coracoclavicular ligament: conoid portion (*F1*) and trapezoid portion (*F2*). (*G*) Coracoacromial ligament.

is not directly located at the joint, it does provide stability to that joint and allows the scapula to be suspended from the clavicle. It connects the scapula to the clavicle by attaching to the inferior surface of the lateral end of the clavicle and the superior surface of the coracoid process of the scapula. The ligament is divided into a lateral trapezoid portion and the deeper medial conoid portion. Together they prevent backward motion of the scapula, and individually they limit the rotation of the scapula.

The **coracoacromial ligament** does not actually cross the acromioclavicular joint, but rather forms an arch over the head of the humerus. It attaches laterally on the superior surface of the coracoid process and runs up and out to the inferior surface of the acromial process. It makes a roof over the head of the humerus and serves as a protective arch providing support to the head when an upward force is transmitted along the humerus (Fig. 7–8).

Joint Motions

As mentioned, motions of the shoulder girdle are elevation and depression, protraction and retraction, and upward and downward rotation (Fig. 7–9). Because these motions can be seen best by looking at the scapula, these motions are commonly described as either *shoulder girdle* or *scapular motion*. For example, shoulder girdle protraction and retraction is synonymous with scapular abduction and adduction, and scapular rotation is the same as shoulder girdle rotation.

Elevation/depression and protraction/retraction are essentially linear motions. All points of the scapula move up and down along the thorax and away from and toward the vertebral column in parallel lines. Angular motion occurs during upward and downward rotation of the scapula. Because of the triangular shape of the scapula, one side moves one way while another side moves in an opposite or dif-

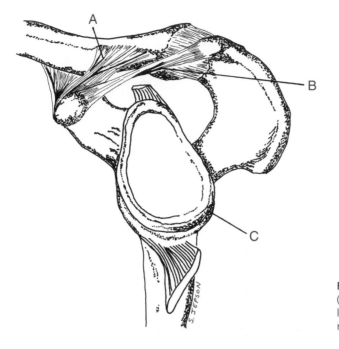

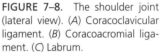

FIGURE 7–8. The shoulder joint (lateral view). (*A*) Coracoclavicular ligament. (*B*) Coracoacromial ligament. (*C*) Labrum.

ferent direction. During upward rotation, the inferior angle of the scapula rotates up and away from the vertebral column, while downward rotation is the return to the resting position. For example, when the inferior angle rotates up and out, the superior angle moves down, and the glenoid fossa moves up and in. Therefore, it is important to have a point of reference to define this rotation. The inferior angle is that reference point (Fig. 7–10).

Another scapular motion should be mentioned—scapular tilt (see Fig. 7–9*D*). Scapular tilt occurs when the shoulder joint goes into hyperextension. The superior end of the scapula tilts forward and the inferior end tilts posteriorly. Examples of these combined motions would be in the "wind-up" or pre-release phase of a softball pitch, a bowling delivery, or a racing dive in swimming.

COMPANION MOTIONS OF THE SHOULDER JOINT
AND SHOULDER GIRDLE

During the linear movements of elevation/depression and protraction/retraction, it is possible to move the shoulder girdle (clavicle and scapula) up, down, forward, or backward without moving the humerus. However, shoulder joint motions must accompany the angular motions of upward and downward rotation. To rotate the scapula upward, you must also flex or abduct the shoulder joint. Stated another way, when there is flexion or abduction of the shoulder joint, the scapula must also rotate upward. When there is extension or adduction of the shoulder joint, the scapula returns to anatomical position, or rotates downward. Table 7–1 lists the shoulder girdle motions that must occur during various shoulder joint motions. Because of the complex and interrelated activities of the shoulder girdle and the shoulder joint, it is difficult to discuss the function of one without discussing activities of the other. Impairment at one joint will also impair function at the other.

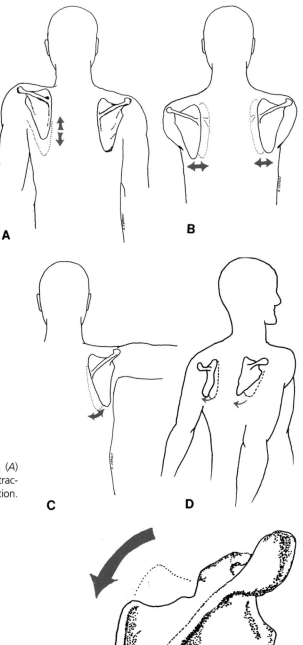

FIGURE 7–9. Shoulder girdle motions. (*A*) Elevation/depression. (*B*) Protraction/retraction. (*C*) Upward rotation/downward rotation. (*D*) Scapular tilt.

FIGURE 7–10. Scapular motion during upward rotation

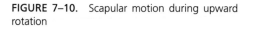

TABLE 7–1	COMPANION MOTIONS OF THE SHOULDER JOINT AND SHOULDER GIRDLE

Shoulder Joint	Shoulder Girdle
Flexion	Upward rotation; protraction
Extension	Downward rotation; retraction
Hyperextension	Scapular tilt
Abduction	Upward rotation
Abduction	Downward rotation
Medial rotation	Protraction
Lateral rotation	Retraction
Horizontal abduction	Retraction
Horizontal abduction	Protraction

SCAPULOHUMERAL RHYTHM

Scapulohumeral rhythm is a concept that further describes the movement relationship between the shoulder girdle and shoulder joint. The first 30 degrees of shoulder joint motion is pure shoulder joint motion. However, after that, for every 2 degrees of shoulder flexion or abduction that occurs, the scapula must upwardly rotate 1 degree. This 2:1 ratio is known as scapulohumeral rhythm.

It is possible to demonstrate that the first part of shoulder joint motion occurs only at that joint, but further motion must be accompanied by shoulder girdle motion. With a person in the anatomical position, stabilize the scapula by putting the heel of your hand against the axillary border to prevent rotation. Instruct the person to abduct the shoulder joint. Notice that the individual is only able to abduct a short distance before motion is impaired.

Muscles of the Shoulder Girdle

ANGLE OF PULL

As discussed in Chapter 4, several factors determine the role that a muscle will play in a particular joint motion. Determining whether a muscle has a major role (prime mover), a minor role (assisting mover), or no role at all will depend on such factors as its size, angle of pull, the joint motions possible, and the location of the muscle in relation to the joint axis. Angle of pull is usually a major factor. Most muscles pull at a diagonal. As discussed in Chapter 6 regarding torque, most muscles have a diagonal line of pull. That diagonal line of pull is the resultant force of a vertical force and a horizontal force. In the case of the shoulder girdle, muscles with a greater vertical angle of pull will be effective in pulling the scapula up or down (elevating or depressing the scapula). Muscles with a greater horizontal pull will be more effective in pulling the scapula in or out (protracting or retracting). Muscles with a more equal horizontal and vertical pull will have a role in both motions (see Fig. 7–4). For example, the levator scapula has a stronger vertical component, the middle trapezius has a stronger horizontal component, whereas the rhomboids have a more equal pull in both directions. As you will see when these muscles are described later in this chapter, the levator scapula is a prime mover in scapular elevation, the middle trapezius is a prime mover in retraction, and the rhomboids are a prime mover in both elevation and retraction.

MUSCLE DESCRIPTIONS

There are five muscles primarily responsible for moving the scapula. Each muscle will be discussed with particular emphasis on its location and function. This will be followed by a summary of its proximal attachment (0, origin), distal attachment (I, insertion), and joint motions in which it is a prime mover (A, action). This listing is given for clarity and is not intended to be the only description. The student is encouraged to visualize the attachments and describe them using proper terminology instead of memorizing these listings. The nerve (N), which innervates the muscle, as well as the spinal cord level of that innervation, are also given.

The muscles of the shoulder girdle are the:

Trapezius
Levator scapulae
Rhomboids
Serratus anterior
Pectoralis minor

The **trapezius muscle** (Fig. 7–11) is a large superficial muscle, which is diamond shaped when looking at both right and left sides. Functionally, it is usually di-

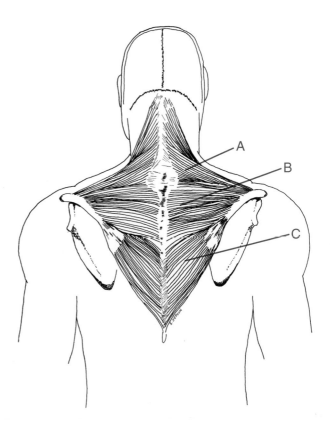

FIGURE 7–11. The trapezius muscle.
A Upper trapezius
B Middle trapezius
C Lower trapezius

vided into three parts: upper, middle, and lower. The reason for this separation is that there are three different lines of pull (up, in, down) resulting in different muscle actions.

The **upper trapezius muscle** (Fig. 7–12) originates from the occipital protuberance and the nuchal ligament of the upper cervical vertebra. The nuchal ligament attaches to the spinous processes of the cervical vertebra. The upper trapezius inserts on the lateral end of the clavicle and acromion process. Because its diagonal line of pull is more vertical (up) than horizontal (in), it is a prime mover in scapular elevation and upward rotation and only an assisting mover in scapular retraction.

The **middle trapezius muscle** (Fig. 7–13) originates from the nuchal ligament of the lower cervical vertebra and spinous process of the upper thoracic vertebra and inserts on the medial aspect of the acromion process and along the scapular spine. Its line of pull is horizontal, which makes it very effective at scapular retraction. Because the line of pull passes just above the axis for upward rotation, its role in scapular upward rotation is only assistive.

The **lower trapezius muscle** (Fig. 7–14) originates from the spinous processes of the middle and lower thoracic vertebrae and inserts on the base of the scapular spine. Its diagonal line of pull is more down (vertical) than in (horizontal), making it effective in depression and upward rotation of the scapula and only assistive in retraction.

All three parts of the trapezius muscle work together (synergists) to retract the scapula. Remember, however, that the middle trapezius muscle is the prime mover and the upper and lower trapezius muscles can only assist. The upper and lower trapezius muscles are antagonistic to each other in elevation/depression and agonistic in upward rotation. To visualize the upward rotation component of these muscles, think of the scapula as a steering wheel (Fig. 7–15). In this example, a right scapula is used. Tie a ribbon at the bottom of the wheel to represent the inferior angle of the scapula. Put your right hand at the 2-o'clock position representing the up-

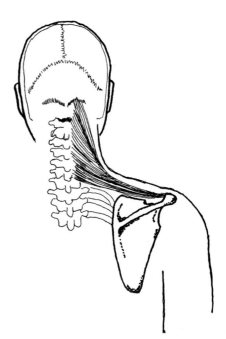

FIGURE 7–12. The upper trapezius muscle.

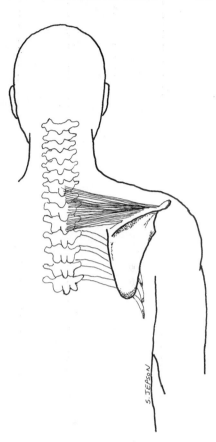

FIGURE 7–13.   The middle trapezius muscle.

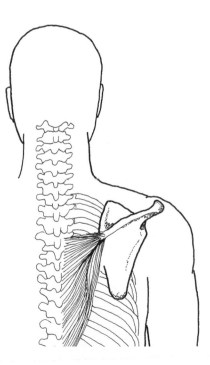

FIGURE 7–14.   The lower trapezius muscle.

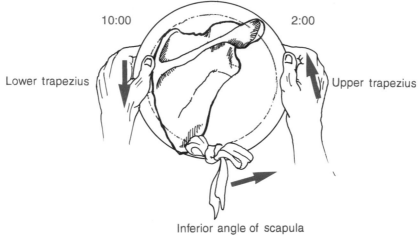

10:00   2:00

Lower trapezius   Upper trapezius

Inferior angle of scapula

FIGURE 7–15. Rotational movement of the right scapula.

per trapezius attachment, and put your left hand at the 10-o'clock position, representing the lower trapezius attachment. Turn the wheel to the left and note that the ribbon moves upward toward the right. In the case of the scapula, the upper trapezius muscle (right hand) moves up and in, the lower trapezius muscle (left hand) moves down and in. This combined effort causes the inferior angle to move up and out (upward rotation).

Upper Trapezius Muscle

(O)	Occipital bone, nuchal ligament on cervical spinous processes
(I)	Outer third of clavicle, acromion process
(A)	Scapular elevation and upward rotation
(N)	Spinal accessory (cranial nerve XI), C3 and C4 sensory component

Middle Trapezius Muscle

(O)	Spinous processes of C7 through T3
(I)	Scapular spine
(A)	Scapular retraction
(N)	Spinal accessory (cranial nerve XI), C3 and C4 sensory component

Lower Trapezius Muscle

(O)	Spinous processes of middle and lower thoracic vertebrae
(I)	Base of the scapular spine
(A)	Scapular depression and upward rotation
(N)	Spinal accessory (cranial nerve XI), C3 and C4 sensory component

The **levator scapula muscle** is named for its function of scapular elevation. It is covered entirely by the trapezius muscle. It arises from the transverse processes of C1 through C4 and attaches on the vertebral border of the scapula between the superior angle and the spine (Fig. 7–16). Its diagonal line of pull is mostly, vertical; therefore, it is a prime mover in scapular elevation and only a secondary mover in

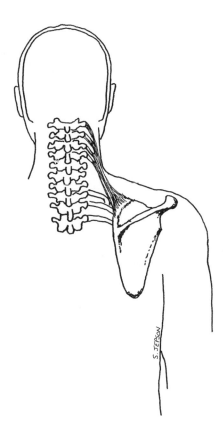

S. JEPSON

FIGURE 7–16.   The levator scapula muscle.

retraction. It is also a prime mover in downward rotation. Visualize the steering wheel with your hand in the 10-o'clock position. Pull up (turning the wheel to the right) and notice that the inferior angle (ribbon) moves to the left (downward rotation). Keep in mind that downward rotation is the return to anatomical position from an upwardly rotated position.

Levator Scapula Muscle	
(O)	Transverse processes of first four cervical vertebrae
(I)	Vertebral border of scapula between the superior angle and spine
(A)	Scapular elevation and downward rotation
(N)	Third and fourth cervical nerves and dorsal scapular nerve (C5)

The **rhomboids** are actually two muscles: rhomboid major and rhomboid minor. However, because it is anatomically difficult to separate these two muscles and because functionally they have the same actions, they are commonly considered together as one muscle. They derive their name from their shape. This geometric shape is basically a rectangle that has been skewed so that the sides have oblique angles instead of right angles. The rhomboid muscles lie under the trapezius muscle and can be palpated when the trapezius muscle is relaxed. They originate from the nuchal ligament and spinous processes of C7 through T5 and insert on the vertebral border of the scapula below the levator scapula muscle between the spine and the inferior angle (Fig. 7–17). Because their oblique line of pull has a good horizontal

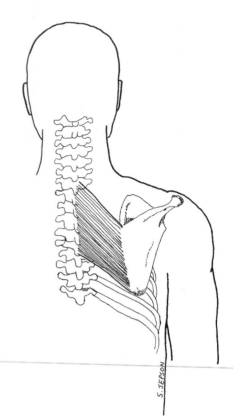

FIGURE 7–17. The rhomboid muscle.

and vertical component, they are a prime mover in retraction and elevation. Like the levator scapula muscle, they downwardly rotate the scapula.

Rhomboid Muscles	
(O)	Spinous processes of C7 through T5
(I)	Vertebral border of scapula between the spine and inferior angle
(A)	Scapular retraction, elevation, and downward rotation
(N)	Dorsal scapular nerve (C5)

It is impossible to raise your arm above your head without the action of the **serratus anterior muscle.** This muscle gets its name from the serrated, or saw-tooth, pattern of attachment on the anterolateral side of the thorax. It is superficial at this point and may be palpated when the arm is overhead. The muscle runs posteriorly to pass between the scapula and the rib cage. It attaches on the anterior surface of the scapula along the vertebral border between the superior and inferior angles (Fig. 7–18). Because it has a nearly horizontal line of pull outward, it is a prime mover in scapular protraction. Its lower fibers pulling outward on the lower part of the scapula are effective in upwardly rotating the scapula. These fibers join with the upper and lower trapezius muscles to form a force couple rotating the scapula upward. Another function of this muscle is to keep the vertebral border of the scapula against the rib cage. Without this muscle the vertebral border lifts away from the rib cage, which is called "winging of the scapula" (Fig. 7–19).

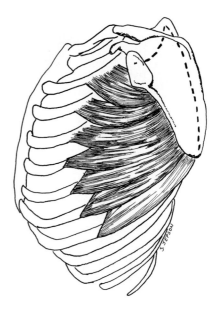

FIGURE 7–18. The serratus anterior muscle.

Serratus Anterior Muscle
(O) Lateral surface of the upper eight ribs
(I) Vertebral border of the scapula, anterior surface
(A) Scapular protraction and upward rotation
(N) Long thoracic nerve (C5, C6, C7)

FORCE COUPLES

A **force couple** is defined as muscles pulling in different directions to accomplish the same motion. In the case of the shoulder girdle, the upper trapezius muscle pulls up, the lower trapezius muscle pulls down, and the lower fibers of the serratus anterior muscle pull out (Fig. 7–20). The net effect is that the scapula is rotated upwardly.

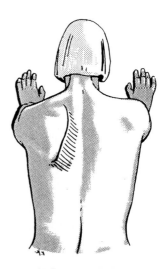

FIGURE 7–19. Winging of the scapula. This woman's left serratus anterior muscle is paralyzed. When she pushes against the wall with both hands, her left scapula rises away from the rib cage, standing out like a small wing. (From Moore, KL: Clinically Oriented Anatomy, ed 3. Williams & Wilkins, Baltimore, 1992, p 525, with permission.)

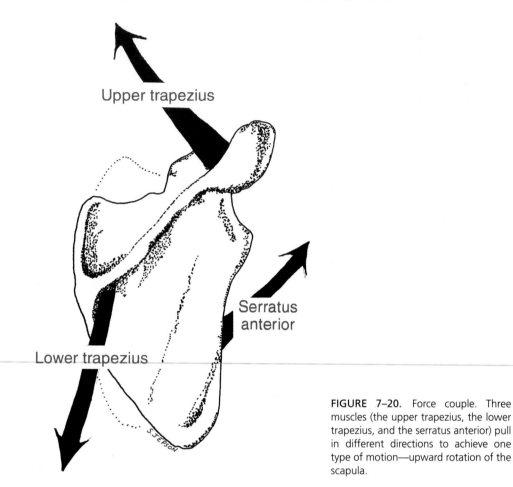

FIGURE 7–20. Force couple. Three muscles (the upper trapezius, the lower trapezius, and the serratus anterior) pull in different directions to achieve one type of motion—upward rotation of the scapula.

The **pectoralis minor muscle** lies deep to the pectoralis major muscle and is the only shoulder girdle muscle located entirely on the anterior surface of the body. It arises from the anterior surface of the third through fifth ribs near the costal cartilages and runs upward to its attachment on the coracoid process of the scapula (Fig. 7–21). Its diagonal line of pull is mostly vertical (down), making it a prime mover in scapular depression and downward rotation. Although it is rather easy to see the depression action, the downward rotation is less obvious because the muscle is on the anterior surface while the scapula moves on the posterior surface. Visualize the steering wheel again with the ribbon (inferior angle of the scapula) rotated up to the right. Place your hand in the 2-o'clock position (coracoid process) and pull down. Notice that the ribbon (inferior angle) moves downward toward the left (downward rotation).

Pectoralis Minor Muscle

(O)	Anterior surface, third through fifth ribs
(I)	Coracoid process of the scapula
(A)	Scapular depression, protraction, and downward rotation
(N)	Medial pectoral nerve (C8, T1)

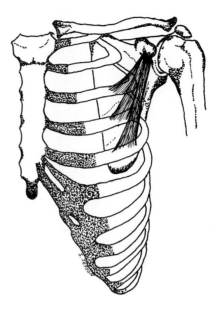

FIGURE 7–21.   The pectoralis minor muscle.

Downward rotation is another example of a force couple. The combined effect of the pectoralis minor muscle pulling down, the rhomboid muscles pulling in, and the levator scapular muscle pulling up is to downwardly rotate the scapula (Fig. 7–22). This motion is accomplished when the shoulder joint is forcefully extended, as when chopping wood or paddling a canoe. Downward rotation of the scapula must accompany extension of the shoulder joint. Table 7–2 summarizes the actions of the prime movers of the shoulder girdle.

REVERSAL OF MUSCLE ACTION

The actions of the shoulder girdle muscles have been described moving insertion toward the origin. However, if the insertion is stabilized, the origin will move. As discussed in Chapter 4, this is called **reversal of muscle action.** This allows some of the shoulder girdle muscles to have assistive roles in other joints, primarily the head and neck.

Because of its attachment on the occiput and cervical vertebrae, the **upper trapezius** plays a role in moving the head and neck. When the shoulder girdle is stabilized, the upper trapezius can assist in extending the head and neck, laterally bending it to the same side (ipsilateral) and rotating it to the opposite side (contralateral).

With the shoulder girdle stabilized, the **lower trapezius** can reverse its action and assist in elevating the trunk. This is particularly useful during crutch walking. With the crutches planted on the floor in front, the person swings the body through. The lower origin on the vertebral column moves toward the higher attachment on the scapula, thus raising the body as it swings through the crutches.

When the scapula is stabilized, the **levator scapula** can move the neck. It can assist the splenius cervicis, a neck muscle, in rotating and laterally bending the neck ipsilaterally.

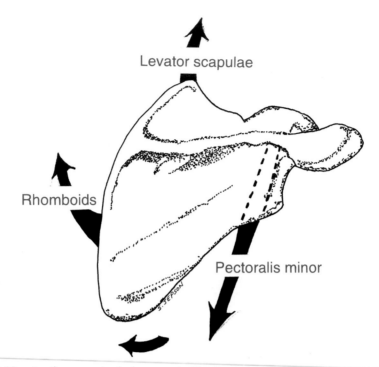

FIGURE 7–22. Another example of a force couple. The rhomboid, levator scapula, and pectoralis muscles during downward rotation of the scapula.

TABLE 7–2	**PRIME MOVERS OF THE SHOULDER GIRDLE**
Action	**Muscles**
Retraction	Middle trapezius, rhomboids
Protraction	Serratus anterior, pectoralis minor
Elevation	Upper trapezius, levator scapula, rhomboids
Depression	Lower trapezius, pectoralis minor
Upward rotation	Upper and lower trapezius
	Serratus anterior (lower fibers)
Downward rotation	Rhomboids, levator scapulae, pectoralis minor

TABLE 7–3	**INNERVATION OF THE MUSCLES OF THE SHOULDER GIRDLE**	
Muscle	**Nerve**	**Spinal Segment**
Trapezius	Cranial nerve XI	C3, C4
Levator scapula	Dorsal Scapular	C3, C4, C5
Rhomboids	Dorsal Scapular	C5
Serratus anterior	Long Thoracic	C5, C6, C7
Pectoralis minor	Medial Pectoral	C8, T1

TABLE 7–4	SEGMENTAL INNERVATION OF SHOULDER GIRDLE MUSCLES						
Spinal Cord Level	**C3**	**C4**	**C5**	**C6**	**C7**	**C8**	**T1**
Trapezius	x	x					
Levator Scapula	x	x	x				
Rhomboids			x				
Serratus Anterior			x	x	x		
Pectoralis Minor						x	x

SUMMARY OF MUSCLE INNERVATION

The shoulder girdle gets its innervation fairly high off the spinal cord from a variety of sources proximal to the terminal nerves of the brachial plexus. The eleventh cranial (spinal accessory) nerve innervates the trapezius muscle with sensory innervation from C3 and C4. The third and fourth cervical nerves innervate the levator scapula muscle with partial innervation by the dorsal scapular nerve coming from C5. The serratus anterior muscle is innervated by the long thoracic nerve, which is made up of branches of C5 through C7 (see Fig. 5–24), and the rhomboid muscles are innervated by a branch of the anterior ramus to C5. The pectoralis minor muscle receives innervation from the medial pectoral nerve, which branches off the medial cord of the brachial plexus. Table 7–3 summarizes the innervation of these muscles and Table 7–4 gives the spinal cord level of innervation for each muscle.

REVIEW QUESTIONS

1. Explain the differences among the terms shoulder girdle, shoulder joint, and shoulder complex.

2. Given that the scapula is shaped somewhat like a triangle, how can you tell if the scapula is rotating upward or downward?

3. Which shoulder girdle motions are more linear? Which are more angular?

4. What is scapulohumeral rhythm? What is its importance to physical therapy?

5. Why is the trapezius muscle usually referred to and described as consisting of three different muscles, whereas the two rhomboid muscles (major and minor) are referred to and described as one?

6. To raise your hand over your head requires the combined action of which muscles?

7. What is the term used to describe this combined action? Define the term.

8. What shoulder girdle muscle(s) lies entirely on the anterior surface of the trunk?

9. What muscles attach to the anterior portion of the scapula?

10. Starting at the inferior angle and going clockwise, name the shoulder girdle muscles that attach to the posterior surface of the scapula.

Shoulder Joint

The shoulder joint is a ball-and-socket joint with movement in all three planes and around all three axes (Fig. 8–1). The humeral head articulating with the glenoid fossa of the scapula makes up the shoulder joint. The shoulder joint is one of the most movable joints in the body and, consequently, one of the least stable.

Joint Motions

There are four groups of motions possible at the shoulder joint (Fig. 8–2): flexion, extension, and hyperextension; abduction and adduction; medial and lateral rotation; and horizontal abduction and adduction. Flexion, extension, and hyperextension occur in the sagittal plane around the frontal axis. Flexion is from 0 to 180 degrees, and extension is the return to the anatomical position. There are approximately 45 degrees of hyperextension possible from anatomical position. *Abduction* and *adduction* occur in the frontal plane around the sagittal axis with 180 degrees of motion possible. *Medial* and *lateral rotation* occur in the transverse plane around the vertical axis. Sometimes the terms *internal* and *external* are used in place of *medial* and *lateral,* respectively. From a neutral position, it is possible to move 90 degrees in each direction. *Horizontal abduction* and *horizontal adduction* also occur in the transverse plane around the vertical axis. The starting position for these motions is 90 degrees of shoulder abduction. There are approximately 30 degrees of

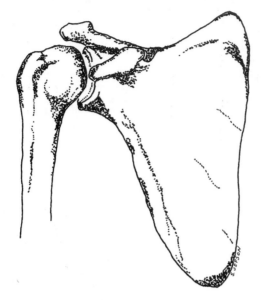

FIGURE 8–1.   The shoulder joint.

horizontal abduction (backward motion) and approximately 120 degrees of horizontal adduction. *Circumduction* is a term used to describe the arc or circle of motion possible at the shoulder. Because it is really only a combination of all the shoulder motions, the term *circumduction* will not be used here.

Bones and Landmarks

The scapula and many of its landmarks have been described earlier with the shoulder girdle. The following are landmarks of the **scapula** that you should know when talking about the shoulder joint (Fig. 8–3).

Glenoid fossa	A shallow, somewhat egg-shaped socket on the superior end, lateral side; articulates with the humerus
Glenoid labrum	Fibrocartilaginous ring attached to the rim of the glenoid fossa, which deeepens the articular cavity
Subscapular fossa	Includes most of area on the anterior (costal) surface, providing attachment for the subscapularis muscle
Infraspinous fossa	Below the spine, providing attachment for the infraspinatus muscle
Supraspinous fossa	Above the spine, providing attachment for the supraspinatus muscle
Axillary lutenal border	Providing attachment for the teres major and minor muscles
Acromion process	Broad, flat area on superior lateral aspect, providing attachment for the middle deltoid muscle

The **humerus** is the longest and largest bone of the upper extremity (Fig. 8–4). The important landmarks are as follows:

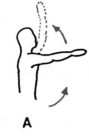
A

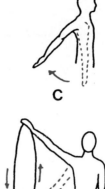
B

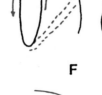
C

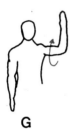
D

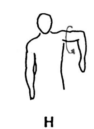
E

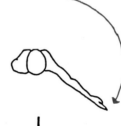
F

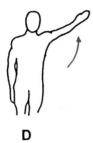
G

H

I

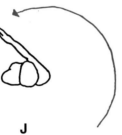
J

FIGURE 8–2. Shoulder joint motions.

A	Flexion	**F**	Circumduction
B	Extension	**G**	Lateral rotation
C	Hyperextension	**H**	Medial rotation
D	Abduction	**I**	Horizontal abduction
E	Adduction	**J**	Horizontal adduction

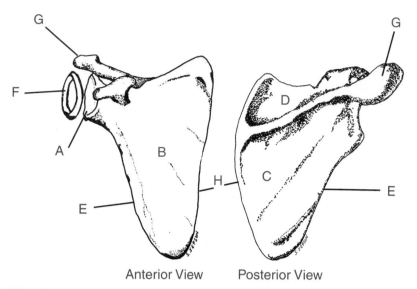

Anterior View   Posterior View

FIGURE 8–3. The right scapula. (*A*) Glenoid fossa. (*B*) Subscapular fossa. (*C*) Infraspinous fossa. (*D*) Supraspinous fossa. (*E*) Axillary border. (*F*) Labrum. (*G*) Acromion process. (*H*) Vertebral border.

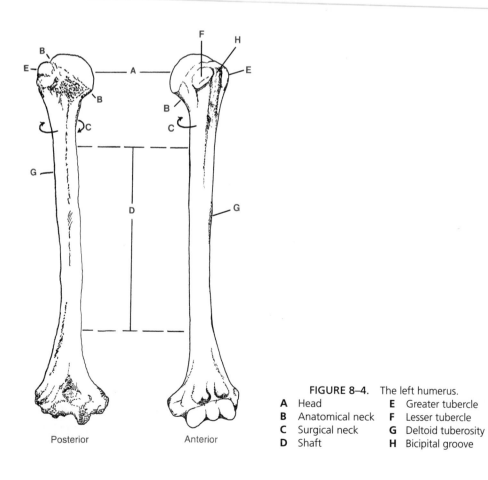

Posterior   Anterior

FIGURE 8–4. The left humerus.

A	Head	**E**	Greater tubercle
B	Anatomical neck	**F**	Lesser tubercle
C	Surgical neck	**G**	Deltoid tuberosity
D	Shaft	**H**	Bicipital groove

Head	Semi-rounded proximal end; articulates with the scapula
Surgical neck	Slightly constricted area just below tubercles where the head meets the body
Anatomical neck	Circumferential groove separating the head from the tubercle
Shaft	Or "body"; the area between the surgical neck proximally and the epicondyles distally
Greater tubercle	Large projection lateral to head and lesser tubercle; provides attachment for the supraspinatus, infraspinatus, and teres minor muscles
Lesser tubercle	Smaller projection on the anterior surface, medial to the greater tubercle; provides attachment for the subscapularis muscle
Deltoid tuberosity	On the lateral side near the midpoint; not usually a well-defined landmark
Bicipital groove	Also called the "intertubercular groove"; the longitudinal groove between the tubercles, containing the tendon of the long head of the biceps
Bicipital ridges	Also called the lateral and medial lips of the bicipital groove, or the crests of the greater and lesser tubercles respectively. The lateral lip (crest of the greater tubercle) provides attachment for the pectoralis major, and the medial lip (crest of the lesser tubercle) provides attachment for the latissimus dorsi and teres major

Ligaments and Other Structures

The **joint capsule** is a thin-walled, spacious container that attaches around the rim of the glenoid fossa of the scapula and anatomical neck of the humerus (Figs. 8–5 and 8–6). It is formed by an outer fibrous membrane and an inner synovial membrane. With the arm hanging at the side, the superior portion of the capsule is taut, and the inferior part is slack. When the shoulder is abducted, the opposite occurs with the inferior portion taut and the superior part slack. The superior, middle, and inferior glenohumeral ligaments reinforce the anterior portion of the capsule. These are not well-defined ligaments but actually pleated folds of the capsule.

The **coracohumeral ligament** attaches from the lateral side of the coracoid process and spans the joint anteriorly to the medial side of the greater tubercle (see Figs. 8–5 and 8–6). It strengthens the upper part of the joint capsule.

The **glenoid labrum** is a fibrous ring that surrounds the rim of the glenoid fossa (see Figs. 8–3 and 8–7). Its function is to deepen the articular cavity.

There are several bursae in the shoulder joint area. The subdeltoid bursa is large and located between the deltoid muscle and the joint capsule. The subacromial bursa lies below the acromion and coracoacromial ligament, between them and the joint capsule, and is frequently continuous with the subdeltoid bursa.

The **rotator cuff** is the tendinous band formed by the blending together of the tendinous insertions of the subscapularis, supraspinatus, infraspinatus, and teres minor muscles. These muscles help to keep the head of the humerus "rotating" against

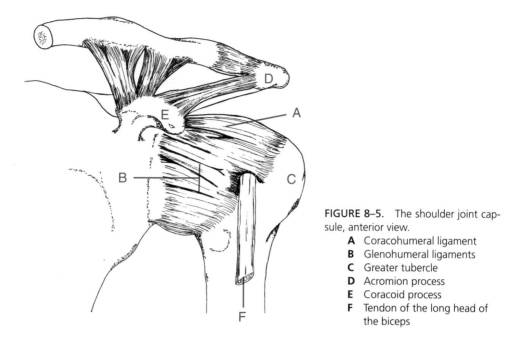

FIGURE 8–5.   The shoulder joint capsule, anterior view.
A Coracohumeral ligament
B Glenohumeral ligaments
C Greater tubercle
D Acromion process
E Coracoid process
F Tendon of the long head of the biceps

the glenoid fossa during joint motion. This rotating motion is what inspired the term rotator cuff, not the muscular action of medial or lateral rotation.

The **thoracolumbar fascia** (lumbar aponeurosis) is a superficial fibrous sheet attaching to the spinous processes of the lower thoracic and lumbar vertebra, the supraspinal ligament, and the posterior part of the iliac crest, covering the sacrospinalis muscle; it provides a very broad attachment for the latissimus dorsi muscle.

As mentioned, the shoulder joint allows a great deal of motion, which also makes it a rather unstable joint. Several features contribute to the stability that this joint does have. The fairly shallow glenoid fossa is made deeper by the glenoid

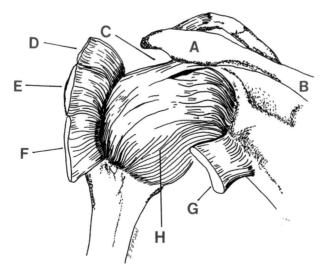

FIGURE 8–6.   Left shoulder joint, posterior view, muscles cut away.
A Acromion
B Scapular spine
C Coracohumeral ligament
D Supraspinatus muscles (cut away)
E Infraspinatus muscle (cut away)
F Teres minor muscle (cut away)
G Triceps muscle (cut away)
H Capsule

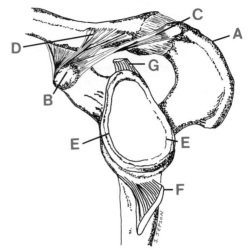

FIGURE 8–7. The left shoulder joint, lateral view.
  A Acromion process
  B Coracoid process
  C Coracoacromial ligament
  D Coracoclavicular ligament
  E Glenoid labrum
  F Triceps muscle (cut away)
  G Biceps muscle (cut away)

labrum. The fossa is positioned in an anterior, lateral, and upward direction. This upward direction provides some stability to the joint. The joint is held intact by the joint capsule reinforced by the coracohumeral and glenohumeral ligaments. Because the capsule completely surrounds the joint, it creates a partial vacuum, which helps hold the head against the fossa. The rotator cuff muscles hold the joint surfaces together during joint motion. It is mostly the shoulder muscles that keep the joint from subluxing, or partially dislocating. An individual who has had a stroke and has lost function in the involved extremity often develops a subluxed shoulder. The lack of a deep socket for the humeral head to fit into, the loss of muscle tone, the weight of the extremity, and gravity all contribute to joint subluxation.

Muscles of the Shoulder Joint

The muscles that span the shoulder joint are as follows:

> Deltoid
> Supraspinatus
> Pectoralis major
> Latissimus dorsi
> Teres major
> Infraspinatus
> Teres minor
> Subscapularis
> Coracobrachialis
> Biceps brachii
> Triceps brachii, long head

The **deltoid muscle** is a superficial muscle covering the shoulder joint on three sides, giving the shoulder its characteristic rounded shape. The name "deltoid" describes its triangular shape (Fig. 8–8). Functionally, this muscle is separated into three parts: anterior, middle, and posterior.

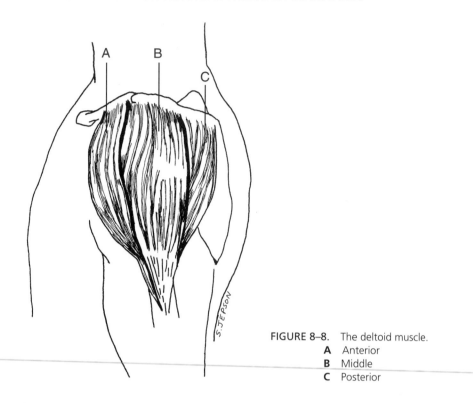

FIGURE 8–8. The deltoid muscle.
A Anterior
B Middle
C Posterior

The **anterior deltoid muscle** attaches on the outer third of the clavicle and runs down and out to the deltoid tuberosity, which is located on the lateral aspect of the humerus near the midpoint. It spans the joint on the anterior surface at an oblique angle. Therefore, it is effective in abduction, flexion, and medial rotation. When the arm is at shoulder level, the line of pull is mostly horizontal and, therefore, an effective horizontal adductor.

The **middle deltoid muscle** attaches on the lateral side of the acromion process and runs directly down to the deltoid tuberosity. Because its vertical line of pull is lateral to the joint axis, it is most effective in abducting the shoulder joint.

The **posterior deltoid muscle** attaches to the spine of the scapula and runs obliquely down to its attachment with the anterior and middle fibers on the deltoid tuberosity. Because its oblique line of pull is posterior to the joint axis, it is a strong shoulder abductor, extensor, hyperextensor, and lateral rotator. When the arm is at shoulder level, the line of pull is mostly horizontal, making it an effective horizontal abductor.

There is a concept called the "inchworm effect" that describes the action of the shoulder girdle and the deltoid muscles, especially the middle deltoid muscle, during shoulder abduction. If only the humerus moved during abduction, the middle deltoid muscle would quickly run out of contractile power as it approached 90 degrees. However, the middle deltoid muscle is effective throughout the entire range. Remember that for every 2 degrees the shoulder joint abducts, the shoulder girdle upwardly rotates 1 degree (scapulohumeral rhythm; see Chap. 7). With this upward rotation of the scapula, the origin of the deltoid muscle (the acromion process, lateral end of the clavicle, and the scapular spine) moves away from the insertion on the humerus. This lengthens the muscle, restoring its contractile potential, and allows it to continue to effectively contract throughout its entire range.

Anterior Deltoid Muscle

(O)	Lateral third of the clavicle
(I)	Deltoid tuberosity
(A)	Shoulder abduction, flexion, medial rotation, and horizontal adduction
(N)	Axillary nerve (C5, C6)

Middle Deltoid Muscle

(O)	Acromion process
(I)	Deltoid tuberosity (same as anterior deltoid muscle)
(A)	Shoulder abduction
(N)	Axillary nerve (C5, C6)

Posterior Deltoid Muscle

(O)	Spine of scapula
(I)	Deltoid tuberosity (same as anterior deltoid muscle)
(A)	Shoulder abduction, extension, hyperextension, lateral rotation, horizontal abduction
(N)	Axillary nerve (C5, C6)

As its name implies, the **supraspinatus muscle** (Fig. 8–9) lies above the spine of the scapula. It passes underneath the acromion process to attach on the greater tuberosity. The portion located in the supraspinous fossa is deep to the trapezius muscle above and to the deltoid muscle laterally. Early kinesiology studies suggested that the supraspinatus muscle was most effective in only initiating shoulder abduction. However, electromyography studies have since shown that it is active throughout abduction. In addition to its joint movement function, the supraspinatus muscle is very important in stabilizing the head of the humerus against the glenoid fossa.

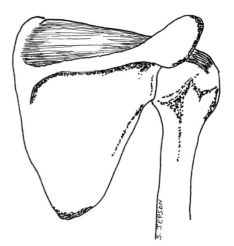

FIGURE 8–9. The supraspinatus muscle.

Supraspinatus Muscle

(O)	Supraspinous fossa of the scapula
(I)	Greater tubercle of the humerus
(A)	Shoulder abduction
(N)	Suprascapular nerve (C5, C6)

The **pectoralis major muscle** (Fig. 8–10) is a large muscle of the chest as its name implies (*pectus* means "breast" or "chest"). It is superficial except for its distal attachment lying under the deltoid muscle. Because this muscle crosses the joint on the anterior surface from medial to lateral, it is effective in adduction and medial rotation of the shoulder joint.

This muscle, because of its proximal attachments and different lines of pull, is often separated into a clavicular and sternal portion. The **clavicular portion** attaches to the medial third of the clavicle. The clavicular portion has a more vertical line of pull when the shoulder is extended, making it very effective at flexing the

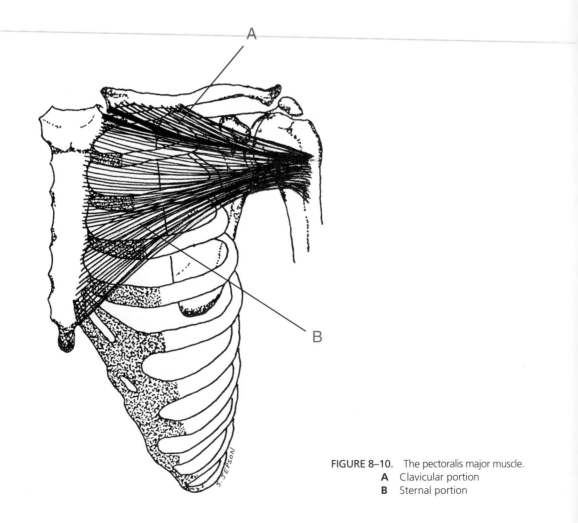

FIGURE 8–10.   The pectoralis major muscle.
A   Clavicular portion
B   Sternal portion

shoulder during the first part of the range. As the shoulder approaches 90 degrees (shoulder level), the line of pull is no longer vertical; thus, this portion of the pectoralis major muscle is no longer effective. The **sternal portion** attaches to the sternum and costal cartilages of the first six ribs. It has a more vertical line of pull when the shoulder is in full flexion and loses effectiveness as the shoulder approaches 90 degrees of extension. Both portions of the pectoralis major muscle are effective in the first parts of motion in the sagittal plane (clavicular portion for flexion, sternal portion for extension). They are, therefore, antagonistic to each other in flexion and extension, but agonists in shoulder adduction, medial rotation, and horizontal adduction.

Pectoralis Major Muscle, Clavicular Portion

(O)	Medial third of clavicle
(I)	Lateral lip of bicipital groove of humerus
(A)	Shoulder flexion to approximately 90 degrees

Pectoralis Major Muscle, Sternal Portion

(O)	Sternum, costal cartilage of first six ribs
(I)	Lateral lip of bicipital groove of humerus (same as clavicular portion)
(A)	Shoulder extension to approximately 90 degrees

Pectoralis Major Muscle, Clavicular and Sternal Portions

(A)	Shoulder adduction, medial rotation, and horizontal adduction
(N)	Lateral and medial pectoral nerve (C5, C6, C7, C8, T1)

The **latissimus dorsi muscle** (Fig. 8–11), as its name implies (in Latin *latissimus* means "widest," *dorsi* means "back" or "posterior"), is a broad, sheetlike muscle located on the back. It is mostly superficial except for a small portion covered posteriorly by the lower trapezius muscle and distally as it passes through the axilla to attach on the proximal, anterior, and medial surfaces of the humerus. Because of its attachment on the ilium and sacrum, it is able to elevate the pelvis if the arms are stabilized. This action occurs during crutch walking when the arms are stabilized on the crutch handles. This closed chain activity is a good example of "reversal of muscle function" where the proximal (origin) attachment pulls toward the distal (insertion) attachment, instead of the more common distal attachment pulling toward the proximal. The latissimus dorsi muscle is a strong agonist in extension, adduction, and medial rotation of the shoulder because it crosses the shoulder joint inferior and medial to the joint axes.

Latissimus Dorsi Muscle

(O)	Spinous processes of T7 through L5 (via dorsolumbar fascia), posterior surface of sacrum, iliac crest, and lower three ribs
(I)	Medial lip of bicipital groove of humerus
(A)	Shoulder extension, adduction, medial rotation, hyperextension
(N)	Thoracodorsal nerve (C6, C7, C8)

Teres means "long and round" in Latin, and the **teres major muscle** (Fig. 8–12) has its proximal attachment on the axillary border just below the teres minor mus-

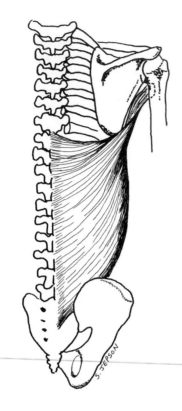

FIGURE 8–11.   The latissimus dorsi muscle.

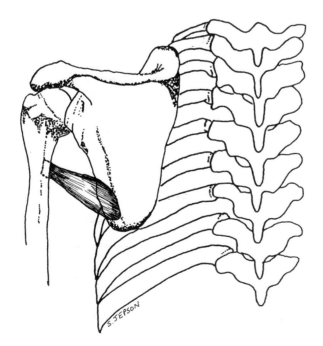

FIGURE 8–12.   The teres major muscle. Note that the humeral attachment is on the anterior surface.

cle. They are both superficial at this point. The teres major muscle travels with the latissimus dorsi muscle through the axilla, to where they attach close together on the anterior medial surface of the humerus near the proximal end. The teres major muscle is often referred to as the "little helper" of the latissimus dorsi muscle because it does everything that the latissimus dorsi muscle does except hyperextension, and because it is much smaller in size. Although the teres major muscle is a prime mover in extension, adduction, and medial rotation, its much smaller size makes it certainly less effective than the latissimus dorsi.

Teres Major Muscle

(O)	Axillary border of scapula near the inferior angle
(I)	Crest below lesser tubercle next to the latissimus dorsi muscle attachment
(A)	Shoulder extension, adduction, and medial rotation
(N)	Subscapular nerve (C5, C6)

As its name implies, the **infraspinatus muscle** (Fig. 8–13) lies below the spine of the scapula. Most of the muscle is superficial; however, the trapezius and deltoid muscles cover portions of it. The infraspinatus muscle's distal attachment is just inferior to the attachment of the supraspinatus muscle. Although some authors refer to the ability of the infraspinatus muscle to extend the shoulder joint, its more horizontal line of pull must be recognized. Therefore, its extension action is assistive at best.

Infraspinatus Muscle

(O)	Infraspinous fossa of scapula
(I)	Greater tubercle of humerus
(A)	Shoulder lateral rotation, horizontal abduction
(N)	Suprascapular nerve (C5, C6)

The **teres minor muscle** (see Fig. 8–13) is closely related to the infraspinatus muscle in both anatomical location and function. Both are mostly superficial with portions covered by the trapezius and the deltoid muscles. Both the teres major and teres minor muscles attach on the axillary border of the scapula and run obliquely up and outward to attach on the humerus. However, the teres minor muscle attaches posteriorly whereas

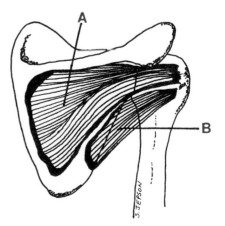

FIGURE 8–13. (*A*) The infraspinatus muscle. (*B*) The teres minor muscle.

the teres major muscle passes through the axilla to attach anteriorly. The long head of the triceps muscle passing between them in the axilla (Fig. 8–14) separates them.

Teres Minor Muscle

(O)	Axillary border of scapula
(I)	Greater tubercle of humerus
(A)	Shoulder lateral rotation, horizontal abduction
(N)	Axillary nerve (C5, C6)

If you observe the attachments of the supraspinatus, infraspinatus, and teres minor muscles, you will notice that they are essentially in a line (Fig. 8–15). For this reason, they are collectively referred to as the *SIT muscles*. These three muscles plus the subscapularis are referred to as the rotator cuff.

The **subscapularis muscle** (Fig. 8–16) gets its name from its location, which can be slightly misleading. *Sub* means "under" in Latin. The subscapularis muscle is located deep on the "underside" of the scapula, lying next to the rib cage. This underside is actually the anterior, or costal, surface. From this attachment on the anterior surface of the scapula, the subscapularis muscle runs laterally to cross the shoulder joint anteriorly and attach on the lesser tubercle of the humerus. This distal attachment blends into a common tendinous sheath with the other rotator cuff muscles to cover the humeral head and hold the head against the glenoid fossa.

Subscapularis Muscle

(O)	Subscapular fossa of the scapula
(I)	Tubercle of the humerus
(A)	Shoulder medial rotation
(N)	Subscapular nerve (C5, C6)

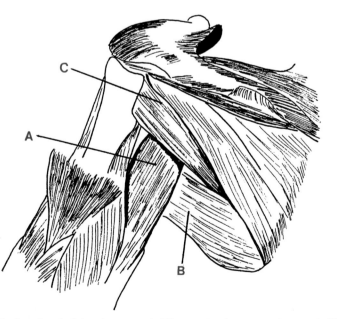

FIGURE 8–14. The long head of the triceps muscle (*A*) separates the teres major muscle (*B*) and teres minor muscle (*C*) at the axilla.

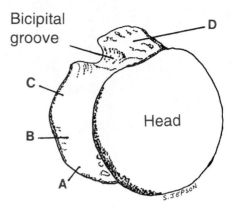

Bicipital groove

Head

FIGURE 8–15. This superior view of the proximal end of the left humerus shows the attachments of the teres minor muscle (*A*), the infraspinatus muscle (*B*), the supraspinatus muscle (*C*), and the subscapularis muscle (*D*). The four muscles are collectively referred to as the rotator cuff.

The **coracobrachialis muscle** (Fig. 8–17) derives its name from its attachments on the coracoid process and the humerus, or arm (in Latin, "brachium"). It has an almost vertical line of pull quite close to the joint axis. Therefore, most of its force is directed back into the joint, thus stabilizing the head against the glenoid fossa. Some authors refer to the ability of this muscle to flex and adduct the shoulder. However, because its vertical line of pull is so close to the joint axes, these actions are assistive at best.

Coracobrachialis Muscle	
(O)	Coracoid process of the scapula
(I)	Medial surface of the humerus near the midpoint
(A)	Stabilizes the shoulder joint
(N)	Musculocutaneous nerve (C6, C7)

The biceps and triceps muscles are two-joint muscles that cross both the shoulder and the elbow. Their actions at the shoulder joint are assistive at best. Because their main functions are at the elbow, they will be discussed in Chapter 9.

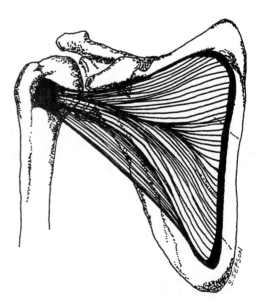

FIGURE 8–16. The subscapularis muscle.

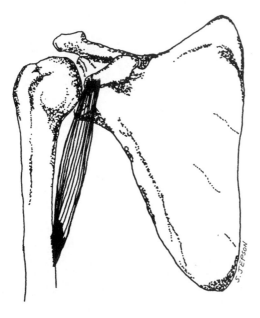

FIGURE 8–17.   The coracobrachialis muscle.

GLENOHUMERAL MOVEMENT

The movement of the humeral head on the glenoid fossa must be given some additional attention. Notice that the humeral head has more articular surface than does the glenoid fossa (Fig. 8–18*A*). If the humeral head simply rotates in the glenoid fossa, it would run

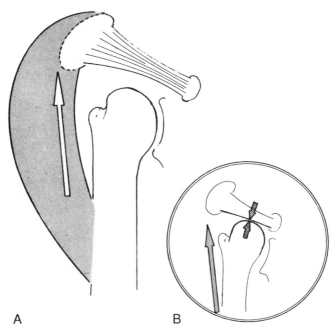

A   B

FIGURE 8–18.   Articular surface of glenohumeral joint and isolated function of deltoid muscle. (*A*) The attachment of the deltoid muscle on the humeral shaft gives the muscle an upward direction of pull, as indicated by the arrow. (*B*) The deltoid muscle's isolated action is that of elevation, impinging the humeral head directly up under the coracoacromial arch. (From Cailliet, R: Shoulder Pain, ed 3. FA Davis, Philadelphia, 1991, p 28, with permission.)

out of articular surface before much abduction has occurred. Also, the vertical pull of the deltoid muscle would pull the head up against the acromion process (Fig. 8–18*B*).

It is the arthrokinematic motions of glide, spin, and roll that keep the head of the humerus articulating with the glenoid fossa (see Chap. 21 for a detailed description of these terms). As abduction occurs, the humeral head rolls across the glenoid fossa. At the same time, the head glides inferiorly, keeping the head of the humerus articulating with the glenoid fossa. This is accomplished by the rotator cuff muscles (Fig. 8–19). The supraspinatus muscle, in addition to abducting the shoulder joint, pulls the humeral head into the glenoid fossa. The other rotator cuff muscles (subscapularis, infraspinatus, and teres minor) pull the head in and downward against the glenoid fossa. The glenoid labrum serves to slightly deepen the glenoid fossa, making the joint surfaces more congruent.

Another feature of shoulder abduction is that complete range of motion can be accomplished only if the shoulder joint is also laterally rotated. Try this on yourself. Start with your arm at your side (shoulder adduction) and in medial rotation; abduct your shoulder, and notice how much motion you can comfortably achieve.

Next, repeat the motion with your shoulder in a neutral position between medial and lateral rotation (fundamental position), and notice how much motion you can comfortably accomplish. Finally, repeat the motion with your shoulder in a laterally rotated position. It is this laterally rotated position that should allow the most comfortable shoulder motion because the greater tubercle is being rotated from under the acromion process, allowing full abduction. The greater tubercle in the medially rotated or neutral position runs into the acromion process overhead.

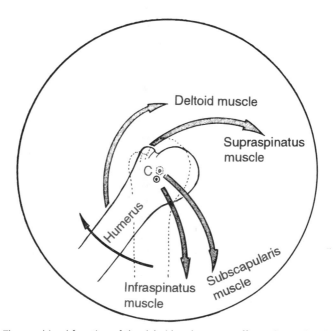

FIGURE 8–19.   The combined function of the deltoid and rotator cuff muscles at the glenohumeral joint results in abduction of the humerus. (Adapted from Cailliet, R: Shoulder Pain, ed 3. FA Davis, Philadelphia, 1991, p 31.)

TABLE 8–1	PRIME MOVERS OF THE SHOULDER JOINT
Action	**Muscles**
Flexion	Anterior deltoid, pectoralis major (clavicular)*
Extension	Posterior deltoid, latissimus dorsi, teres major, pectoralis major (sternal)*
Hyperextension	Latissimus dorsi, posterior deltoid
Abduction	Deltoid, supraspinatus
Adduction	Pectoralis major, teres major, latissimus dorsi
Horizontal abduction	Posterior deltoid, infraspinatus, teres minor
Horizontal adduction	Pectoralis major, anterior deltoid
Lateral rotation	Infraspinatus, teres minor, posterior deltoid
Medial rotation	Latissimus dorsi, teres major, subscapularis, pectoralis major, anterior deltoid

*To approximately 90 degrees.

SUMMARY OF MUSCLE ACTION

The actions of the shoulder joint muscles are summarized in Table 8–1.

SUMMARY OF MUSCLE INNERVATION

Muscles of the shoulder joint receive innervation from various branches high on the brachial plexus (see Fig. 5–24). Tables 8–2 and 8–3 summarize the segmental and nerve innervation of the muscles of the shoulder joint. It should be noted that there is some discrepancy among various sources regarding spinal cord level of innervation.

TABLE 8–2	INNERVATION OF THE MUSCLES OF THE SHOULDER JOINT		
Muscle	**Nerve**	**Plexus Portion**	**Segment**
Subscapularis	Upper subscapular	Superior trunk	$C_5 C_6$
Teres major	Lower subscapular	Posterior cord	C_5, C_6, C_7
Pectoralis major	Lateral pectoral	Lateral cord	C_5, C_6, C_7
	Medial pectoral	Medial cord	$C_8, T1$
Latissimus dorsi	Thoracodorsal	Posterior cord	C_6, C_7, C_8
Supraspinatus	Suprascapular	Superior trunk	C_5, C_6
Infraspinatus	Suprascapular	Superior trunk	C_5, C_6
Deltoid	Axillary		C_5, C_6
Teres minor	Axillary		C_5, C_6
Coracobrachialis	Musculocutaneous		C_6, C_7
Biceps	Musculocutaneous		C_5, C_6
Triceps	Radial		C_7, C_8

TABLE 8–3	**SEGMENTAL INNERVATION OF SHOULDER JOINT**					
Spinal Cord Level	**C4**	**C5**	**C6**	**C7**	**C8**	**T1**
Supraspinatus		x	x			
Infraspinatus		x	x			
Teres Minor		x	x			
Subscapularis		x	x			
Teres Major		x	x			
Deltoid		x	x			
Biceps		x	x			
Pectoralis Major		x	x	x	x	x
Coracobrachialis			x	x		
Latissimus Dorsi			x	x	x	
Triceps				x	x	

REVIEW QUESTIONS

1. There are four sets of motions that occur at the shoulder joint. Which of these occur:

    a. in the frontal plane around the sagittal axis?

    b. in the transverse plane around the vertical axis?

    c. in the sagittal plane around the frontal axis?

2. Describe circumduction and the motions involved.

3. Is the infraspinous fossa or the subscapular fossa on the anterior surface of the scapula?

4. Which two fossas does the spine of the scapula divide?

5. What landmarks can be used to determine if an unattached humerus bone is a right or left one?

6. What muscle(s) is (are) involved in the rotator cuff?

7. Why are the muscles in question 6 called "rotator cuff muscles"?

8. Which shoulder joint muscle(s) attaches on the anterior surface of the scapula?

9. Which shoulder joint muscle(s) attaches on the posterior surface of the scapula?

10. Which shoulder joint muscle(s) does not attach on the scapula?

11. Which shoulder joint muscle(s) does not attach on the humerus?

12. Which portion of the pectoralis major is effective in shoulder flexion? Is it more effective at 20°or at 80°? Why?

Elbow

Joint Structure and Motions

The elbow complex is made of three bones, three ligaments, two joints, and one capsule. The articulation of the humerus with the ulna and radius is commonly called the **elbow joint** (Fig. 9–1). On the humerus, the trochlea articulates with the trochlear notch of the ulna and the capitulum articulates with the head of the radius. The elbow is a uniaxial hinge joint that allows only flexion and extension (Fig. 9–2). There are approximately 145 degrees of flexion measured from the 0-degree position of extension (Lehmkuhl, p 403).

There is no active hyperextension at the elbow as there is at the shoulder joint. This motion is blocked by the olecranon process of the ulna fitting into the olecranon fossa of the humerus. Some individuals may be able to hyperextend a few degrees, but this is due to a laxity of ligaments rather than bony structure.

The articulation between the radius and ulna is known as the **radioulnar joint** (Fig. 9–3). They articulate with each other at both ends. At the proximal end, the head of the radius pivots within the radial notch of the ulna, forming the **superior** or **proximal radioulnar joint.** At the distal end, the ulnar notch of the radius rotating around the head of the ulna forms the **inferior,** or **distal, radioulnar joint.** They are considered together as one joint (Brunnstrom, 1983 p 403). The radioulnar joint is a pivot joint, which is uniaxial (allowing only pronation and supination of the forearm) (Fig. 9–4). Measured from the neutral or midposition, there are approximately 90 degrees of supination and 80 degrees of pronation.

When pronation and supination occur, the radius moves around the ulna (Fig. 9–5). The ulna does not rotate. It is locked in place by its bony shape at the proximal end. You can confirm this on yourself. With your elbow flexed, place the fingers of your other hand on either side of the olecranon process, and then pronate and supinate

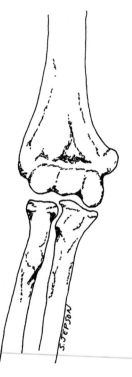

FIGURE 9–1. The right elbow joint.

A   B   **FIGURE 9–2.** Elbow motions. (*A*) Flexion. (*B*) Extension.

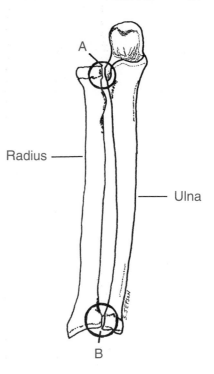

FIGURE 9–3. (*A*) Proximal radioulnar joint. (*B*) Distal radioulnar joint.

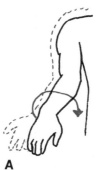 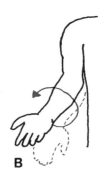

FIGURE 9–4. Forearm motions. (*A*) Pronation. (*B*) Supination.

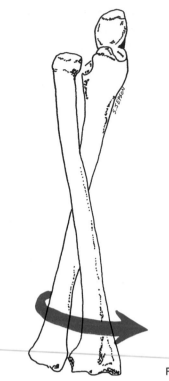

FIGURE 9–5. The radius moves around the ulna.

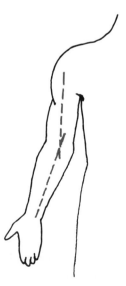

FIGURE 9–6. The carrying angle.

your forearm. Note that the olecranon process did not move. If you put your fingers on the shaft of the ulna, you again will notice that the ulna does not move. This is important to remember when figuring out muscle action. Because only the radius moves, a muscle must attach on the radius to have an effect on pronation or supination.

In the anatomical position, the longitudinal axes of the humerus and forearm form an angle called the **carrying angle** (Fig. 9–6). This angle tends to be greater in women than in men. Normal carrying angle measures approximately 5 degrees in males and between 10 and 15 degrees in females (Hoppenfeld, 1976 p 36). This angle occurs because the distal end of the humerus is not level. The trochlea on the medial side is lower than the capitulum on the lateral side. Therefore, as the ulna and radius rotate about the trochlea and capitulum, they do not do so in a straight line like a typical hinge joint in which the long axis of the lower segment is in line with the long axis of the upper segment. Note, however, that if a line of the long axis of the humerus is extended down the forearm, you will notice that during elbow extension the hand is on the outside of that imaginary line. When the elbow is in flexion, the hand is on the inside. This angle is quite functional in getting your hand to your mouth.

Bones and Landmarks

The bony landmarks on the **scapula** are covered in Chapter 8, but those that are important to elbow function are as follows (Fig. 9–7):

Infraglenoid tubercle	The raised portion on the inferior lip of the glenoid fossa providing attachment of the long head of the triceps muscle
Supraglenoid tubercle	Raised portion on the superior lip of the glenoid fossa, providing attachment for the long head of the biceps muscle
Coracoid process	Provides attachment for the short head of the biceps muscle (Described in Chap. 8)

The distal end of the **humerus** (Fig. 9–8) provides the bony landmarks important to elbow function.

Trochlea	Located on the medial side of the distal end; articulates with the ulna
Capitulum	On the lateral side next to the trochlea; articulates with head of radius
Medial epicondyle	Located on the medial side of the distal end above the trochlea; provides attachment for the pronator teres muscle; larger and more prominent than the lateral epicondyle
Lateral epicondyle	Located on the lateral sides of the distal end above the capitulum; provides attachment for the anconeus and supinator muscles
Lateral supracondylar ridge	Located above the lateral epicondyle; provides attachment for the brachioradialis muscle
Olecranon fossa	Located on the posterior surface between the medial and lateral epicondyles; articulates with the olecranon process of the ulna

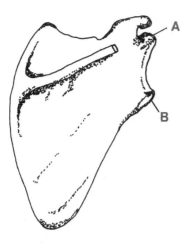

FIGURE 9–7. Attachments for the biceps and triceps muscles. A posterior view with the scapular spine cut away. (*A*) Supraglenoid tubercle. (*B*) Infraglenoid tubercle.

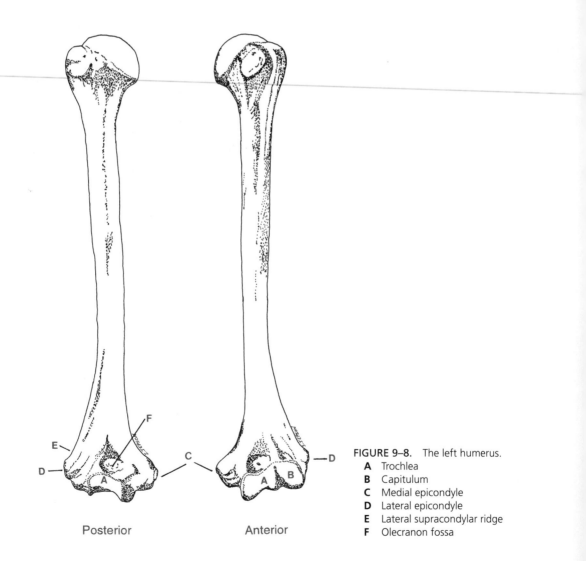

Posterior   Anterior

FIGURE 9–8. The left humerus.
  A Trochlea
  B Capitulum
  C Medial epicondyle
  D Lateral epicondyle
  E Lateral supracondylar ridge
  F Olecranon fossa

The **ulna** is the medial bone of the forearm lying parallel to the radius. The bony landmarks important to elbow function are as follows (Fig. 9–9):

Olecranon process	Located at the proximal end of the ulna, on posterior surface; forms the prominent point of the elbow and provides attachment for the triceps muscle
Trochlear notch	Also called the *semilunar notch;* articulates with the trochlea of the humerus; makes up the anterior surface of the proximal end
Coronoid process	Located just below the trochlear notch; with the ulnar tuberosity provides attachment for the brachialis muscle
Radial notch	Located at the proximal end on the lateral side just distal to the trochlear notch; articulation point for the head of the radius

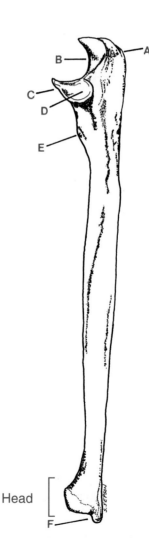

FIGURE 9–9. Left ulna, lateral view.

A	Olecranon process	**D**	Radial notch
B	Trochlear notch	**E**	Ulnar tuberosity
C	Coronoid process	**F**	Styloid process

Head

Ulnar tuberosity	Located below the coronoid process; provides an attachment of the brachialis muscle
Styloid process	At the distal end on the posterior medial surface
Head	At the distal end on the lateral surface; the ulnar notch of the radius pivots around it during pronation and supination

The **radius,** located lateral to the ulna, provides many important bony landmarks for elbow function. They are as follows (Fig. 9–10):

Head	Proximal end; has a cylinder shape with a depression in the superior surface where it articulates with the capitulum of the humerus
Radial tuberosity	Located on the medial side near the proximal end; provides attachment for the biceps muscle
Styloid process	Located on the posterior lateral side of the radius at the distal end; provides attachment for the brachioradialis muscle

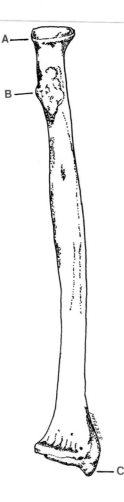

FIGURE 9–10. Left radius, anterior view. (*A*) Head. (*B*) Radial tuberosity. C. Styloid process.

Ligaments and Other Structures

The three ligaments of the elbow are the medial and lateral collateral ligaments and the annular ligament (Fig. 9–11). The **medial collateral ligament** is triangular shaped and spans the medial side of the elbow. It attaches on the medial epicondyle of the humerus and runs obliquely to the medial sides of the coronoid process and olecranon process of the ulna. The **lateral collateral ligament** is also triangular shaped. It attaches proximally on the lateral epicondyle of the humerus and distally on the annular ligament and the lateral side of the ulna. These two ligaments provide a great deal of medial and lateral stability to the elbow. The **annular ligament** attaches anteriorly and posteriorly to the radial notch of the ulna, encompassing the head of the radius and holding it against the ulna.

The **joint capsule** attaches around the distal end of the humerus, encompassing the trochlea and capitulum and the fossas located above them. It attaches around the proximal end of the ulna under the radial notch and coronoid process and around the trochlear notch. It attaches around the radius just under the head. The capsule is strengthened anteriorly and somewhat posteriorly by the annular ligament. The collateral ligaments reinforce the capsule on the sides of the joint.

In addition to the annular ligament, the radioulnar articulations are held together by the **interosseous membrane** (Fig. 9–12). This broad, flat membrane is located between the radius and ulna for most of their length. Not only does this membrane keep the two bones from separating, but also it provides more surface area for attachment of the forearm and wrist muscles.

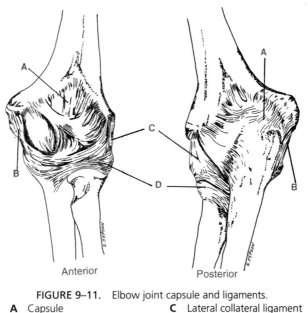

Anterior   Posterior

FIGURE 9–11.   Elbow joint capsule and ligaments.
A Capsule   **C** Lateral collateral ligament
B Medial collateral ligament   **D** Annular ligament

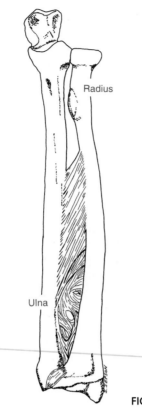

Radius

Ulna

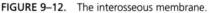

FIGURE 9–12.   The interosseous membrane.

Muscles of the Elbow and Forearm

Muscles of the elbow and forearm are as follows:

Brachialis
Brachioradialis
Biceps
Supinator
Triceps
Anconeus
Pronator teres
Pronator quadratus

The **brachialis muscle** (Fig. 9–13) gets its name from its location (Latin for "arm"). It attaches to the distal half of the humerus on the anterior surface and spans the elbow joint anteriorly to attach on the coronoid process and ulnar tuberosity of the ulna. It lies directly under the biceps muscle. Because the brachialis muscle has no attachment on the radius, it has no possibility of pronation or supination. This muscle is, however, a very strong elbow flexor regardless of the position of the forearm and is therefore sometimes referred to as the "workhorse of the elbow joint."

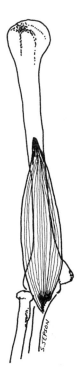

FIGURE 9–13. The brachialis muscle.

Brachialis Muscle

(O)   Distal half of humerus, anterior surface
(I)   Coronoid process and ulnar tuberosity of the ulna
(A)   Elbow flexion
(N)   Musculocutaneous nerve (C5, C6)

As the name of the **biceps brachii muscle** implies, it has two heads and is located on the arm (Fig. 9–14). The muscle is commonly referred to as simply the *biceps*. Both heads attach on the scapula. The **long head** arises from the supraglenoid tubercle and runs over the head of the humerus and out of the joint capsule to descend through the intertubercular (bicipital) groove to join with the **short head** that has come from the coracoid process. Because tendons of both heads cross the shoulder joint anteriorly, the biceps assists in shoulder flexion. However, its main function is at the elbow. After joining, the two heads form a common muscle belly covering the anterior surface of the arm. The biceps muscle tendon crosses the elbow joint to attach on the radial tuberosity. It is the superficial muscle of the anterior arm. Because the biceps brachii muscle spans the elbow joint anteriorly, it is a good elbow flexor, especially in the midrange. Because it attaches obliquely on the radius, it contributes to supination of the forearm.

To understand the supination component of the biceps muscle, think of it as a corkscrew. The tendon crosses the elbow joint anteriorly to attach medially on the radial tuberosity. When the forearm is in pronation, the radial tuberosity is rotated further medially toward the posterior side. In effect, the tendon of the biceps muscle wraps partially around the radius in the pronated position. During supination, the biceps muscle contracts and essentially "unwraps" or "untwists" the forearm (Fig. 9–15).

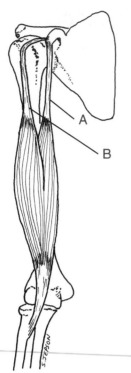

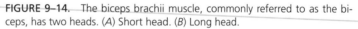

FIGURE 9–14. The biceps brachii muscle, commonly referred to as the biceps, has two heads. (*A*) Short head. (*B*) Long head.

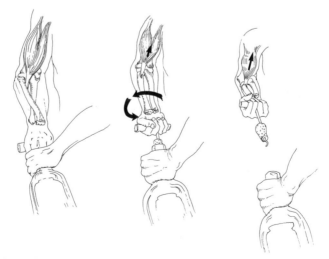

FIGURE 9–15. Supination action of biceps. The action of the biceps as a forearm supinator and elbow flexor is used when pulling a cork out of a bottle with a corkscrew.

It is most effective in supination when the elbow is in approximately 90 degrees of flexion, and it loses its effectiveness as the elbow is extended. This is because at 90 degrees the moment arm of the muscle is greatest; therefore its angular force is also greatest. As the elbow is extended, the moment arm decreases, as does angular force, while the stabilizing force increases (see Chap. 6 for a discussion on torque).

Biceps Brachii Muscle

(O)	Long head, supraglenoid tubercle of scapula
	Short head, coracoid process of scapula
(I)	Radial tuberosity of radius
(A)	Elbow flexion, forearm supination
(N)	Musculocutaneous nerve (C5, C6)

The **brachioradialis muscle** gets its name from its two attachments: one on the humerus (brachii) and the other on the radius (Fig. 9–16). Proximally it is attached slightly above the lateral epicondyle of the humerus on the supracondylar ridge. It crosses the elbow anteriorly and laterally to attach distally near the styloid process of the radius. It is a superficial muscle and easy to identify. Place your hand in your lap in a neutral position between supination and pronation; then give resistance to elbow flexion. The brachioradialis muscle should be quite prominent on the top of your forearm near the elbow. Because of its more lateral attachment, it is most effective as an elbow flexor when the forearm is in a neutral position. This is because its line of pull is quite vertical with essentially no diagonal component and goes through the axis for pronation and supination. The brachioradialis muscle has no real effect in these actions, even though it has an attachment on the radius.

Brachioradialis Muscle

(O)	Lateral supracondylar ridge on the humerus
(I)	Styloid process of the radius
(A)	Elbow flexion
(N)	Radial nerve (C5, C6)

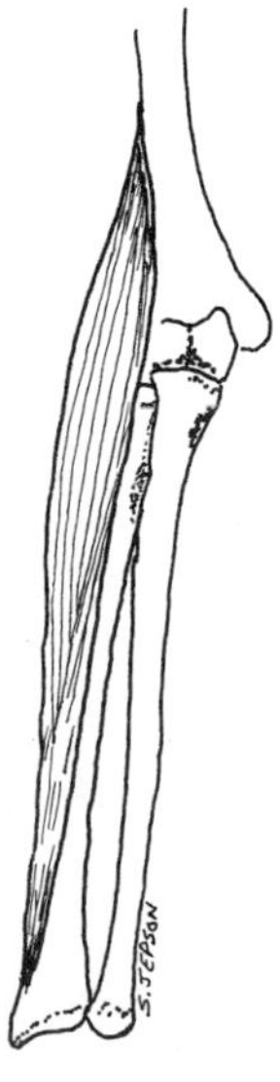

FIGURE 9–16. The brachioradialis muscle.

The **triceps brachii muscle,** commonly called the **triceps,** derives its name from its three heads; this muscle is located on the posterior arm (Fig. 9–17). The **long head** comes from the inferior rim of the glenoid fossa of the scapula and descends between the teres minor muscle and teres major muscle to join the other two heads. The **lateral head** is attached laterally on the posterior surface of the humerus below the greater tubercle. The **medial head** lies deep to the long and lateral heads and is attached below the lateral head to most of the posterior surface. The three heads come together to form the muscle belly. The triceps muscle tendon crosses the elbow posteriorly to attach to the olecranon process of the ulna. The triceps muscle makes up the entire muscle mass of the posterior arm. Because it spans the elbow quite vertically, it is very effective in elbow extension. Because it has no attachment on the radius, it can play no role in pronation or supination.

Triceps Muscle

(O)	Long head: Infraglenoid tubercle of scapula
	Lateral head: Inferior to greater tubercle on posterior humerus
	Medial head: Posterior surface of humerus
(I)	Olecranon process of ulna
(A)	Elbow extension
(N)	Radial nerve (C7, C8)

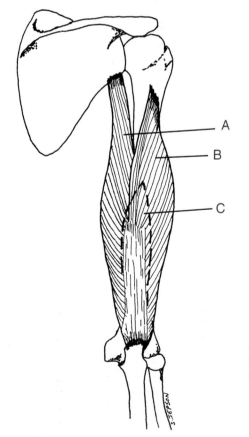

FIGURE 9–17.   The triceps brachii muscle, commonly referred to as the triceps, has three heads.
A   Long head
B   Lateral head
C   Medial head—dotted line indicates that muscle lies deep to the other two heads.

The **anconeus muscle** is a very small muscle that attaches beside the much larger triceps muscle (Fig. 9–18). It attaches proximally to the posterior surface of the lateral epicondyle and then spans the elbow posteriorly to attach laterally and inferior to the olecranon process. It is a small muscle in comparison to the triceps muscle, and it would therefore be foolish to say that the anconeus plays any significant role in elbow extension. Perhaps Carlin 1975 has explained its role best: the anconeus lies on top of the annular ligament and attaches to part of it. When the anconeus contracts, it pulls on the ligament and keeps the ligament from being pinched in the olecranon fossa during elbow extension.

Anconeus Muscle

(O)	Lateral epicondyle of humerus
(I)	Lateral and inferior to olecranon process of ulna
(A)	Not a prime mover in any joint action; assists in elbow extension
(N)	Radial nerve (C7, C8)

The **pronator teres muscle** (Fig. 9–19) gets its name partially from its action (pronation) and partially from its cordlike shape (*teres,* from the Latin). It is a superficial muscle; it crosses the elbow but is covered by the brachioradialis muscle at its distal attachment. Proximally, it attaches on the medial epicondyle of the humerus and the medial aspect of the coronoid process of the ulna. It crosses the anterior surface of the elbow, running diagonally to attach distally on the lateral surface of the radius at about the midpoint.

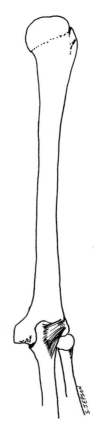

FIGURE 9–18. The anconeus muscle.

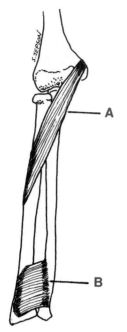

FIGURE 9–19. (*A*) The pronator teres muscle. (*B*) The pronator quadratus muscle.

Pronator Teres Muscle

(O)	Medial epicondyle of humerus and coronoid process of ulna
(I)	Lateral aspect of radius at its midpoint
(A)	Forearm pronation, assistive in elbow flexion
(N)	Median nerve (C6, C7)

The **pronator quadratus muscle** (see Fig. 9–19) also gets its name from its action (pronation) and partially from its shape (quadratus). It is a small, flat, quadrilateral muscle located deep on the anterior surface of the distal forearm; therefore, it cannot be palpated. It attaches from the distal fourth of the ulna to the distal fourth of the radius. It has a horizontal line of pull, and it works with the pronator teres muscle to pronate the forearm.

Pronator Quadratus Muscle

(O)	Distal fourth of ulna
(I)	Distal fourth of radius
(A)	Forearm pronation
(N)	Median nerve (C8, T1)

The **supinator muscle** (Fig. 9–20) is a deep muscle that wraps around the elbow joint laterally from the posterior surface to the anterior surface. It attaches posteriorly to the lateral epicondyle and adjacent surface of the ulna. It crosses the elbow joint laterally to wrap around the proximal end of the radius to attach distally on the proximal anterior surface of the radius. It combines with the biceps muscle to be a prime mover in forearm supination (Fig. 9–21).

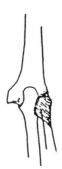

FIGURE 9–20. The supinator muscle.

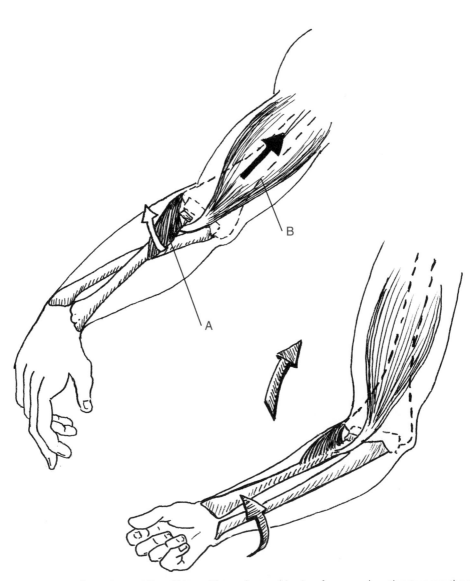

FIGURE 9–21. The supinator (*A*) and biceps (*B*) muscles combine in a force couple action to move the radius around the ulna from a pronated position into forearm supination.

TABLE 9–1	PRIME MOVERS OF THE ELBOW JOINT
Flexion	Biceps, brachialis, and brachioradialis
Extension	Triceps
Pronation	Pronator teres and pronator quadratus
Supination	Biceps and supinator

Supinator Muscle

(O)	Lateral epicondyle of humerus and adjacent ulna
(I)	Anterior surface of the proximal radius
(A)	Forearm supination
(N)	Radial nerve (C6)

SUMMARY OF MUSCLE ACTION

Table 9–1 summarizes the muscle action of the prime movers of the elbow and forearm.

SUMMARY OF MUSCLE INNERVATION

Terminal nerves of the brachial plexus innervate all muscles of the elbow. The musculocutaneous nerve innervates muscles of the anterior arm involved with elbow flexion. The radial nerve travels through the axilla and around the middle portion of the humerus to innervate the posterior surface of the arm, forearm, and hand. It is responsible for all elbow extension. The median nerve descends the arm anteriorly, sending branches to the pronator muscles. Table 9–2 summarizes the innervation of elbow joint musculature. Table 9–3 summarizes the segmental innervation. Please note that there is some discrepancy among various sources regarding spinal cord level of innervation.

TABLE 9–2	INNERVATION OF THE MUSCLES OF THE ELBOW JOINT	
Muscle	**Nerve**	**Spinal Segment**
Brachialis	Musculocutaneous	C5, C6
Biceps	Musculocutaneous	C5, C6
Brachioradialis	Radial	C5, C6, C7
Triceps	Radial	C6, C7, C8
Aconeus	Radial	C7, C8, T1
Pronator teres	Median	C7, C8, T1
Pronator quadratus	Median	C8, T1
Supinator	Radial	C6

TABLE 9–3	SEGMENTAL INNERVATION OF THE ELBOW JOINT				
Spinal Cord Level	**C5**	**C6**	**C7**	**C8**	**T1**
Biceps	x	x			
Brachialis	x	x			
Brachioradialis	x	x			
Supinator		x			
Pronator teres		x	x		
Triceps			x	x	
Anconeus			x	x	x
Pronator quadratus				x	x

REVIEW QUESTIONS

1. What motions are referred to as forearm motions?

2. What joint(s) and bones are involved in forearm motions?

3. What joint(s) and bones are involved in elbow motions?

4. Describe the joints in questions 2 and 3:

	Forearm	*Elbow*
a. Number of axes:		
b. Shape of joint:		
c. Type of motion allowed:		

5. If you were handed an unattached ulna, how could you tell what side of the body it belonged to?

6. Name the ligament that:
   a. Stabilizes the lateral side of the elbow
   b. Stabilizes the medial side of the elbow
   c. Stabilizes the radius and allows it to rotate

7. Which muscles discussed in this chapter are two-joint muscles?

8. For a muscle to act in supination or pronation of the forearm, to which bone must it attach?

9. Which muscle(s) lies anterior to the elbow joint?

10. Which muscle(s) lies posterior to the elbow joint?

11. Which elbow or forearm muscle(s) does not attach to the humerus?

12. Which muscles connect the scapula to the ulna and/or radius?

13. Which muscles connect the humerus and ulna?

14. Which muscles connect the humerus and radius?

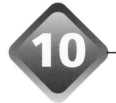

Wrist

Joint Structure

The wrist joint is perhaps one of the most complex joints of the body. The wrist joint is actually made up of two joints: the radiocarpal joint and the midcarpal joint. The **radiocarpal joint** (Fig. 10–1) consists of the distal end of the radius and the radioulnar disk proximally and the scaphoid, lunate, and triquetrum distally. Because an articular disk is located between the ulna and the proximal row of carpals, the ulna is not considered part of this joint. The pisiform, located in the proximal row of carpal bones, does not articulate with the disk because it is more anterior to the triquetrum. Therefore, it is not considered part of this joint, either. As a synovial joint, the radiocarpal joint is classified as a **condyloid joint,** with the concave distal end of the radius and the articular disk articulating with the convex scaphoid, lunate, and triquetrum.

The radiocarpal joint is also classified as a biaxial joint allowing flexion and extension, plus radial deviation and ulnar deviation. The combination of all four of these motions is called *circumduction*. There is no rotation at the wrist.

The **midcarpal, or intercarpal, joints** (see Fig. 10–1) occur between the two rows of carpal bones and contribute to wrist motion. Their shape is **irregular** and are classified as **plane joints.** They are nonaxial joints that allow gliding motions, which collectively contribute to radiocarpal joint motion.

The **carpometacarpal (CMC) joints** occur between the distal row of carpal bones and the proximal end of the metacarpal bones (see Fig. 10–1). Because they have a more direct function in the movement of the hand, they will be discussed in more detail in Chapter 11.

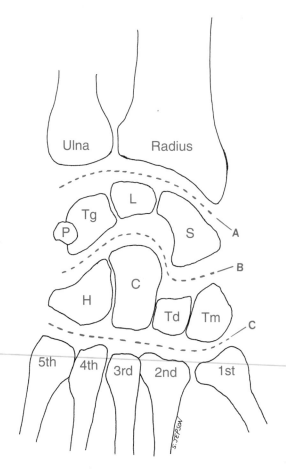

FIGURE 10–1. The joints of the left wrist, anterior view. (*A*) Radiocarpal joint. (*B*) Midcarpal joint. (*C*) Carpometacarpal joint.

Joint Motions

When discussing wrist motion, several terms are frequently used. *Wrist flexion* and *palmar flexion* are synonymous terms as are *extension, hyperextension,* and *dorsiflexion.* Approximately midway between flexion and extension, putting the hand in a straight line with the forearm, is referred to as *neutral position. Extension* is the return from *flexion.* Movement beyond the neutral position would be *hyperextension.* However, the most commonly used terms are *flexion, neutral,* and *extension,* and will be used here. You should, nevertheless, be familiar with these other terms, which are summarized in Table 10–1.

Flexion and extension occur in the sagittal plane around the frontal axis. There are approximately 90 degrees of flexion and 70 degrees of extension. Radial and ulnar deviation occur in the frontal plane around the sagittal axis. There are approximately 25 degrees of radial deviation and 35 degrees of ulnar deviation. These motions are illustrated in Figure 10–2.

TABLE 10–1	COMPARISON OF WRIST JOINT TERMINOLOGY*	
Preferred Terminology	**Alternate Terminology**	**Motion or Position**
Flexion	Flexion, palmar flexion	Anterior from anatomical position
Neutral	Extension, neutral	Anatomical position
Extension	Hyperextension, dorsiflexion	Posterior from anatomical position
Radial deviation	Abduction	Lateral from anatomical position
Ulnar deviation	Adduction	Medial from anatomical position

*Bold print indicates which terms are used in this book.

Bones and Landmarks

The **carpal bones** consist of two rows of four bones each (Fig. 10–3). Starting on the thumb side of the proximal row are the **scaphoid, lunate, triquetrum,** and **pisiform.** In the distal row, lateral to medial, are the **trapezium, trapezoid, capitate,** and **hamate.** These are short bones arranged in an arch with the concavity on the anterior (palmar surface) side, and the convexity on the posterior side. This arched arrangement contributes greatly to the ability of the thumb to oppose.

The bony landmarks for the wrist are as follows:

Styloid process — Distal projection on the lateral side of the radius and distal medial posterior side of the ulna, providing attachment for the collateral ligaments

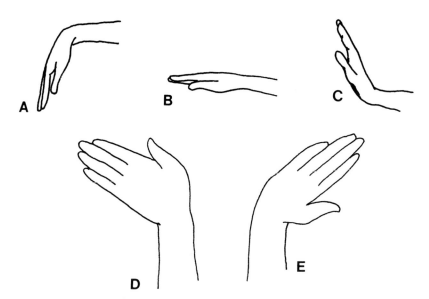

FIGURE 10–2. Joint motions of the wrist. (*A*) Flexion. (*B*) Neutral position. (*C*) Extension. (*D*) Ulnar deviation. (*E*) Radial deviation.

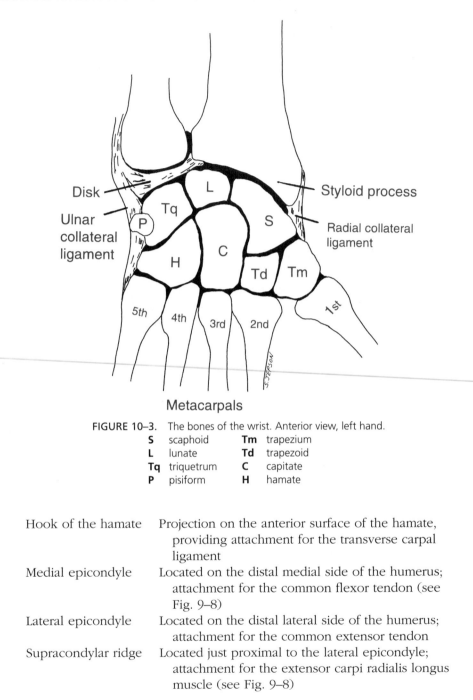

FIGURE 10–3. The bones of the wrist. Anterior view, left hand.

S	scaphoid	**Tm**	trapezium
L	lunate	**Td**	trapezoid
Tq	triquetrum	**C**	capitate
P	pisiform	**H**	hamate

Hook of the hamate	Projection on the anterior surface of the hamate, providing attachment for the transverse carpal ligament
Medial epicondyle	Located on the distal medial side of the humerus; attachment for the common flexor tendon (see Fig. 9–8)
Lateral epicondyle	Located on the distal lateral side of the humerus; attachment for the common extensor tendon
Supracondylar ridge	Located just proximal to the lateral epicondyle; attachment for the extensor carpi radialis longus muscle (see Fig. 9–8)

Ligaments and Other Structures

There are basically four ligaments of the radiocarpal joint that provide the major support of the wrist. In addition, there are numerous smaller ligaments supporting the intercarpal joints. The **radial collateral ligament** attaches to the styloid process of the radius and to the scaphoid and trapezium bones. The **ulnar collateral ligament**

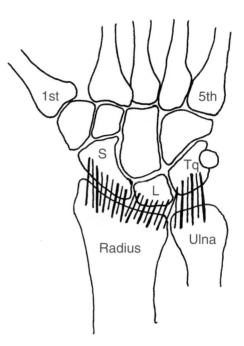

FIGURE 10–4. Anterior wrist (left) ligament. palmar radiocarpal.

S scaphoid   **L** lunate   **Tq** triquetrum

attaches to the styloid process of the ulna and to the pisiform and triquetrum. These ligaments provide lateral and medial support respectively to the wrist joint. They are illustrated in Figures 10–3, 10–4, and 10–5.

The **palmar radiocarpal ligament** is a thick, tough ligament that limits wrist extension. It is a broad band attaching from the anterior surface of the distal radius and ulna to the anterior surface of the scaphoid, lunate, and triquetrum (see Fig. 10–4). It is perhaps more important to wrist function than its counterpart, the dorsal radiocarpal ligament, because most activities of the hand occur with the wrist extended, as opposed to being flexed. Therefore, the palmar radiocarpal ligament is also more apt to be stretched or sprained.

The **dorsal radiocarpal ligament** attaches from the posterior surface of the distal radius to the same surface of the scaphoid, lunate, and triquetrum (see Fig. 10–5). This ligament limits the amount of flexion allowed at the wrist. Because forces causing excessive flexion are not as great as those causing excessive extension, this ligament is not as strong as the palmar radiocarpal ligament.

A joint capsule, which encloses the radiocarpal joint, is reinforced by the radial and ulnar collateral ligaments and by the palmar and dorsal radiocarpal ligaments. The **articular disk** (see Fig. 10–3) is located on the distal end of the ulna and articulates with the triquetrum and lunate bones. It not only acts as a shock absorber, but also as filler between the distal ulna and its adjacent carpal bones—the disk fills the gap created because the ulna and its styloid process do not extend as far distally as the radius and its styloid process.

The **palmar fascia** is a relatively thick, triangular-shaped fascia located superficially in the palm of the hand (Fig. 10–6). It is also called the *palmar aponeurosis*. It covers the tendons of the extrinsic muscles and provides some protection to the structures in the palm. The palmar fascia serves as the distal attachment of the palmaris longus, which blends into this fascia, as does the flexor retinaculum.

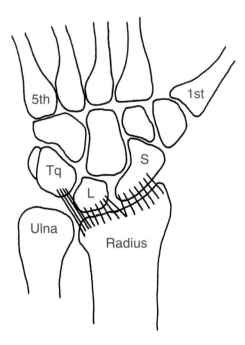

FIGURE 10–5. Posterior wrist (left) ligament: dorsal radiocarpal.
S scaphoid **L** lunate **Tq** triquetrum

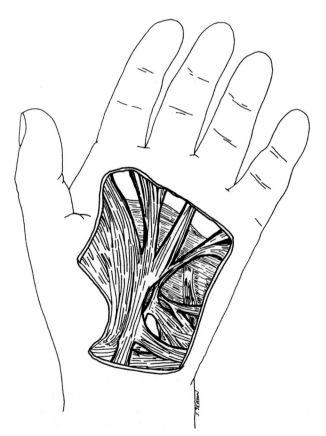

FIGURE 10–6. Palmar fascia.

Muscles of the Wrist

The muscles spanning and having a primary function at the wrist will be discussed here; the muscles that cross the wrist but have a more significant function at the thumb or fingers will be discussed later. The muscles to be discussed in this section are as follows:

ANTERIOR	**POSTERIOR**
Flexor carpi ulnaris	Extensor carpi radialis longus
Flexor carpi radialis	Extensor carpi radialis brevis
Palmaris longus	Extensor carpi ulnaris

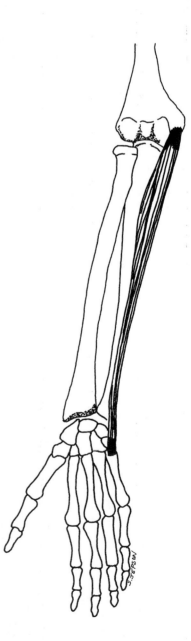

FIGURE 10–7. The flexor carpi ulnaris muscle.

You can make some general statements about the proximal muscle attachments of the wrist muscles. First, the flexors attach on the medical epicondyle and the extensors attach on the lateral epicondyle. Second, the distal attachment for all of the wrist muscles is a metacarpal. Third, the names of the muscles tell generally what their action is (flexor, extensor), that they act on the wrist (*carpi* means "wrist"), and on what side of the wrist the distal attachment (radialis means "radial," *ulnaris* means "ulnar") is located. Their names will also describe if the muscle functions in ulnar or radial deviation.

The **flexor carpi ulnaris muscle** is a superficial muscle running along the ulnar, slightly anterior, side of the forearm (Fig. 10–7). Its proximal attachment is mostly on the medial epicondyle of the humerus, and its distal attachment is the base of the fifth metacarpal and pisiform bone. It is the only wrist muscle attaching to a carpal bone. It is a prime mover in wrist flexion and ulnar deviation.

Flexor Carpi Ulnaris Muscle

(O)	Medial epicondyle of humerus
(I)	Pisiform, and base of fifth metacarpal
(A)	Wrist flexion, ulnar deviation
(N)	Ulnar nerve (C8, T1)

The **flexor carpi radialis muscle** is also a relatively superficial muscle running from the medial epicondyle diagonally across the anterior forearm to attach laterally at the base of the second and third metacarpals (Fig. 10–8). It is a prime mover in wrist flexion and radial deviation.

Flexor Carpi Radialis Muscle

(O)	Medial epicondyle of the humerus
(I)	Base of second and third metacarpals
(A)	Wrist flexion, radial deviation
(N)	Median nerve (C6, C7)

The **palmaris longus muscle** is also a superficial muscle running down the anterior surface of the forearm from the common flexor attachment of the medial epicondyle to attach in the midline to the palmar fascia (Fig. 10–9). It is easily identified in the midline at the base of the wrist, especially against slight resistance to wrist flexion. This muscle is rather unique because it only has one bony attachment. This muscle is missing in approximately 21 percent of individuals, either unilaterally or bilaterally (Moore, 1985 p 698). Because the palmaris longus muscle is quite small, its absence does not result in any real loss of strength. Although it is in an ideal position to flex the wrist; however, because of its size, it is assistive at best.

Palmaris Longus Muscle

(O)	Medial epicondyle of humerus
(I)	Palmar fascia
(A)	Assistive in wrist flexion
(N)	Median nerve (C6, C7)

On the posterior side of the wrist is the **extensor carpi radialis longus muscle.** This muscle is mostly superficial (Fig. 10–10). It attaches proximally just above

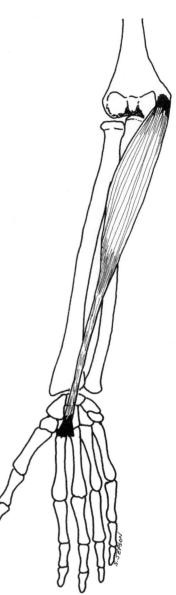

FIGURE 10–8.   The flexor carpi radialis muscle.

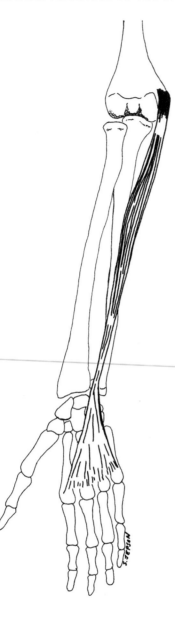

FIGURE 10–9.   The palmaris longus muscle.

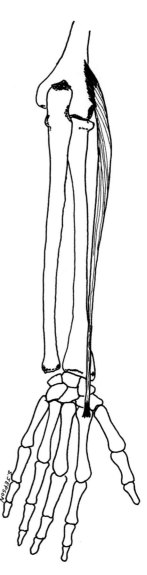

FIGURE 10–10.   The extensor carpi radialis longus muscle.

the lateral epicondyle on the lateral supracondylar ridge. It then runs down the lateral posterior side of the forearm, under two tendons that go to the thumb, and then under the extensor retinaculum to attach at the base of the second metacarpal. It is a prime mover in wrist extension and radial deviation.

Extensor Carpi Radialis Longus Muscle	
(O)	Supracondylar ridge of humerus
(I)	Base of second metacarpal
(A)	Wrist extension, radial deviation
(N)	Radial nerve (C6, C7)

Because the extensor carpi radialis muscle also has "longus" in its name, this implies that there is a "brevis." The **extensor carpi radialis brevis muscle** lies next to the extensor carpi radialis longus muscle (Fig. 10–11). It arises from the common

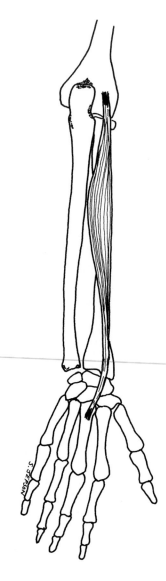

FIGURE 10–11. The extensor carpi radialis brevis muscle.

extensor tendon on the lateral epicondyle. Like the "longus," it passes under two tendons that go to the thumb and then under the extensor retinaculum. Its distal attachment is at the base of the third metacarpal. Because its attachment is close to the axis of motion for radial and ulnar deviation, it is only assistive in radial deviation. It is, however, a prime mover in wrist extension.

Extensor Carpi Radialis Brevis Muscle

(O)	Lateral epicondyle of humerus
(I)	Base of third metacarpal
(A)	Wrist extension
(N)	Radial nerve (C6, C7)

The **extensor carpi ulnaris muscle** is also a superficial muscle arising from the common extensor tendon on the lateral epicondyle (Fig. 10–12). It runs down

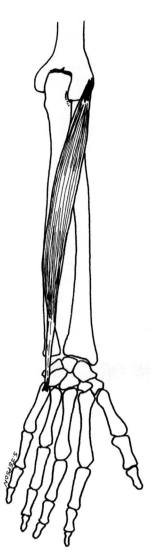

FIGURE 10–12.   The extensor carpi ulnaris muscle.

the medial side of the posterior forearm to attach at the base of the fifth metacarpal. It is a prime mover in wrist extension and ulnar deviation.

Extensor Carpi Ulnaris Muscle	
(O)	Lateral epicondyle of humerus
(I)	Base of fifth metacarpal
(A)	Wrist extension, ulnar deviation
(N)	Radial nerve (C6, C7, C8)

SUMMARY OF MUSCLE ACTION

Table 10–2 summarizes the muscle action of the prime movers of the wrist.

TABLE 10–2	PRIME MOVERS OF THE WRIST
Active	**Muscles**
Flexion	Flexor carpi radialis, flexor carpi ulnaris
Extension	Extensor carpi radialis longus and brevis, extensor carpi ulnaris
Radial deviation	Flexor carpi radialis, extensor carpi radialis longus
Ulnar deviation	Flexor carpi ulnaris, extensor carpi ulnaris

SUMMARY OF MUSCLE INNERVATION

Innervation of the wrist muscles is quite straightforward. If it is a posterior muscle, the radial nerve innervates it. If it is an anterior muscle on the thumb side, the median nerve innervates it, and if on the ulnar side, it is innervated by the ulnar nerve. Tables 10–3 and 10–4 summarize the innervation of the muscles of the wrist. There is some variation among sources regarding segmental innervation.

TABLE 10–3	INNERVATION OF THE MUSCLES OF THE WRIST	
Muscle	**Nerve**	**Spinal Segment**
Extensor carpi radialis longus	Radial	C6, C7
Extensor carpi radialis brevis	Radial	C6, C7
Extensor carpi ulnaris	Radial	C6, C7, C8
Flexor carpi radialis	Median	C6, C7
Palmaris longus	Median	C6, C7
Flexor carpi ulnaris	Ulnar	C8, T1

TABLE 10–4	SEGMENTAL INNERVATION OF THE WRIST JOINT			
Spinal Cord Level	**C6**	**C7**	**C8**	**T1**
Extensor carpi radialis longus	x	x		
Extensor carpi radialis brevis	x	x		
Extensor carpi ulnaris	x	x	x	
Palmaris longus	x	x		
Flexor carpi radialis	x	x		
Flexor carpi ulnaris			x	x

REVIEW QUESTIONS

1. Name the bones of the wrist joint.

2. Which wrist motions occur in:

   a. the sagittal plane around the frontal axis?

   b. the frontal plane around the sagittal axis?

   c. the transverse plane around the vertical axis?

3. Describe the wrist joints:

	Radiocarpal	*Intercarpal*
a. Number of axes:	_____	_____
b. Shape of joint	_____	_____
c. Type of motion allowed	_____	_____

4. Which muscle(s) attaches on the medial epicondyle of the humerus?

5. Which muscle(s) attaches on the lateral epicondyle of the humerus?

6. If you were shown a drawing of only a wrist joint, how could you tell if it were the posterior or anterior view?

7. Which muscles cross the wrist on the radial side?

8. Which muscles cross the wrist on the ulnar side?

9. Which muscle, if present, is very easy to identify but has little functional importance?

10. Starting on the anterior surface of the ulnar side and moving in the direction of the radial side, name the muscles that span the wrist. Go completely around the wrist.

Hand

The hand is the distal end of the upper extremity. It is made up of the thumb and finger metacarpals and phalanges. The hand is the key point of function for the upper extremity. We use our hand to accomplish an inexhaustible number of activities, ranging from very simple to quite complex tasks. The main purpose of the other joints of the upper extremity is to place the hand in various positions to accomplish these tasks. Not only is the hand extremely useful and versatile, it is also quite complex. This chapter will deal only with the hand's more basic structures and functions.

Joints and Motions of the Thumb

The first digit, the thumb, has three joints: the carpometacarpal (CMC) joint, metacarpophalangeal (MCP) joint, and interphalangeal (IP) joint (Fig. 11–1). The CMC joint is made up of the trapezium bone articulating with the base of the first metacarpal (Fig. 11–2). It is a saddle joint with both joint surfaces being both concave and convex. Sometimes the CMC joint is described as a modified ball-and-socket joint, implying that it has motion in all three planes. If you look at your thumb in anatomical position, you will notice that the pad is perpendicular to the palm. When you oppose your thumb, the pad is facing, or parallel to, the palm. Clearly, rotation has occurred. However, if you try to rotate the thumb without any other joint movement,

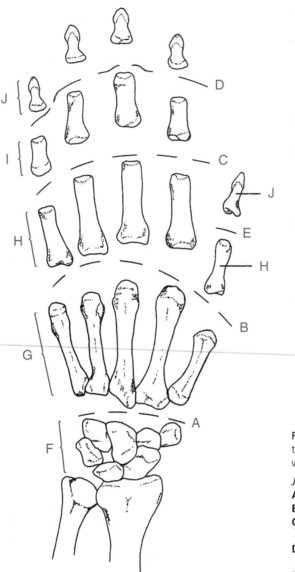

FIGURE 11–1. Joints of the hand. Note that each finger has a DIP and PIP joint, whereas the thumb only has an IP joint.

Joints		*Bones*	
A	CMC joints	**F**	Carpals
B	MCP joints	**G**	Metacarpals
C	PIP joints	**H**	Proximal phalanges
D	DIP joints	**I**	Middle phalanges
E	IP joint	**J**	Distal phalanges

you will find that impossible. The rotation at the CMC joint is a passive motion, not a voluntary one, which occurs as a result of the shape of the joint. This type of motion is commonly referred to as an **accessory movement** (a movement that accompanies the active movement and is essential to normal motion).

The CMC joint of the thumb allows more mobility than the CMC joints of the other four fingers, yet also provides as much stability. This is unusual. It allows flexion and extension, abduction and adduction, and opposition and reposition (Fig. 11–3). Thumb motions differ from the usual way we name joint motions. Flexion and extension occur in a plane *parallel* to the palm. Abduction and adduction occur in a plane *perpendicular* to the palm. In other words, with the forearm supinated and the palm facing up, the thumb moving side to side across the palm is flexion and extension. The thumb moving up toward the ceiling, away from the palm, is ab-

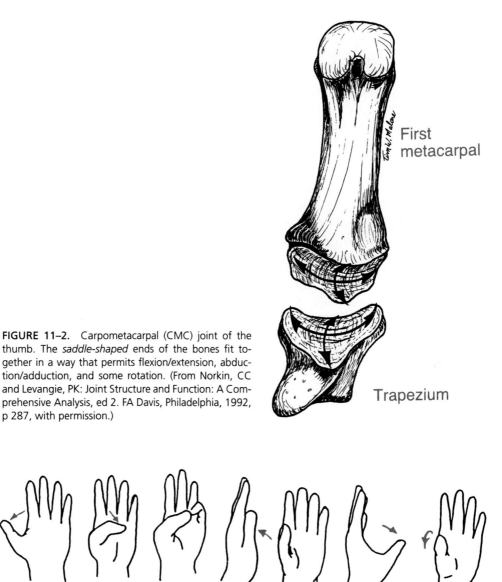

FIGURE 11–2. Carpometacarpal (CMC) joint of the thumb. The *saddle-shaped* ends of the bones fit together in a way that permits flexion/extension, abduction/adduction, and some rotation. (From Norkin, CC and Levangie, PK: Joint Structure and Function: A Comprehensive Analysis, ed 2. FA Davis, Philadelphia, 1992, p 287, with permission.)

First metacarpal

Trapezium

A   B   C   D   E

FIGURE 11–3. Motions of the thumb. (*A*) Extension and reposition. (*B*) Flexion. (*C*) Opposition. (*D*) Adduction. (*E*) Abduction.

duction, and its return is adduction. Opposition is a combination of flexion, abduction, with "built in" accessory motion of rotation; reposition is the return to anatomical position. For this reason, the CMC joint is usually considered a "modified" biaxial joint.

As discussed, the CMC joint of the thumb is quite mobile; the MCP joint and the IP joint, however, are not. The MCP joint is a hinge joint that allows only flexion and extension and is therefore a uniaxial joint. The IP joint, the only phalangeal joint, also allows only flexion and extension.

Joints and Motions of the Fingers

The second, third, fourth, and fifth digits, commonly known as the *index, middle, ring,* and *little fingers,* respectively, have four joints each. These joints are the CMC joint, MCP joint, proximal interphalangeal (PIP) joint, and distal interphalangeal (DIP) joint (see Fig. 11–1).

The CMC joints are classified as nonaxial plane (irregular) synovial joints that provide more stability than mobility. The trapezium articulates with the base of the first metacarpal as described previously in the discussion of the thumb joint. The trapezoid articulates with the second metacarpal, the capitate with the third metacarpal, and the hamate with the fourth and fifth metacarpals (Fig. 11–4). The fifth CMC joint is the most mobile of the fingers and allows for a small amount of fifth finger opposition. It does not allow as much opposition as the thumb (the first CMC joint). The fourth CMC joint is slightly mobile, but the second and third CMC joints are not.

This can be demonstrated by looking at your knuckles with your forearm supinated and your elbow flexed. Note that with a relaxed fist, the MCP joints are essentially in a straight line. When you make a tight fist, the fifth MCP joint moves a great deal and the fourth MCP joint moves to a lesser extent, while the second and third MCP joints remain stationary. This MCP movement actually is initiated at the CMC joints.

The MCP joints of the fingers are biaxial condyloid joints. The rounded heads of the metacarpals articulate with the base of the proximal phalanges, which have a concave shape (see Fig. 11–1). These are commonly referred to as the "knuckles." The motions allowed at these joints are flexion, extension, and hyperextension plus abduction and adduction (Fig. 11–5). The middle finger is the point of reference for abduction and adduction. Abduction occurs when the second, fourth, and fifth fingers move away from the middle finger, and when the middle finger moves in either direction. Adduction is the return from abduction and occurs with the second, fourth, and fifth fingers. There is no adduction of the middle finger, only abduction occurring in either direction.

There are two interphalangeal joints in the fingers. The PIP joint occurs between the proximal and middle phalange, and the DIP joint occurs between the middle and distal phalanges. They are uniaxial hinge joints and allow only flexion and extension.

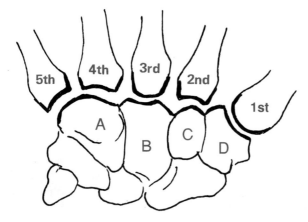

FIGURE 11–4. The carpometacarpal (CMC) joints of the thumb and fingers. (From Norkin, CC and Levangie, PK: Joint Structure and Function: A Comprehensive Analysis, ed 2. FA Davis, Philadelphia, 1992, p 273, with permission.)
HA Hamate   **CA** Capitate
TD Trapezoid   **TM** Trapezium

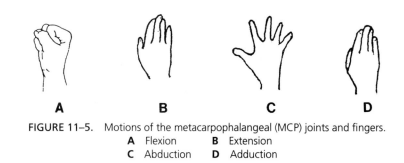

FIGURE 11–5.   Motions of the metacarpophalangeal (MCP) joints and fingers.
A Flexion   **B** Extension
C Abduction   **D** Adduction

Bones and Landmarks

Although the thumb and fingers have essentially the same bony structure, there is one major difference. The thumb has two phalanges, whereas the fingers each have three. This feature makes the thumb shorter, allowing opposition to be more functional.

Therefore, the hand, made up of the thumb and four fingers, has five metacarpals, five proximal phalanges, five distal phalanges, but only four middle phalanges (see Fig. 11–1). There are no significant landmarks on these bones other than the bone ends. The proximal end of the metacarpals and phalanges is called the base, and the distal end is called the head. There is one landmark on the forearm, which, although not distinct, is sometimes referred to when describing muscle attachments.

Oblique line   Located on the anterior surface from below the tuberosity, running diagonally to approximately midradius.

Ligaments and Other Structures

Although there are numerous structures in the hand, only a few of those more commonly referred to will be described here. The flexor retinaculum ligament is a fibrous band that spans the wrist on the anterior surface of the wrist in a mediolateral direction (Fig. 11–6). It is made up of two parts that formerly were known as the *palmar carpal ligament* and the *transverse carpal ligament*. Currently, they are grouped together as the *flexor retinaculum*. Because of their clinical significance, they will be individually described. The **palmar carpal ligament** is more proximal and superficial than the transverse carpal ligament. Its distal fibers do blend with the transverse carpal ligament. The palmar carpal ligament attaches to the styloid process of the radius and ulna and crosses over the flexor muscles. Its main function is to hold these tendons close to the wrist, thus preventing the tendons from pulling away from the wrist when the wrist flexes.

The **transverse carpal ligament** lies deeper and more distally (Fig. 11–7). It attaches to the pisiform and hook of the hamate on the medial side and to the scaphoid and trapezium bones laterally. It arches over the carpal bones forming a tunnel through which the long finger flexor tendons and the median nerve pass. This ligament is often surgically cut to relieve the symptoms of carpal tunnel syndrome.

The **extensor retinaculum ligament** is a fibrous band traversing the wrist on

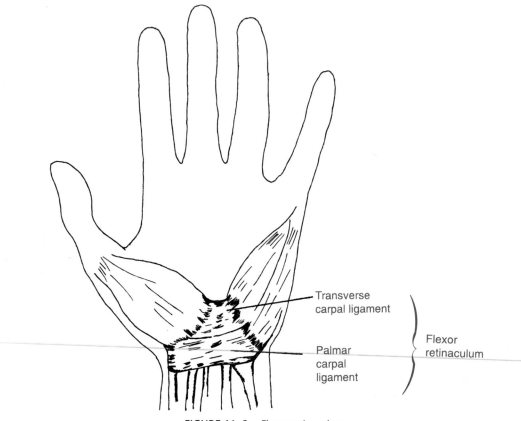

FIGURE 11–6. Flexor retinaculum.

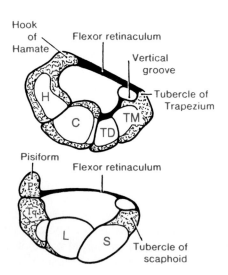

FIGURE 11–7. Distal (*top*) and proximal (*bottom*) rows of carpal bones showing the transverse carpal ligament portion of the flexor retinaculum, which stretches between the ends of the concavity of the carpal bones and forms an osseofibrous carpal tunnel. (From Moore, KL: Clinically Oriented Anatomy, ed 3. Williams & Wilkins, Baltimore, 1992, p 561, 570, with permission.)

H	Hamate	**P**	Pisiform
C	Capitate	**Tq**	Triquetrum
TD	Trapezoid	**L**	Lunate
TM	Trapezium	**S**	Scaphoid

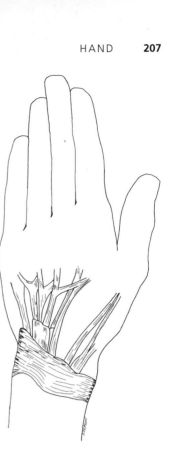

FIGURE 11–8. Extensor retinaculum.

the posterior side in a mediolateral direction (Fig. 11–8). It attaches to the styloid process of the ulna medially, and to the triquetrum, pisiform, and lateral side of the radius. It holds the extensor tendons close to the wrist, especially during wrist extension.

The **extensor expansion ligament,** also called the **extensor hood,** (Fig. 11–9) is a small triangular-shaped aponeurosis located on the dorsum and sides of the proximal phalanx of the fingers. It is a continuation of the extensor digitorum tendon. It is wider at its base over the MCP joint, actually wrapping over the sides somewhat. As it approaches the PIP joint, it is joined by tendons of the lumbricales and interossei muscles. It narrows toward its distal end at the base of the distal phalanx. The extensor digitorum, lumbricales, and interossei muscles form an attachment to the middle and/or distal phalanx by way of this expansion.

When the hand is relaxed, the palm assumes a cupped position. This palmar concavity is due to the arrangement of the bony skeleton reinforced by ligaments. There are three arches that are responsible for this shape (Fig. 11–10). The **proximal carpal arch** is formed by the proximal end of the metacarpals (base) and carpal bones and is maintained by the flexor retinaculum (see Fig. 11–7). The shallower **distal carpal arch** is made up of the metacarpal heads. The **longitudinal arch** begins at the wrist and runs the length of the metacarpal and phalanges for each digit. These arches contribute to the function of various types of grasp described at the end of this chapter.

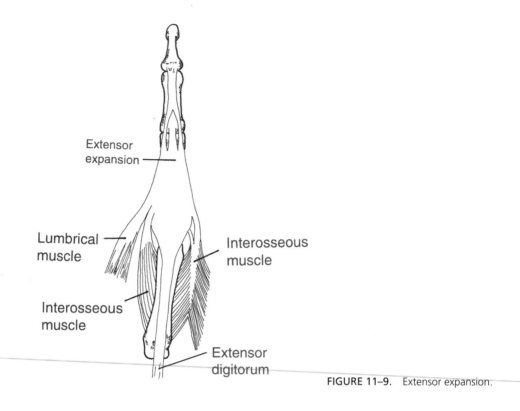

FIGURE 11–9. Extensor expansion.

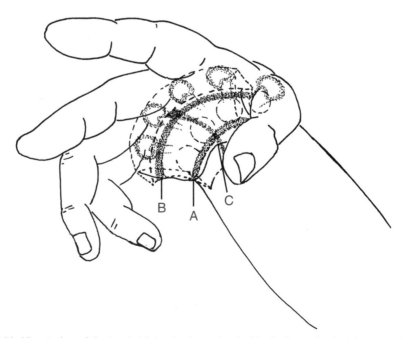

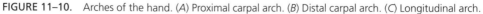

FIGURE 11–10. Arches of the hand. (*A*) Proximal carpal arch. (*B*) Distal carpal arch. (*C*) Longitudinal arch.

Muscles of the Thumb and Fingers

EXTRINSIC MUSCLES

Besides the wrist muscles previously described, several other muscles not only span the wrist but also cross the joints in the hand as well. These muscles are called **extrinsic muscles** of the hand because their proximal attachment is above the wrist joint. They have an assistive role in wrist function, but their primary function is at the thumb or finger. They are as follows:

ANTERIOR	POSTERIOR
Flexor digitorum superficialis	Extensor digitorum
Flexor digitorum profundus	Extensor digiti minimi
	Extensor indicis
Flexor pollicis longus	Abductor pollicis longus
	Extensor pollicis longus
	Extensor pollicis brevis

The **flexor digitorum superficialis** muscle lies deep to the wrist flexors and palmaris longus muscle (Fig. 11–11). Its broad proximal attachment is part of the common flexor tendon on the medial epicondyle of the humerus. It also has an attachment on the coronoid process of the ulna and the oblique line of the radius. It divides into four tendons and crosses the wrist with one tendon then going to each finger (Fig. 11–12). Its distal attachment splits into two parts and attaches on each side of the middle phalanx of each finger. Its action is to flex the MCP and PIP joints of the second through fifth fingers.

Flexor Digitorum Superficialis Muscle	
(O)	Common flexor tendon, coronoid process, and radius
(I)	Sides of the middle phalanx of the four fingers
(A)	Flexes the MCP and PIP joints of the fingers
(N)	Median nerve (C7, C8, T1)

The **flexor digitorum profundus muscle** lies deep to the flexor digitorum superficialis muscle, as they traverse the forearm and hand together (Fig. 11–13). The profundus muscle has its proximal attachment on the ulna on the anterior and medial surfaces from the coronoid process to approximately three-fourths of the way down the ulna. It runs beneath the flexor digitorum superficialis muscle until the superficialis tendon splits into two parts at its distal attachment. The profundus muscle passes through this split and continues distally to attach at the base of the distal phalanx of the second through fifth fingers (see Fig. 11–12).

Flexor Digitorum Profundus Muscle	
(O)	Upper three-fourths of the ulna
(I)	Distal phalanx of the four fingers
(A)	Flexes all three joints of the fingers
(N)	Median and ulnar nerves (C8, T1)

The **extensor digitorum muscle** is a superficial muscle on the posterior forearm and hand (Fig. 11–14). It attaches proximally to the lateral epicondyle of the humerus as part of the common extensor tendon. It passes under the extensor reti-

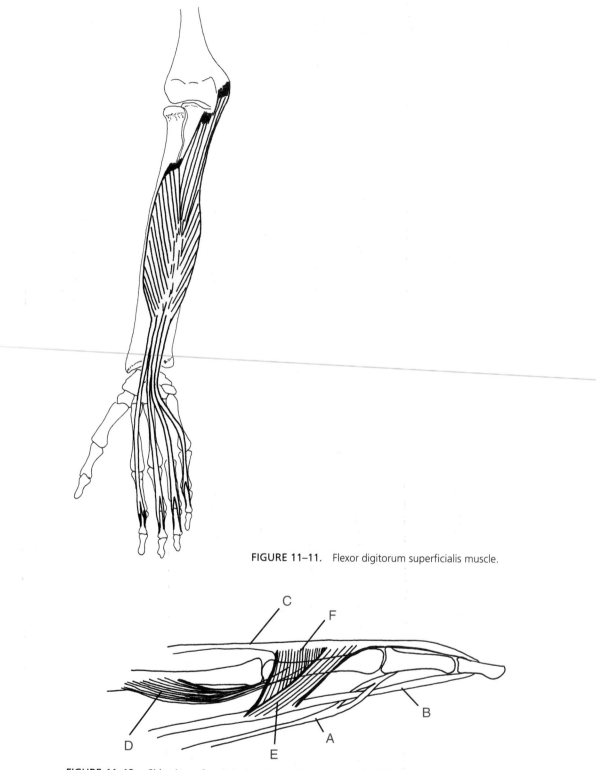

FIGURE 11–11. Flexor digitorum superficialis muscle.

FIGURE 11–12. Side view of a digit showing tendon relationship. (*A*) Flexor digitorum superficialis. (*B*) Flexor digitorum profundus. (*C*) Extensor digitorum. (*D*) Palmar interossous. (*E*) Lumbrical. (*F*) Extensor expansion.

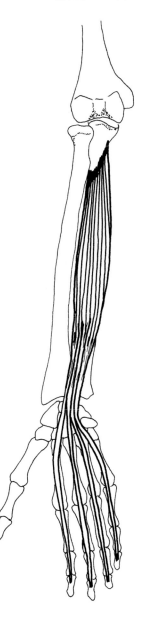

FIGURE 11–13.   Flexor digitorum profundus muscle.

naculum to attach distally on the distal phalanx of the second through fifth fingers via the extensor expansion (see Fig. 11–12). In the area of the metacarpals are interconnecting bands joining the four extensor digitorum tendons. These interconnecting bands limit independent finger extension. The extensor digitorum muscle is the only common extensor muscle of the fingers. It extends the MCP, PIP, and DIP joints of the second, third, fourth, and fifth fingers.

Extensor Digitorum Muscle

(O)	Lateral epicondyle of the humerus
(I)	Base of distal phalanx of the second through fifth fingers
(A)	Extends all three joints of the fingers
(N)	Radial nerve (C6, C7, C8)

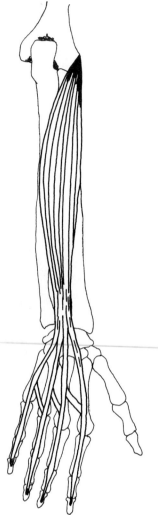

FIGURE 11–14. Extensor digitorum muscle.

The **extensor indicis muscle** is a deep muscle that has its proximal attachment on the posterior surface of the distal ulna (Fig. 11–15). It crosses the wrist under the extensor retinaculum medial to the extensor digitorum muscle and attaches into the extensor expansion, with the extensor digitorum muscle. It extends the MCP, PIP, and DIP joints of the index finger.

Extensor Indicis Muscle	
(O)	Distal ulna
(I)	Base of distal phalanx of the second finger
(A)	Extends all joints of the second finger
(N)	Radial nerve (C6, C7, C8)

The **extensor digiti minimi muscle** is a long, narrow muscle (Fig. 11–16) that is deep to the extensor digitorum and extensor carpi ulnaris muscles near its proximal attachment, but it becomes superficial before crossing the wrist. It comes off the

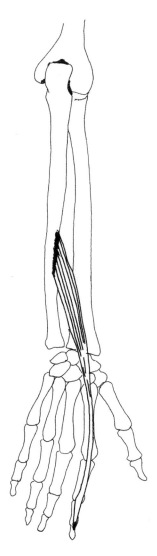

FIGURE 11–15. Extensor indicis muscle.

common extensor tendon on the lateral epicondyle of the humerus, crosses the wrist under the extensor retinaculum, and attaches to the base of the distal phalanx of the fifth finger via the extensor expansion. It is a prime mover in extending the MCP, PIP, and DIP joints of the fifth finger.

Extensor Digiti Minimi Muscle	
(O)	Lateral epicondyle of humerus
(I)	Base of distal phalanx of fifth finger
(A)	Extends all joints of fifth finger
(N)	Radial nerve (C6, C7, C8)

It is rather easy to distinguish the muscles having a function on the thumb because *pollicis* means "thumb" in Latin. The extrinsic muscles of the thumb are the following:

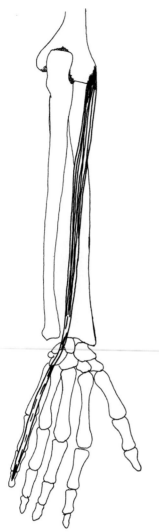

FIGURE 11–16. Extensor digiti minimi muscle.

Flexor pollicis longus
Abductor pollicis longus
Extensor pollicis longus
Extensor pollicis brevis

The **flexor pollicis longus muscle** is a deep muscle that has its proximal attachment on the anterior surface of the radius and interosseous membrane and its distal attachment at the base of the distal phalanx of the thumb (Fig. 11–17). It is a prime mover in flexion of all three joints of the thumb.

Flexor Pollicis Longus Muscle

(O)	Radius, anterior surface
(I)	Distal phalanx of thumb
(A)	Flexes all joints of the thumb
(N)	Median nerve (C8, T1)

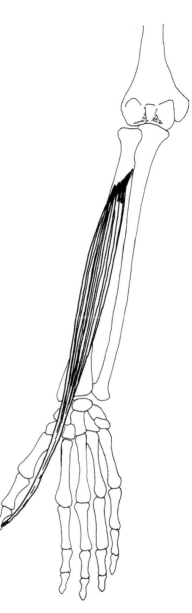

FIGURE 11–17.   Flexor pollicis longus muscle.

The **abductor pollicis longus muscle** is located deep on the posterior fore-arm (Fig. 11–18). It attaches to the radius just distal to the supinator, the interosseous membrane, and the middle portion of the ulna. It becomes superficial just proximal to crossing the wrist and attaches to the base of the first metacarpal on the radial side. It effectively abducts the thumb at the CMC joint even though it is attached only to the metacarpal because the distal joints (MCP and IP) allow only flexion and ex-tension. Therefore, the thumb moves as one unit in the direction of abduction and adduction. Similarly, adducting the metacarpal also adducts the entire thumb. There-fore, in this text, when referring to thumb abduction, adduction, opposition, and reposition, it is implied that the action occurs at the CMC joint.

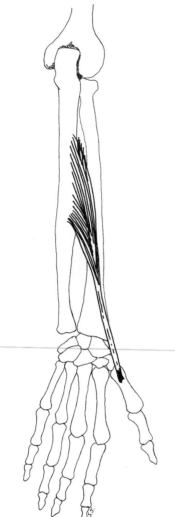

FIGURE 11–18. Abductor pollicis longus muscle.

Abductor Pollicis Longus Muscle

(O)	Posterior radius, interosseous membrane, middle ulna
(I)	Base of the first metacarpal
(A)	Abducts thumb
(N)	Radial nerve

The **extensor pollicis brevis muscle** is also located deep on the posterior forearm and spans the wrist just medial to the abductor pollicis longus muscle. Its proximal attachment is on the posterior radius near the distal end and just below the abductor pollicis longus muscle. Its distal attachment is on the posterior surface at the base of the thumb's proximal phalanx (Fig. 11–19). It functions to extend the MCP joint of the thumb.

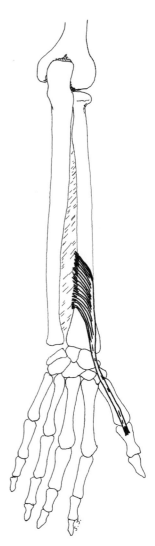

FIGURE 11–19.   Extensor pollicis brevis muscle.

Extensor Pollicis Brevis Muscle

(O)	Posterior distal radius
(I)	Base of the proximal phalanx of thumb
(A)	Extends MCP joint of thumb
(N)	Radial nerve (C6, C7)

The **extensor pollicis longus muscle** is located near the two previously mentioned muscles deep on the posterior forearm. Its proximal attachment is on the middle third of the ulna and interosseous membrane (Fig. 11–20). Like the other two muscles, it becomes superficial just before crossing the wrist. Its distal attachment is at the base of the distal phalanx of the thumb on the posterior side. It functions to extend the CMC, MCP, and IP joints of the thumb.

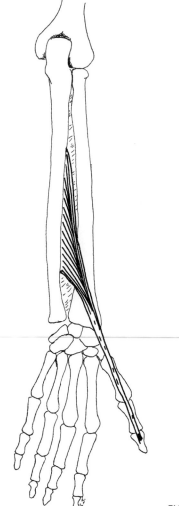

FIGURE 11–20. Extensor pollicis longus muscle.

Extensor Pollicis Longus Muscle

(O)	Middle posterior ulna and interosseous membrane
(I)	Base of distal phalanx of thumb
(A)	Extends all joints of the thumb
(N)	Radial nerve (C6, C7, C8)

If you extend your thumb, you will notice that a depression is formed between what appears to be two tendons. Actually, there are three tendons. The abductor pollicis longus and extensor pollicis brevis muscles form the lateral border, and the extensor pollicis longus muscle forms the medial border. This depression is called the **anatomical snuffbox** (Fig. 11–21).

This concludes our discussion of the extrinsic muscles of the hand. In review, the extrinsic muscles have their proximal attachment above the wrist and their distal attachment on the hand. Because they cross the wrist, they could have a function

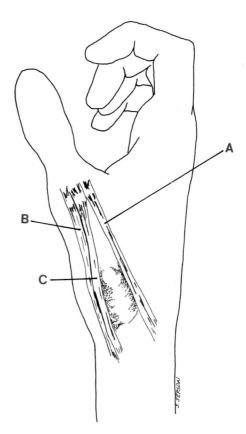

FIGURE 11–21. Anatomical snuff box. *(A)* Extensor pollicis longus muscle. *(B)* Abductor pollicis longus muscles. *(C)* Extensor pollicis brevis muscle.

there; however, any wrist function is usually assistive at best with their prime function of these muscles being to move the fingers or thumb.

INTRINSIC MUSCLES

Intrinsic muscles have their proximal attachment at, or distal to, the carpal bones, and have a function on the thumb or fingers. These muscles are responsible for the fine motor control and precision movement of the hand. The intrinsic muscles can be further divided into the thenar, hypothenar, and palm muscles. The **thenar muscles** are those muscles that function to move the thumb. They form the thenar eminence, or ball of the thumb. The **hypothenar muscles,** forming the hypothenar eminence, act primarily on the little finger. The **deep palm muscles** are located deep in the palm of the hand between the thenar and hypothenar muscles. They have some of the more intricate motions that usually involve multiple muscles. These muscles are the adductor pollicis, the interossei (of which there are four dorsal and four palmar), and the lumbricales (of which there are also four muscles). Table 11–1 summarizes the three groups of intrinsic muscles.

In the thenar group, the **flexor pollicis brevis muscle** is a relatively superficial muscle. It attaches proximally to the trapezium and the flexor retinaculum, and distally to the base of the proximal phalanx of the thumb (Fig. 11–22). In older texts, this muscle is described as having two parts: a lateral superficial part (described here) and a medial deep part. In more recent literature, this medial part is often consid-

TABLE 11–1	INTRINSIC MUSCLES OF THE HAND	
Thenar	**Hypothenar**	**Deep Palm**
Flexor pollicis brevis	Flexor digiti minimi	Adductor pollicis
Abductor pollicis brevis	Abductor digiti minimi	Interossei
Opponens pollicis	Opponens digiti minimi	Lumbricales

ered a separate muscle—the first palmar interossei, and this is the terminology used here. Thus, the flexor pollicis muscle has one part, and its primary action is to flex the MCP joint of the thumb. Because it crosses the CMC joint it also flexes that joint, but its role is more assistive.

Flexor Pollicis Brevis Muscle

(O)	Trapezium and flexor retinaculum
(I)	Proximal phalanx
(A)	Flexes the CMC and MCP joints of thumb
(N)	Median nerve (C6, C7)

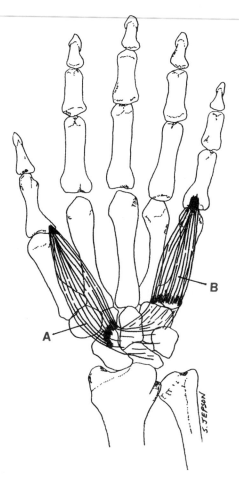

FIGURE 11–22. (*A*) Flexor pollicis brevis muscle. (*B*) Flexor digiti minimi muscle.

The **abductor pollicis brevis muscle** lies just lateral to the flexor pollicis brevis muscle. It attaches proximally to the flexor retinaculum, scaphoid, and trapezium, and distally to the base of the proximal phalanx of the thumb (Fig. 11–23). It acts to abduct the CMC joint of the thumb.

Abductor Pollicis Brevis Muscle

(O)	Scaphoid, trapezium, and flexor retinaculum
(I)	Proximal phalanx
(A)	Abducts the thumb
(N)	Median nerve (C6, C7)

The **opponens pollicis muscle** lies deep to the abductor pollicis brevis muscle. It attaches proximally to the trapezium and flexor retinaculum and distally to the entire lateral surface of the first metacarpal (Fig. 11–24). Its primary function is to oppose the CMC joint of the thumb. Remember, this action occurs at the CMC joint.

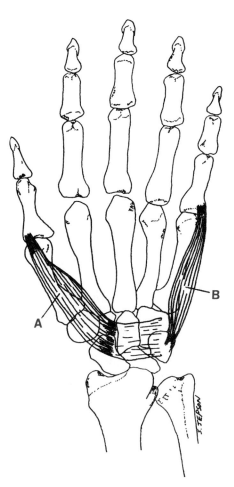

FIGURE 11–23. *(A)* Abductor pollicis brevis muscle. *(B)* Abductor digiti minimi muscle.

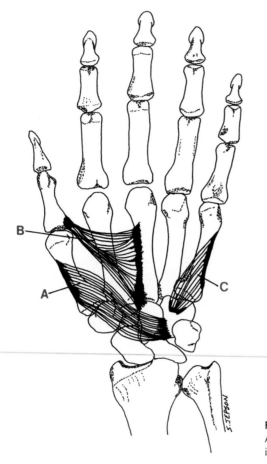

FIGURE 11–24. (*A*) Opponens pollicis muscle. (*B*) Adductor pollicis muscle. (*C*) Opponens digiti minimi muscle.

Opponens Pollicis Muscle

(O)	Trapezium and flexor retinaculum
(I)	First metacarpal
(A)	Opposes the thumb
(N)	Median nerve (C6, C7)

Thumb opposition is perhaps the most important function of the hand. Because it is a combination of flexion, abduction, and rotation of the thumb, other muscles, such as the flexor pollicis brevis and abductor pollicis muscles, assist in this function.

The **adductor pollicis muscle** is a thumb muscle, although it is not usually considered part of the thenar group. This is probably because it is located deep and does not make up the muscle bulk of the thenar eminence. This concept will be discussed in more detail later in this chapter. It has its proximal attachments on the capitate, base of the second metacarpal, and the palmar surface of the third metacarpal. Its distal attachment is at the base of the proximal phalanx of the thumb (see Fig. 11–24). As its name implies, its function is to adduct the thumb (at the CMC joint).

Adductor Pollicis Muscle

(O)   Capitate, base of the second metacarpal, palmar surface of the
          third metacarpal
(I)   Base of proximal phalanx of thumb
(A)   Adducts thumb
(N)   Ulnar nerve (C8, T1)

The counterpart to the thenar muscle group is the hypothenar group. The **flexor digiti minimi muscle** serves the same function on the little finger as the flexor pollicis brevis does on the thumb. It is attached proximally to the hook of the hamate and the flexor retinaculum, and distally to the base of the proximal phalanx of the little finger (see Fig. 11–22). It flexes the MCP joint of that finger. Remember, although most thumb motion occurs at the CMC joint, most finger motion occurs at the MCP joint.

Flexor Digiti Minimi Muscle

(O)   Hamate and flexor retinaculum
(I)   Base of proximal phalanx of the fifth finger
(A)   Flexes CMC and MCP joints of the fifth finger
(N)   Ulnar nerve (C8, T1)

The **abductor digiti minimi muscle** lies superficially just medial to the flexor digiti minimi muscle on the ulnar border of the hypothenar eminence. It attaches proximally to the pisiform and to the tendon of the flexor carpi ulnaris muscle and distally to the base of the proximal phalanx of the fifth finger (see Fig. 11–23). It abducts the MCP joint of that finger.

Abductor Digiti Minimi Muscle

(O)   Pisiform and tendon of flexor carpi ulnaris
(I)   Proximal phalanx of fifth finger
(A)   Abducts the MCP joint of the fifth finger
(N)   Ulnar nerve (C8, T1)

The **opponens digiti minimi muscle** lies deep to the other hypothenar muscles. Its proximal attachments, the hook of the hamate and the flexor retinaculum, are similar to the proximal attachments of the flexor digiti minimi muscle. Distally, it attaches to the ulnar border of the fifth metacarpal (see Fig. 11–24). It primarily opposes the CMC joint of the fifth finger.

Opponens Digiti Minimi Muscle

(O)   Hamate and flexor retinaculum
(I)   Fifth metacarpal
(A)   Opposes the fifth finger
(N)   Ulnar nerve (C8, T1)

The muscles located in the area between the thenar and hypothenar muscle groups are often called the deep palm group, or the *intermediate group*. The adductor pollicis muscle is sometimes placed in this group because it is located deep within the palm. Other sources will place it with the thenar group because of its action on the thumb. Here it is placed in the deep palm group for perhaps no other reason than to discuss the intrinsic muscles in groups of three. In any event, it was described with the thenar muscles.

There are four **dorsal interossei** muscles. They each attach proximally to two adjacent metacarpals and distally at the base of the proximal phalanx (Fig. 11–25). Table 11–2 summarizes the attachments and actions of each of the dorsal interossei muscles. The ulnar nerve innervates all dorsal interossei muscles.

Dorsal Interossei	
(O)	Adjacent metacarpals
(I)	Base of proximal phalanx
(A)	Abduct fingers at MCP joint
(N)	Ulnar nerve (C8, T1)

The **palmar interossei** muscles are an interesting group of muscles with some controversy as to whether there are three or four of them. Most of the older texts describe three. These texts also describe the flexor pollicis brevis muscle as having two parts: a medial part coming from the flexor retinaculum and attaching to the base of the proximal phalanx of the thumb, and a lateral part coming from the first metacarpal bone and attaching on the proximal phalanx. Each part has a different innervation. A branch of the median nerve innervates the lateral portion. The medial portion gets its nerve supply from a branch of the ulnar nerve, as do the palmar interossei muscles.

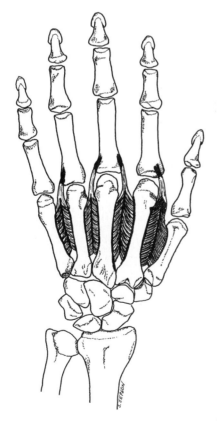

FIGURE 11–25. Dorsal interossei muscles of the hand.

TABLE 11–2	DORSAL INTEROSSEI MUSCLES OF THE HAND		
Muscle	**Proximal Attachment**	**Distal Attachment**	**Action**
First	First and second metacarpals	Lateral side of index finger	Abduct index finger
Second	Second and third metacarpals	Lateral side of middle finger	Abduct middle finger laterally
Third	Third and fourth metacarpals	Medial side of middle finger	Abduct middle finger medially
Fourth	Fourth and fifth metacarpals	Medial side of ring finger	Abduct ring finger

More recent texts, however, list the flexor pollicis brevis muscle as having only one part (lateral part) with innervation from the median nerve. These sources have renamed the medial head as the first palmar interosseous muscle. This muscle has the same attachments and nerve supply as the other palmar interossei muscles, so it makes sense to group these muscles together. Although this appears to be a logical way to present these muscles (and how they will be presented here), you should be aware of the discrepancies.

The palmar interossei muscles, like the dorsal interossei muscles, are four in number. They attach proximally to the palmar surface of the first, second, fourth, and fifth metacarpals. Distally, they attach to the base of the proximal phalanx of the same finger as the proximal attachment (Fig. 11–26). These attachments are summarized in Table 11–3. Like the dorsal interossei muscles, the palmar interossei muscles are innervated by the ulnar nerve.

Palmar Interossei Muscles

(O)	Respective muscles
(I)	Base of respective proximal phalanx
(A)	Adduct fingers at MCP joint
(N)	Ulnar nerve (C8, T1)

As mentioned, the middle finger is the point of reference for abduction and adduction. Movement away from the middle finger is abduction, and movement toward it is adduction. Note that the middle finger abducts in two directions and therefore does not adduct.

The last muscle group to be discussed is rather unique. The **lumbrical muscles,** of which there are four, have no bony attachment. They are located quite deep and attach only to tendons. Proximally, they attach to the tendon of the flexor digitorum profundus muscle, spanning the MCP joint anteriorly (see Fig. 11–12). They then pass posteriorly at the proximal phalange to attach to the tendinous expansion of the extensor digitorum muscle (Fig. 11–27). Their action is to flex the MCP joint and extend the PIP and DIP joints of the second through fifth fingers. This combined motion is referred to as the "table-top position."

Lumbrical Muscles

(O)	Tendon of the flexor digitorum profundus muscle
(I)	Tendon of the extensor digitorum muscle
(A)	Flex the MCP joint while extending the IP joints
(N)	First and second lumbrical muscles: medial nerve Third and fourth lumbrical muscles: ulnar nerve (C6, C7, C8)

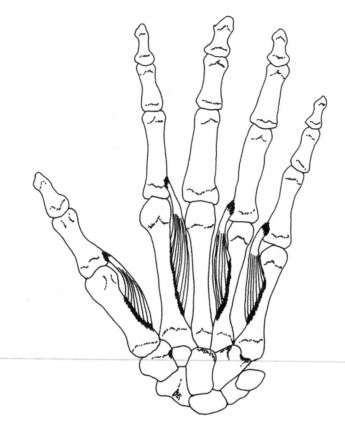

FIGURE 11–26. Palmar interossei muscles of the hand.

SUMMARY OF MUSCLE ACTIONS

The actions of the prime movers of the hand are summarized in Table 11–4.

SUMMARY OF MUSCLE INNERVATION

Innervation of the hand is almost as straightforward as the wrist; however, a few exceptions must be discussed. As with the wrist, muscles on the posterior surface of the hand are innervated mostly by the radial nerve. Muscles on the thumb side are supplied primarily by the median nerve, and the ulnar side by the ulnar nerve.

The adductor pollicis muscle appears to be the exception; it is innervated by the ulnar nerve instead of the median nerve like all the other thumb (pollicis) muscles.

TABLE 11–3	PALMAR INTEROSSEI MUSCLES		
Muscles	**Proximal Attachment**	**Distal Attachment**	**Action**
First	First metacarpal	Medial side of thumb	Adduct thumb
Second	Second metacarpal	Medial side of index finger	Adduct index finger
Third	Fourth metacarpal	Lateral side of ring finger	Adduct ring finger
Fourth	Fifth metacarpal	Lateral side of little finger	Adduct little finger

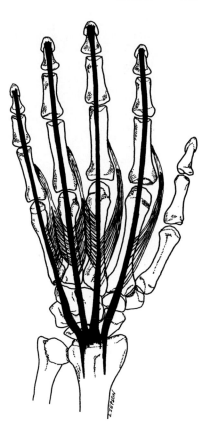

FIGURE 11–27. Lumbricales muscles.

However, remember that the adductor pollicis muscle attaches in the middle of the palm to the third metacarpal (see Fig. 11–24). It is here that the ulnar nerve changes directions and runs toward the thumb. As it does, it sends branches to the adductor pollicis and dorsal and palmar interossei muscles (see Fig. 5–29). The flexor digitorum profundus muscle receives its innervation from both the median and ulnar nerve, as do the lumbrical muscles. This does not seem surprising, because the lumbrical muscles have their proximal attachment on the tendons of the flexor digitorum profundus muscle. Table 11–5 further summarizes hand muscle innervation. One can see from the table that injury to the lower cervical vertebrae will affect all hand function. Table 11–6 summarizes the segmental innervation. Note that there is some discrepancy among various sources regarding spinal cord level of innervation.

Hand Function

The human hand performs many functions. The primary function of the hand is grasp, or *prehension*. This means the hand is adapted to hold or manipulate objects. There are also many nonprehensile hand functions, such as expressing emotions, scratching, using a fist as a club, and using the open palm, as in pushing down on an armrest to assist in standing. Because no manipulative movement occurs with these types of activities, no further description of nonprehensile function will be made here.

With prehension (grasping or holding an object) how the hand is used depends on the size, shape, and weight of the object, how that object will be used, and the in-

TABLE 11–4	PRIME MOVERS OF THE HAND	
Action	**Joint**	**Muscle**
	THUMB	
Flexion	CMC, MCP	Flexor pollicis brevis
	IP (MCP, CMC)	Flexor pollicis longus
Extension	CMC, MCP	Extensor pollicis brevis
	IP (MCP, CMC)	Extensor pollicis longus
Abduction	CMC	Abductor pollicis brevis
	CMC	Abductor pollicis longus
Adduction	CMC	Adductor pollicis
Opposition	CMC	Opponens pollicis
	FINGER	
Flexion	MCP	Lumbricales, flexor digitorum superficialis, flexor digitorum profundus
	PIP	Flexor digitorum superficialis, flexor digitorum profundus
	DIP	Flexor digitorum profundus
Extension	MCP	Extensor digitorum, extensor indicis, extensor digiti minimi
	PIP and DIP	Lumbricales, extensor digitorum, extensor digiti minimi, extensor indicis
Abduction	MCP	Dorsal interossei, abductor digiti minimi
Adduction	MCP	Palmar interossei
Opposition (fifth)	CMC	Opponens digiti minimi

volvement of the proximal segments of the upper extremity. Generally speaking, the shoulder girdle and shoulder joint place the hand in space. The elbow allows the hand to move closer or farther away from the body, especially the face. The wrist provides stability while the hand is manipulating objects and is important in the tenodesis action described in Chapter 4. Although much attention tends to be placed on the grasping aspect of hand function, release is equally important. Release is the role of the MP and IP extensors. Without the ability to release, the hand's grasp function is greatly diminished.

Of paramount importance to hand function is sensation. Without intact sensation, an individual must compensate with visual clues to find items, know what is being held, and how hard the object is being grasped. For example, if you were presented with a laundry bag full of clothes and told to find the small box of soap, you could feel around inside the bag until locating the soap. However, if your hand's sensation were not intact, you would have to empty the bag and visually search for the box. A person with an upper extremity amputation who uses a prosthetic device is a good example of having hand function without sensation. That person would need visual feedback to find the soap and to know if the terminal device had grasped it. Hand sensation is provided by the radial, ulnar, and median nerves. Figure 11–28 shows the pattern of sensory distribution. This distribution varies somewhat with authors.

TABLE 11–5	INNERVATION OF THE MUSCLES OF THE HAND

Muscle	Nerve	Spinal Segment
Extensor digitorum	Radial	C6, C7, C8
Extensor indicis	Radial	C6, C7, C8
Extensor digiti minimi	Radial	C6, C7, C8
Extensor pollicis longus	Radial	C6, C7, C8
Extensor pollicis brevis	Radial	C6, C7
Abductor pollicis longus	Radial	C6, C7
Flexor digitorum superficialis	Median	C7, C8, T1
Flexor digitorum profundus	Median	C8, T1
	Ulnar	C8, T1
Flexor pollicis longus	Median	C8, T1
Flexor pollicis brevis	Median	C6, C7
Abductor pollicis brevis	Median	C6, C7
Opponens pollicis	Median	C6, C7
Lumbricales 1 and 2	Median	C6, C7
Lumbricales 3 and 4	Ulnar	C8
Flexor digiti minimi	Ulnar	C8, T1
Abductor digiti minimi	Ulnar	C8, T1
Opponens digiti minimi	Ulnar	C8, T1
Adductor pollicis	Ulnar	C8, T1
Dorsal and palmar interossei	Ulnar	C8, T1

TABLE 11–6	SEGMENTAL INNERVATION OF THE HAND

Spinal cord level	C6	C7	C8	T1
Extensor digitorum	X	X	X	
Extensor indicis	X	X	X	
Extensor digiti minimi	X	X	X	
Extensor pollicis longus	X	X	X	
Extensor pollicis brevis	X	X		
Abductor pollicis longus	X	X		
Abductor pollicis brevis	X	X		
Flexor pollicis brevis	X	X		
Opponens pollicis	X	X		
Flexor digitorum superficialis		X	X	X
Flexor digitorum profundus			X	X
Flexor pollicis longus			X	X
Lumbricales			X	X
Flexor digiti minimi			X	X
Abductor digiti minimi			X	X
Opponens digiti minimi			X	X
Adductor pollicis			X	X
Dorsal and palmar interossei			X	X

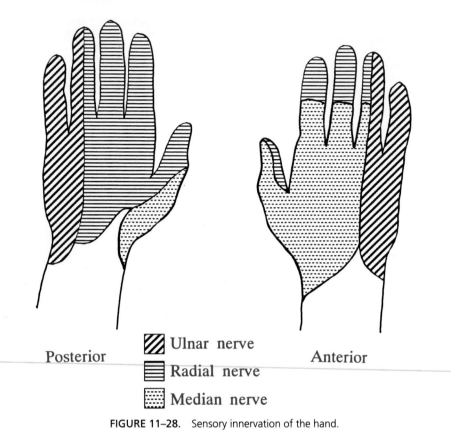

Ulnar nerve

Radial nerve

Median nerve

Posterior

Anterior

FIGURE 11-28.   Sensory innervation of the hand.

There is an optimal position for the wrist and hand for the hand to be most effective in terms of strength and precision. This position is called the **functional position of the hand.** In this position the wrist is in a slightly extended position, the MCP and PIP joints of the fingers are slightly flexed, and the thumb is in opposition. Figure 11–29 illustrates this position. Maintenance of the thenar web is vital to thumb opposition.

GRASP

There are basically two types of prehension: power grips and precision grips. The activity dictates which grip is needed. A **power grip** is used when an object needs to be held forcefully while being moved about by more proximal joint muscles (holding a hammer or door knob) (Fig. 11–30). Often a power grip involves an isometric

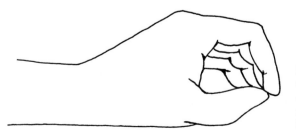

FIGURE 11–29. Functional position of the wrist and hand. The wrist is in slight extension, the MCP and PIP joints are in some degree of flexion, and the thumb is in opposition.

contraction with no movement occurring between the hand and the object being held. A **precision grip,** often referred to as **precision prehension,** is used when an object needs to be manipulated in a finer type movement such as holding a pen or threading a needle (Fig. 11–31).

Power Grips

A power grip usually involves a significant amount of force and is considered the most powerful grip. The fingers tend to flex around the object in one direction and the thumb wraps around in the opposite direction, providing a counter force to keep the object in contact with the palm and/or fingers. Once the object is firmly set in the hand, it can be moved about in space by more proximal joint musculature. The long finger flexors (extrinsics) grip the object, and the long finger extensors (also extrinsics) assist in holding the wrist in a neutral or slightly extended position. When the thumb is involved, it tends to be in an adducted position.

The three commonly described power grips are cylindrical, spherical, and hook. The **cylindrical grip** (Fig. 11–32) has all the fingers flexed around the object, which usually lies at a right angle to the forearm. The thumb is wrapped around the object in the opposite direction often overlapping the fingers. Examples of a cylindrical grip would be holding a hammer, racquet, or wheelbarrow handle.

A variation of the cylindrical grip has the fingers flexed around a handle in a graded fashion (Fig. 11–33). The fifth finger joints are flexed the most, and the second finger joints are only partly flexed. The thumb lies parallel and against the handle, and the wrist is in slight ulnar deviation. The advantage of this grip over a cylindrical grip is that it allows a forceful, but more controlled, use of the tool. Examples of this type of grip would involve holding a golf club or screwdriver.

A **spherical grip** has all the fingers and thumb adducted around an object, and unlike the cylindrical grip, the fingers are more spread apart. The palm of the hand is often not involved (Fig. 11–34). Activities involving a spherical grip would be holding an apple or doorknob, or picking up a glass by its top.

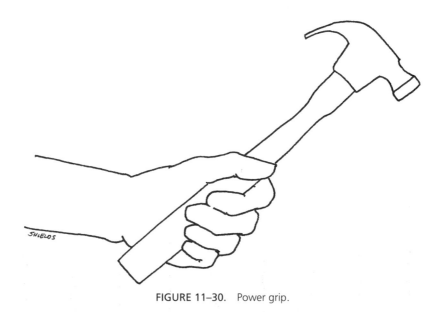

FIGURE 11–30. Power grip.

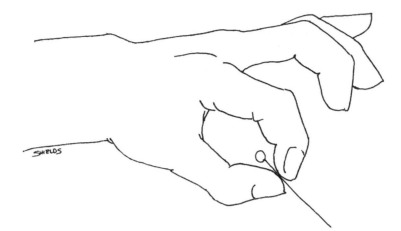

FIGURE 11–31. Precision grip.

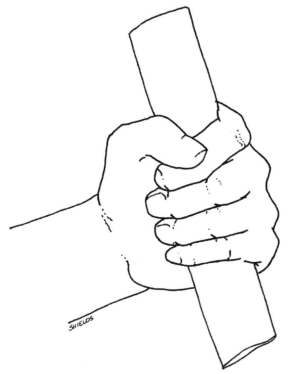

FIGURE 11–32. Cylindrical grip.

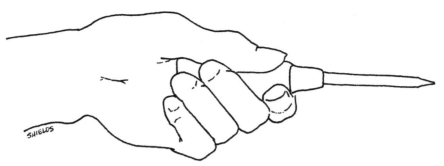

FIGURE 11–33.   Cylindrical grip variation.

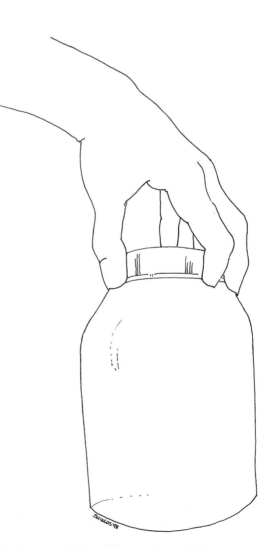

FIGURE 11–34.   Spherical grip.

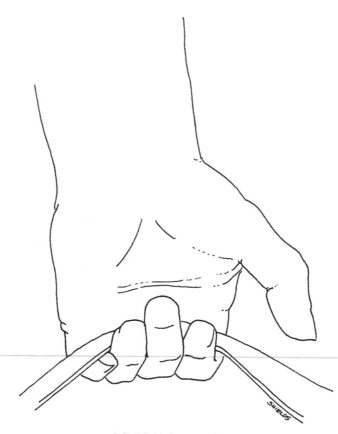

FIGURE 11–35. Hook grip.

The **hook grip** involves the second through fifth fingers flexed around an object in a hooklike manner (Fig. 11–35). The MCP joints are extended, and the PIP and DIP joints are in some degree of flexion. The thumb is usually not involved. Therefore, this is the only power grip possible if a person has a median nerve injury and looses the ability to oppose the thumb. Examples of a hook grip are seen when holding on to a handle, like a suitcase, wagon, or bucket.

Precision Grips

Precision grips tend to hold the object between the tips of the fingers and thumb. The intrinsic muscles are involved along with the extrinsics. The thumb tends to be abducted. These grips provide more fine movement and accuracy. The object is usually small, even fragile. The palm does not tend to be involved, and the proximal joints do not tend to move. There are four commonly recognized types of precision grip.

With the **pad-to-pad grip,** the MCP and PIP joints of the finger(s) are flexed, the thumb is abducted, and the distal joints of both are extended bringing the pads of the finger(s) and thumb together. It may involve the thumb and one finger, usually the index finger, which is called a **pinch grip** (Fig. 11–36). It may also involve the thumb and two fingers, usually the index and middle fingers. This is called a **three-jaw chuck.** If you observe how a power drill holds the drill bit in place, you will see the similarity to this grip (Fig. 11–37). There are three "jaws" pinching in on the drill bit

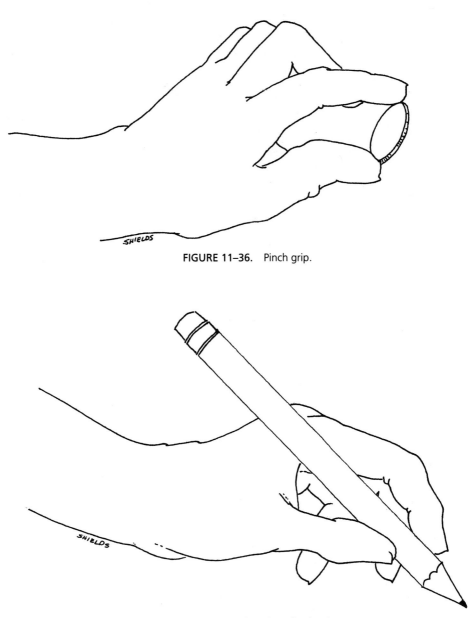

FIGURE 11–36.   Pinch grip.

FIGURE 11–37.   Three-jaw chuck grip.

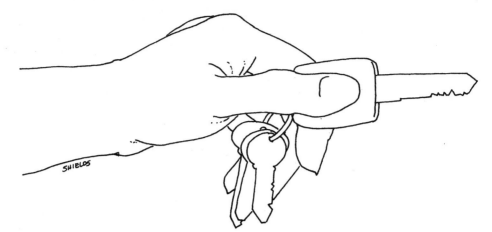

FIGURE 11–38. Pad-to-side grip.

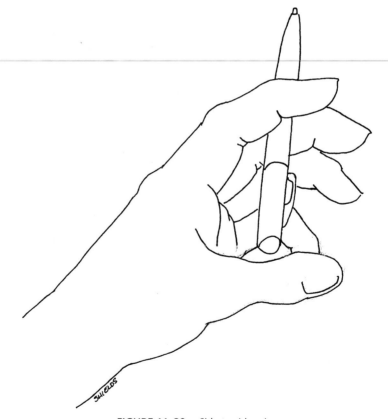

FIGURE 11–39. Side-to-side grip.

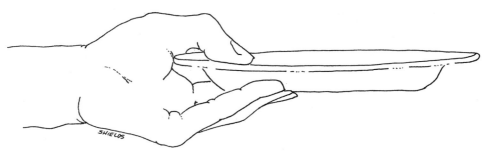

FIGURE 11–40.   Lumbrical grip.

and the entire holding mechanism is called a "chuck." Holding a pen or pencil would be an example of this grip. This is by far the most common precision grip.

Similar to the pad-to-pad grip, the **tip-to-tip grip** involves bringing the tip of the thumb up against the tip of another digit, usually the index finger, to pick up a small object such as a coin or pin (see Fig. 11–31). It is also called **pincer grip.**

The **pad-to-side grip,** also called lateral prehension, has the pad of the extended thumb pressing an object against the radial side of the index finger (Fig. 11–38). This is a strong grip, but allows less fine movements than the other two types. The terminal device of upper extremity prostheses adapts this type of grip. Also, because this grip does not require an opposed thumb, a person who has lost opposition but has retained thumb adduction can grasp and hold small objects.

The **side-to-side grip,** somewhat similar to pad-to-side grip, requires adduction of two fingers, usually the index or middle fingers (Fig. 11–39). It is a weak grip and does not permit much precision. It is perhaps most frequently used holding a cigarette. It is also used to hold an object, like a pencil, between two fingers while using another pencil or pen. Because the thumb is not involved, this grip could be used in the absence of the thumb.

Lumbrical grip, sometimes referred to as the **plate grip,** has the MCP and PIP joints flexed and the DIP joints extended. The thumb opposes the fingers holding an object horizontal (Fig. 11–40). This grip is usually used when something needs to be kept horizontal such as a plate or tray. It is called a lumbrical grip because the action of the lumbrical muscles is to flex the MCP joints while extending the IP joints.

REVIEW QUESTIONS

1. Which finger and thumb motions occur in:
   a. the frontal plane around the sagittal axis?
   b. the sagittal plane around the frontal axis?
   c. the transverse plane around the vertical axis?

2. Compare the thumb and fingers in terms of number of bones and joints.

3. Thumb opposition is a combination of what motions?

4. What is the purpose of the retinaculum?

5. What structures make up the carpal tunnel? Which structures run through the carpal tunnel?

6. What is an extrinsic muscle? List the extrinsic muscles of the hand.

7. What is an intrinsic muscle? List the intrinsic muscles of the hand.

8. Explain the difference between thenar muscles and hypothenar muscles, and give examples of each.

9. What is the "anatomical snuff box"? Which muscles are involved in this structure?

10. What hand muscle does not have a bony attachment? What does it attach to?

11. Identify the type of grip used for the following activities:
    a. holding the handle of a skillet
    b. pulling a little red wagon
    c. picking up a cassette tape
    d. fastening snaps or buttons
    e. carrying a mug by its handle
    f. holding a hand of cards
    g. holding an apple
    h. holding on to a barbell

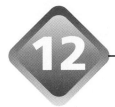

Temporomandibular Joint

Joint Structure and Motions

Bones and Landmarks

Ligaments and Other Structures

Mechanics of Movement

Muscles of the TMJ

Summary of Muscle Action

Summary of Muscle Innervation

Review Question

Joint Structure and Motions

The temporomandibular joint, often referred to as the TMJ, is one of the most frequently used joints in the body. It is used during chewing, swallowing, yawning, talking, and any other activity involving jaw motion. The TMJ is located anterior to the ear and at the posterior superior end of the jaw (Fig. 12–1). It is made up of the articular fossa of the temporal bone superiorly articulating with the condyle of the mandible inferiorly. It is a synovial joint and is best described as having a hingelike shape, although it is not a pure hinge joint because it also allows some gliding motion.

The TMJ is made up of two bones, a disk that divides the joint into two joint spaces, a joint capsule, four ligaments, and four main muscles that create five motions. The joint motions are **mandibular elevation** (closing the mouth), **depression** (opening the mouth), **protraction** (moving the jaw forward), **retraction** (moving the jaw posteriorly), and **lateral deviation** (side-to-side jaw movement) (Fig. 12–2). Protraction is also called protrusion, and retraction is synonymous with retrusion. Retraction is basically the return to anatomical position from a protracted position.

When the mandible is at rest, the condyle of the mandible is seated in the mandibular fossa of the temporal bone. The normal resting position of the mandible is with the lips closed and teeth several millimeters apart. This is maintained by low levels of activity of the temporalis muscles (Basmajian, 1978). The mouth should open far enough for you to be able to put two to three fingers between the front upper and lower teeth.

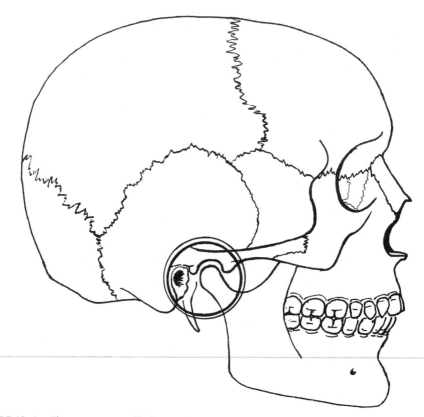

FIGURE 12–1.   The temporomandibular joint (TMJ) can be seen within the circle portion of this drawing.

Bones and Landmarks

The skull consists of two parts: the bones of the large cranium cavity, which encases the brain, and the bones of the face (Fig. 12–3). The TMJ is made up of the mandible, a facial bone articulating with the temporal bone, a cranial bone. Surrounding bones provide an area for muscle and ligament attachment. The following is a description of the bones and landmarks significant to the TMJ.

The **mandible,** or **mandibular bone,** is shaped somewhat like a horseshoe and it articulates with the temporal bone on each side of the face. It consists of a body and two upwardly projecting rami (Figs. 12–4*A* and 12–5*A*). Therefore, although the mandible is considered one bone, each lateral end articulates with a temporal bone, forming two identical joints on either side of the face. The mandible makes up the inferior part of the face and is often referred to as the jaw or lower jaw. Its significant landmarks are as follows:

Angle	Located between the body and ramus, and the joining point of the two landmarks (Figs. 12–4*B* and 12–5*B*).
Body	The horizontal portion of the mandible. The superior surface of the body holds the lower teeth (Figs. 12–4*C* and 12–5*C*).
Condyle	Also called the condylar process. It is the posterior projection on the ramus and it articulates with the temporal bone (Figs. 12–4*D* and 12–5*D*).

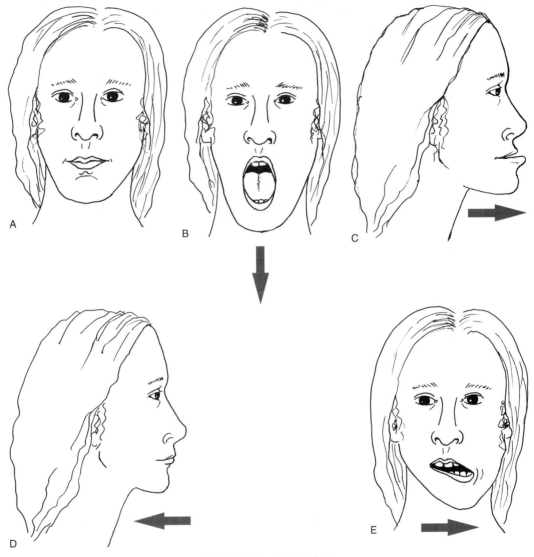

FIGURE 12–2.   TMJ motions.

A Mandibular elevation (return from depression)   **D** Mandibular retraction
B Mandibular depression   **E** Mandibular lateral deviation
C Mandibular protraction

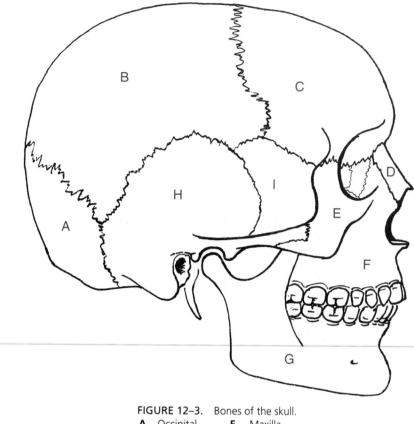

FIGURE 12–3. Bones of the skull.

A	Occipital	**F**	Maxilla
B	Parietal	**G**	Mandible
C	Frontal	**H**	Temporal
D	Nasal	**I**	Sphenoid
E	Zygomatic		

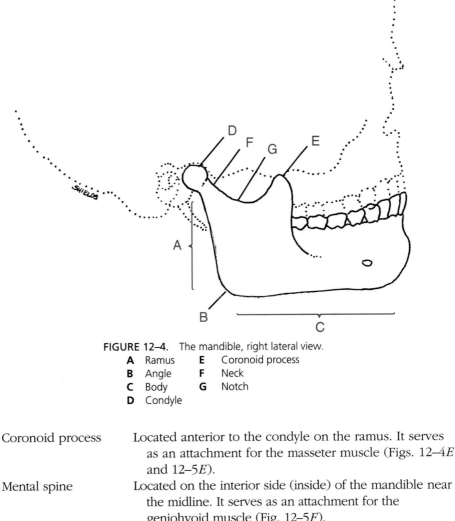

FIGURE 12–4. The mandible, right lateral view.

A	Ramus	**E**	Coronoid process
B	Angle	**F**	Neck
C	Body	**G**	Notch
D	Condyle		

Coronoid process	Located anterior to the condyle on the ramus. It serves as an attachment for the masseter muscle (Figs. 12–4*E* and 12–5*E*).
Mental spine	Located on the interior side (inside) of the mandible near the midline. It serves as an attachment for the geniohyoid muscle (Fig. 12–5*F*).
Neck	Located just inferior to the condyle (Figs. 12–4*F* and 12–5*G*).
Notch	Located between the condyle and coronoid process on the ramus (Figs. 12–4*G* and 12–5*H*).
Ramus	The vertical portion of the mandible from the angle to the condyle (Figs. 12–4*A* and 12–5*A*).

The **temporal bone** is located on the side of the skull posterior to the zygomatic bone, inferior to the parietal bone, posterior to the greater wing of the sphenoid, and anterior to the occipital bone (see Fig. 12–3). The articular portion of the temporal bone is made up of the concave articular (mandibular) fossa in the middle with the convex articular tubercle located anteriorly and the convex postglenoid tubercle located posteriorly (Fig. 12–6). Its main landmarks consist of:

Articular tubercle	Makes up the anterior portion of the articulating surface of the temporal bone. When the mandible is depressed, the condyle of the mandible rests under this landmark.

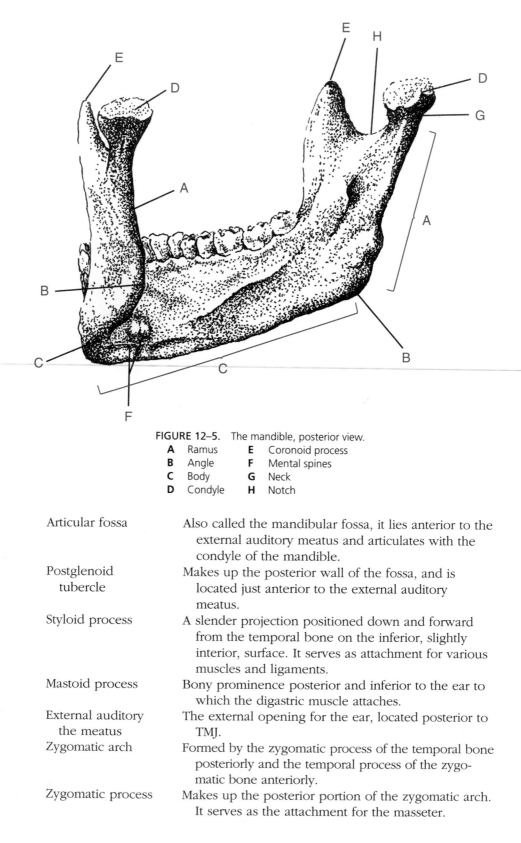

FIGURE 12–5. The mandible, posterior view.

A	Ramus	**E**	Coronoid process
B	Angle	**F**	Mental spines
C	Body	**G**	Neck
D	Condyle	**H**	Notch

Articular fossa	Also called the mandibular fossa, it lies anterior to the external auditory meatus and articulates with the condyle of the mandible.
Postglenoid tubercle	Makes up the posterior wall of the fossa, and is located just anterior to the external auditory meatus.
Styloid process	A slender projection positioned down and forward from the temporal bone on the inferior, slightly interior, surface. It serves as attachment for various muscles and ligaments.
Mastoid process	Bony prominence posterior and inferior to the ear to which the digastric muscle attaches.
External auditory the meatus	The external opening for the ear, located posterior to TMJ.
Zygomatic arch	Formed by the zygomatic process of the temporal bone posteriorly and the temporal process of the zygomatic bone anteriorly.
Zygomatic process	Makes up the posterior portion of the zygomatic arch. It serves as the attachment for the masseter.

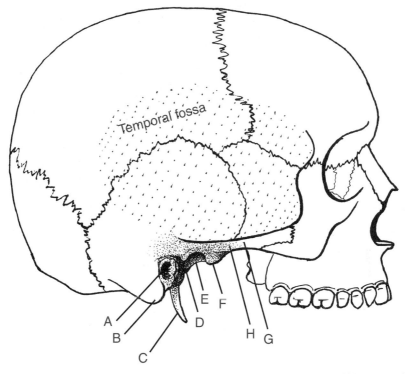

FIGURE 12–6. Temporal bone portion of TMJ, right lateral view with mandible removed.

A	External auditory meatus	**E**	Articular fossa
B	Mastoid process	**F**	Articular tubercle
C	Styloid process	**G**	Zygomatic arch
D	Postglenoid tubercle	**H**	Zygomatic process

Temporal fossa — Bony floor formed by the zygomatic, frontal, parietal, sphenoid, and temporal bones. It contains the temporalis muscle.

The **sphenoid bone** is located at the lateral base of the skull anterior to the temporal bone. It resembles a bat with extended wings (Fig. 12–7). Because of its location, the sphenoid bone connects with six other cranial bones and two facial bones. Only the following external surface features are relevant to TMJ function:

Greater wing — A large bony process located medial to the zygomatic bone and arch, and anterior to the rest of the temporal bone. As part of the temporal fossa, it provides attachment for the temporalis and lateral pterygoid muscles.

Lateral pterygoid plate — Lies deep to the zygomatic arch. It serves as an attachment for the lateral and medial pterygoid muscles.

Spine — Lies deep to the articular fossa of the temporal bone and provides attachment for the sphenomandibular ligament.

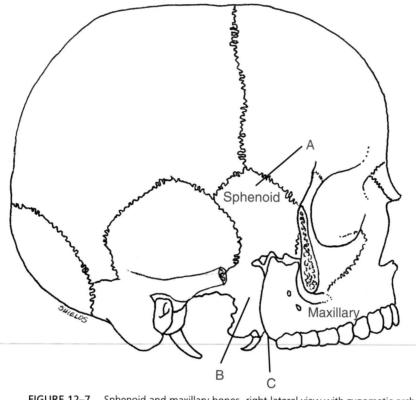

FIGURE 12–7. Sphenoid and maxillary bones, right lateral view with zygomatic arch removed.

Sphenoid bone	*Maxillary bone*
A Greater wing	**C** Tuberosity
B Lateral pterygoid plate	

The **zygomatic bone** forms the prominence of the cheek and contributes the lateral wall and floor of the eye orbit (see Fig. 12–6). The frontal, maxilla, sphenoid, and temporal bones border it. The zygomatic bone, along with the zygomatic process of the temporal bone, forms the zygomatic arch, to which the masseter attaches.

The **maxilla** or **maxillary bone** is commonly called the upper jaw. It is located in the upper part of the face and houses the upper teeth. It connects with the nasal bone superiorly and the zygomatic bone laterally (see Fig. 12–7).

Tuberosity   A rounded projection located on the inferior posterior angle. It serves as attachment for the medial pterygoid.

The **hyoid bone** is a horseshoe shaped bone lying just superior to the thyroid cartilage at about the level of C3. It has no bony articulation, but is suspended from the styloid processes of the temporal bones by the stylohoid ligaments (Fig. 12–8). Its main function is to provide attachment for the tongue muscles. However, it also provides attachment for the suprahyoid and infrahyoid muscles that have an assisting role in mandibular depression.

The **thyroid cartilage** is the largest of the nine cartilages of larynx. It is commonly called the "Adam's apple" and tends to be more prominent in males. It lies just inferior to the hyoid bone at about the level of C3 to C4 (see Fig. 12–8*D*). It provides attachment for the infrahyoid muscles.

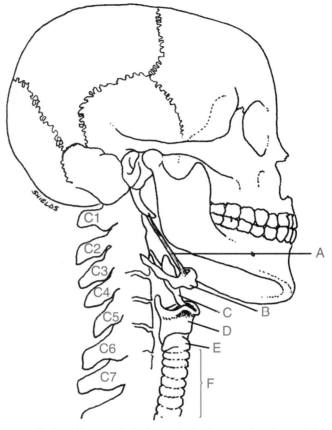

FIGURE 12–8. The hyoid bone with skull, vertebral column, and trachea—right side view.

A	Stylohyoid ligament	**D**	Thyroid cartilage
B	Hyoid bone	**E**	First cricoid ring
C	Epiglottis	**F**	Trachea

Ligaments and Other Structures

The **lateral ligament** is also known as the **temporomandibular ligament.** Anteriorly, it attaches on the neck of the mandibular condyle and disk, and then runs superiorly to the articular tubercle of the temporal bone (Fig. 12–9). It limits downward, posterior, and lateral motion of the mandible.

The **sphenomandibular ligament** attaches to the spine of the sphenoid bone and runs to the middle of the ramus on the internal surface of the mandible (see Figs. 12–9*C* and 12–10*B*). It suspends the mandible and limits excessive anterior motion.

The **stylomandibular ligament** runs from the styloid process of the temporal bone to the posterior inferior border of the ramus of the mandible (see Figs. 12–9*D* and 12–10*C*). It lies between the masseter and medial pterygoid muscles and has a role in limiting excessive anterior motion.

The **stylohyoid ligament** attaches from the styloid process of the temporal bone to the hyoid bone (see Fig. 12–8*A*). Its function is to hold the hyoid bone in place.

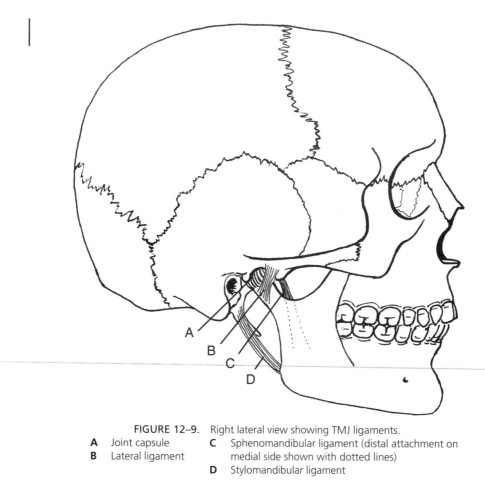

FIGURE 12–9. Right lateral view showing TMJ ligaments.

A Joint capsule   **C** Sphenomandibular ligament (distal attachment on
B Lateral ligament   medial side shown with dotted lines)
                                       D Stylomandibular ligament

The **joint capsule** envelops the TMJ by attaching superiorly to the articular tubercle and borders of the fossa of the temporal bone. Inferiorly, it attaches to the neck of the condyle of the mandible (see Figs. 12–9*A* and 12–10*A*).

The **articular disk** of the TMJ is somewhat similar to the articular disk of the sternoclavicular joint. It is connected circumferentially to the capsule and tendon of the lateral pterygoid (Fig. 12–11). It also divides the joint space into two separate compartments: a larger upper joint space and a smaller lower joint space. The superior surface is both concave and convex to accommodate the shape of the fossa. The inferior surface is concave, accommodating the convex surface of the condyle and allowing the joint to remain congruent (compatible) throughout the motion. The disk's shape and attachments also allow it to rotate in an anterior/posterior direction on the condyle. Because the articular disk is more firmly attached to the mandible than the temporal bone, it allows the disk to move forward with the condyle of the mandible when the mouth opens. It returns posteriorly when the mouth closes.

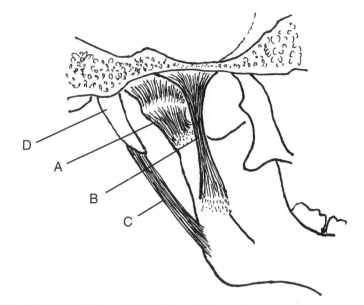

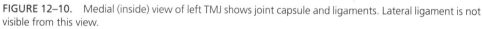

FIGURE 12–10. Medial (inside) view of left TMJ shows joint capsule and ligaments. Lateral ligament is not visible from this view.

A	Joint capsule	**C**	Stylomandibular ligament
B	Sphenomandibular ligament	**D**	Styloid process

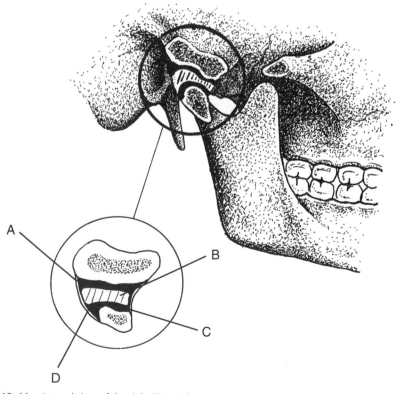

FIGURE 12–11. Lateral view of the right TMJ with zygomatic arch removed and condylar process cut. This shows the relationship of the mandibular condyle, disk, and articular fossa in a closed-jaw position. The articular disk divides the joint space into upper and lower spaces.

A	Upper joint space	**C**	Lower joint space
B	Articular disk	**D**	Articular disk

Mechanics of Movement

Depression of the mandible (opening the jaw) involves two motions (Fig. 12–12). The first part is accomplished by anterior rotation of the mandibular condyle on the disk. The second part of the motion involves a sliding of the disk and condyle forward and downward under the articular tubercle. Elevation of the mandible (closing the jaw) is the reverse action. It involves sliding the disk and condyle posteriorly and superiorly, which rotates the condyle posteriorly on the disk. These movements occur in the sagittal plane.

Protraction and retraction involves anterior/posterior movement in the horizontal plane. There is no rotation. All parts of the mandible move forward and backward the same amount. The mandibular condyle and disk move as one unit against the articular fossa of the temporal bone.

Lateral movement also occurs in the horizontal plane. It involves one condyle rotating in the articular fossa while the other condyle slides forward. To move the mandible toward the left, the left condyle will spin and the right condyle will slide forward (Fig. 12–13). This rotation occurs around a vertical axis.

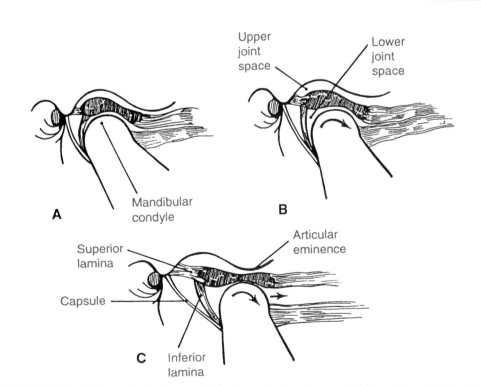

FIGURE 12–12.   Joint motion during mandibular depression (mouth opening). (From Perry, JF, Rohe, DA, and Garcia, OA: The Kinesiology Workbook, ed 2. FA Davis, Philadelphia, 1996, p 168, with permission.)
A   Condyle sitting in articular fossa
B   The condyle first rotates in the mandibular fossa
C   Condyle then glides downward and forward over the articular eminence (tuberosity)

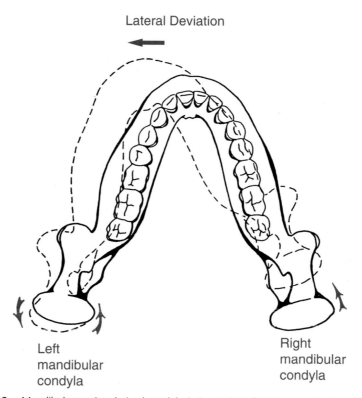

FIGURE 12–13. Mandibular motion during lateral deviation to the left side—superior view. (Adapted from Perry, JF, Rohe, DA, and Garcia, OA: The Kinesiology Workbook, ed 2. FA Davis Company, Philadelphia, 1996, p 175, with permission.)

Muscles of the TMJ

The TMJ is involved in activities such as talking, chewing, biting, swallowing, and yawning. Several muscles come into play, often in a synergistic manner. The muscles primarily involved are listed below. Unless stated otherwise, the action is considered a bilateral action that is occurring at each joint (right and left) simultaneously.

Temporalis	Medial pterygoid
Masseter	Lateral pterygoid

Other muscles involved in TMJ movements are:

Suprahyoid muscles	Infrahyoid muscles
Mylohyoid	Sternohyoid
Geniohyoid	Sternothyroid
Stylohoid	Thyrohyoid
Digastric	Omohyoid

The **temporalis** is a rather broad and fan-shaped muscle that lies in the temporal fossa (Fig. 12–14). Because of its fan shape, the more anterior fibers run almost vertically, the middle fibers are at a diagonal, and the posterior fibers are nearly horizontal. From the temporal fossa, the fibers come together to form a tendon that passes deep to the zygomatic arch to insert on the coronoid process and anterior

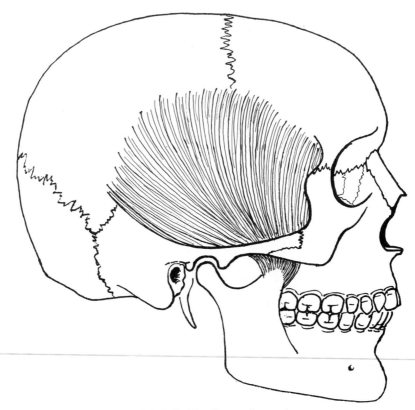

FIGURE 12–14. Temporalis muscle.

border of the ramus of the mandible. Its primary function is to elevate the mandible. Because of the horizontal direction of the posterior fibers, they also retract the jaw. In side-to-side movements, the temporalis contracts on one side, moving the mandible to the same side (ipsilaterally).

Temporalis Muscle	
(O)	Temporal fossa
(I)	Coronoid process and ramus of mandible
(A)	Bilaterally: elevation, retraction (posterior fibers)
	Unilaterally: ipsilateral lateral deviation
(N)	Trigeminal nerve (cranial nerve V)

The powerful **masseter** is a thick, almost quadrilateral-shaped muscle that produces the fullness of the posterior part of the cheek between the mandibular angle and zygomatic arch (Fig. 12–15). It is made up of two parts: the larger, superficial part, and the smaller, deep portion. The superficial part arises from the zygomatic process of the maxilla and inferior border of the zygomatic arch of the temporal bone. The deep part comes from the inferior and medial borders of the zygomatic arch. The two parts run inferiorly and posteriorly, coming together to attach on the angle of the ramus and coronoid process of the mandible. Both parts act as one muscle to elevate the mandible (close the jaw). Acting unilaterally, the masseter is an ipsilateral (same side) lateral deviator.

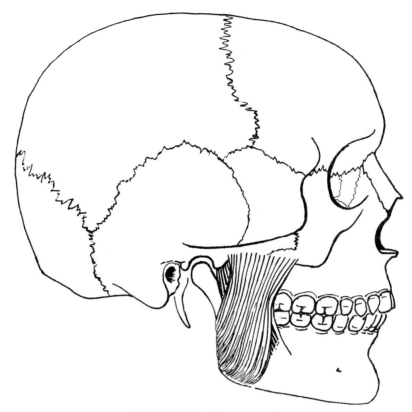

FIGURE 12–15. Masseter muscle.

Masseter Muscle

(O)	Zygomatic arch of temporal bone and zygomatic process of maxilla
(I)	Angle of the ramus and coronoid process of mandible
(A)	Bilaterally: elevation
	Unilaterally: ipsilateral lateral deviation
(N)	Trigeminal nerve (cranial nerve V)

Although it is less powerful, the **medial pterygoid** is very similar to the masseter muscle. It is located on the medial side (inside) of the mandibular ramus (Fig. 12–16); the more superficial masseter is on the lateral side (outside). It arises from the medial side of the lateral pterygoid plate of the sphenoid bone and the tuberosity of the maxilla. It runs inferiorly, laterally, and posteriorly to attach on the medial side of the ramus and angle of the mandible (Fig. 12–17). Its actions are mandibular elevation, protraction, and contralateral (opposite side) lateral deviation.

Medial Pterygoid Muscle

(O)	Lateral pterygoid plate of the sphenoid bone and tuberosity of the maxilla
(I)	Ramus and angle of the mandible
(A)	Bilaterally: elevation, protraction
	Unilaterally: contralateral lateral deviation
(N)	Trigeminal nerve (cranial nerve V)

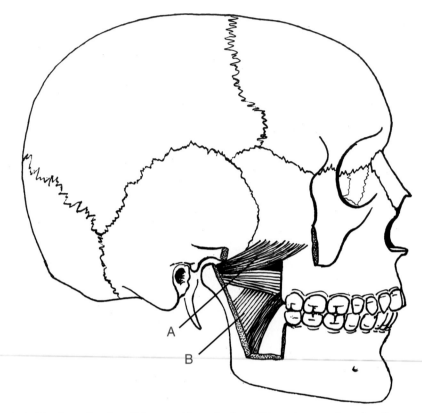

FIGURE 12–16.   Lateral and medial pterygoid muscles (mandible and zygomatic arch cut).
A   Lateral pterygoid muscle
B   Medial pterygoid muscle

The **lateral pterygoid** muscle is short, thick, and somewhat cone-shaped. It has two heads: superior and inferior. The superior part comes off the lateral surface of the greater wing of the sphenoid bone. The inferior, more horizontal part comes off the lateral surface of the lateral pterygoid plate. Both parts run nearly horizontal in a posterior and lateral direction. They attach on the neck of the mandibular condyle, the articular disk, and the capsule (see Figs. 12–16 and 12–17). This muscle depresses, protrudes, and laterally deviates the mandible to the opposite side (contralateral).

Lateral Pterygoid Muscle	
(O)	Lateral pterygoid plate and greater wing of the sphenoid
(I)	Mandibular condyle and articular disk
(A)	Bilaterally: depression, protrusion
	Unilaterally: contralateral lateral deviation
(N)	Trigeminal nerve (cranial nerve V)

The **suprahyoid muscles,** as their name implies, are a group of muscles located above the hyoid bone. They connect the hyoid bone to the skull, primarily to the mandible. Individually, these muscles are known as the mylohyoid, geniohyoid, stylohyoid, and digastric muscles. Although their primary function is to elevate the

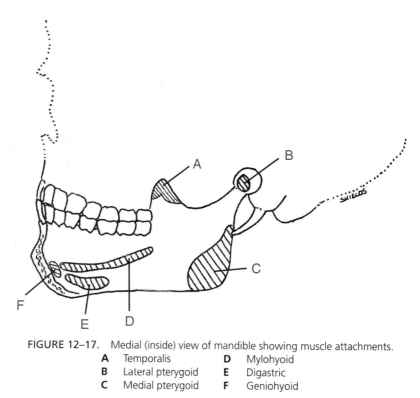

FIGURE 12–17. Medial (inside) view of mandible showing muscle attachments.

A	Temporalis	**D**	Mylohyoid
B	Lateral pterygoid	**E**	Digastric
C	Medial pterygoid	**F**	Geniohyoid

hyoid, they can assist in mandibular depression when the infrahyoid muscles stabilize the hyoid bone. Therefore, these muscles will be described here in terms of their importance to the TMJ only.

The **mylohyoid** is a broad muscle running from the interior (inside) medial part of the mandible to the superior border of the hyoid bone (Figs. 12–18*C* and 12–19*C*). The **geniohyoid** is a narrow muscle located superior to the mylohyoid (Fig. 12–18*D*). It attaches to the mental spine on the inside midline of the mandible and runs down to the hyoid. The **digastric** muscle has two bellies connected in the middle by a tendon (Fig. 12–20). The anterior belly goes from the internal inferior surface of the mandible near the midline posteriorly and inferiorly, where it attaches to the tendinous inscription at the hyoid bone. The tendon is held in place by a fibrous sling attached to the hyoid bone. From this point the posterior belly runs posterior and superior to attach to the mastoid process of the temporal bone. This pulleylike tendon is an example of how a muscle can change its line of pull. The **stylohyoid** is almost parallel to the digastric muscle. It attaches to the styloid process of the temporal bone and goes to the hyoid bone (see Fig. 12–19*E*).

Mylohyoid Muscle

(O)	Interior medial mandible
(I)	Hyoid
(A)	Assists in depressing mandible
(N)	Branch of trigeminal nerve (cranial nerve V)

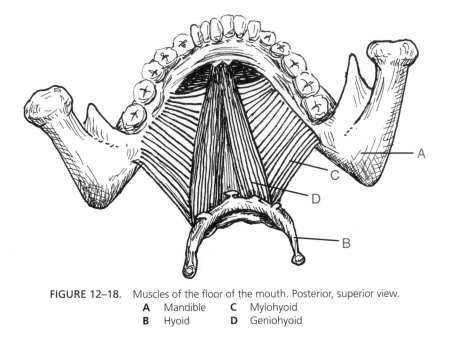

FIGURE 12–18.   Muscles of the floor of the mouth. Posterior, superior view.

A	Mandible	**C**	Mylohyoid
B	Hyoid	**D**	Geniohyoid

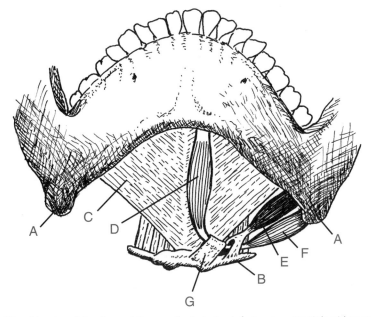

FIGURE 12–19.   Muscles of the floor of the mouth. Anterior, inferior view. Geniohyoid muscle is not visible from this view.

A	Mandible	**E**	Stylohyoid
B	Hyoid	**F**	Posterior digastic
C	Mylohyoid	**G**	Fibrous loop for digastric tendon (pulley)
D	Anterior digastric		

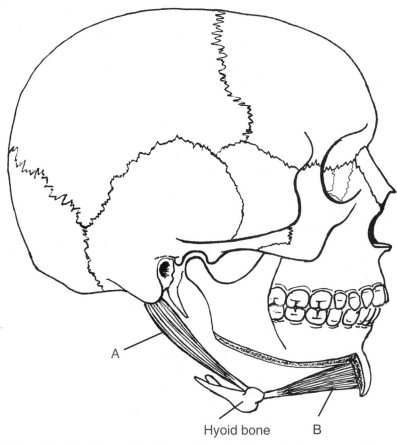

FIGURE 12–20.   The digastric muscle. Right lateral view with the mandible cut away to show anterior attachment.

A Posterior digastric
B Anterior digastric

Geniohyoid Muscle

(O)	Mental spine of mandible
(I)	Hyoid
(A)	Assist in depressing mandible
(N)	Branch of C1 via hypoglossal nerve (cranial nerve XII)

Stylohyoid Muscle

(O)	Styloid process of temporal bone
(I)	Hyoid
(A)	Assist in depressing mandible
(N)	Branch of facial nerve (cranial nerve VII)

Digastric Muscle

(O)   Anterior: internal inferior mandible
          Posterior: mastoid process

(I)   Via pulleylike tendon to hyoid

(A)   Assist in depressing mandible

(N)   Branch of trigeminal nerve (cranial nerve V) and branch of facial
          nerve (cranial nerve VII)

The **infrahyoid muscles,** as their name implies, are located below the hyoid bone and serve to depress it (Fig. 12–21). Individually, these muscles are known as the sternohyoid, sternothyroid, thyrohyoid, and omohyoid muscles. In terms of their effect on the TMJ, they stabilize the hyoid bone, allowing the suprahyoid muscles to depress the mandible. These muscles will be described here in terms of their importance to the TMJ only.

The **sternohyoid** is a thin, narrow muscle that runs vertically next to the midline from the posterior aspect of the medial end of the clavicle, sternoclavicular ligament, and sternal manubrium. It is covered distally by the sternocleidomastoid. It, like all the infrahyoid muscles, attaches to the inferior border of the hyoid bone. The **sternothyroid** is shorter, wider, and lies deep to the sternohyoid. It runs vertically from the sternal manubrium and cartilage of the first rib to the thyroid cartilage. It indirectly pulls down on the hyoid bone by pulling down on the thyroid cartilage, which, in turn, is connected to the hyoid bone via the thyrohyoid muscle. The **thyrohyoid** is a short, rectangular muscle that acts much like a continuation of the sternothyroid muscle. It runs from the thyroid cartilage vertically to the inferior border of the hyoid bone. It serves to close the laryngeal opening, thus preventing food from going into the larynx during swallowing. In terms of the TMJ, it pulls down on the hyoid bone, stabilizing it so that the suprahyoid muscles can assist in depressing the jaw.

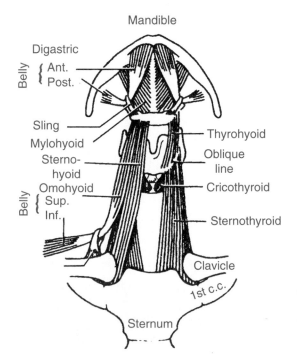

FIGURE 12–21.   Infrahyoid muscles. Anterior view of inferior mandible, hyoid bone, thyroid cartilage, superior sternum, and medial end of clavicle. (From Moore, K: Clinically Oriented Anatomy, ed 2. Williams & Wilkins, Baltimore, 1985, p 1001, with permission.)

The **omohyoid** has two bellies connected by a tendon in between, much like the digastric muscle. The inferior belly comes off the superior border of the scapula and runs mostly horizontally. At the tendinous inscription, the muscle changes direction and the superior belly runs mostly vertically to the inferior border of the hyoid. The tendon is held in place by a fibrous sling attached to the clavicle that allows the muscle to make an almost right-angle turn. This is another example of an internal fixed pulley changing the line of pull of a muscle. This muscle also stabilizes the hyoid bone by pulling down on it.

Sternohyoid Muscle

(O)   Medial end of clavicle, sternoclavicular ligament, and manubrium of sternum
(I)   Inferior border of hyoid bone
(A)   Stabilize hyoid bone
(N)   Branch of hypoglossal nerve (cranial nerve XII) communicating with C1 to C3

Sternothyroid Muscle

(O)   Manubrium of sternum and cartilage of the first rib
(I)   Thyroid cartilage
(A)   Stabilize hyoid bone
(N)   Branch of hypoglossal nerve (cranial nerve XII) communicating with C1 to C3

Thyrohyoid Muscle

(O)   Thyroid cartilage
(I)   Inferior border of hyoid bone
(A)   Stabilize hyoid bone
(N)   Branch of hypoglossal nerve (cranial nerve XII) communicating with C1

Omohyoid Muscle

(O)   Superior border of the scapula
(I)   Inferior border of hyoid bone
(A)   Stabilize hyoid bone
(N)   Branch of hypoglossal (cranial nerve XII) communicating with C1 to C3

TABLE 12–1	PRIME MOVERS OF THE TMJ
Mandibular Action	**Muscle**
Elevation	Temporalis, masseter, medial pterygoid
Depression	Lateral pterygoid
Protraction	Lateral pterygoid, medial pterygoid
Retraction	Temporalis (posterior)
Ipsilateral lateral deviation	Temporalis, masseter
Contralateral lateral deviation	Medial pterygoid, lateral pterygoid

TABLE 12–2	INNERVATION OF TMJ MUSCLES	
Muscle	**Nerve**	**Cranial Nerve Number**
Temporalis	Trigeminal	CN 5
Masseter	Trigeminal	CN 5
Lateral pterygoid	Trigeminal	CN 5
Medial pterygoid	Trigeminal	CN 5
Suprahyoid group		
Mylohyoid	Trigeminal	CN 5
Geniohyoid	C1, hypoglossal	CN 12
Stylohyoid	Facial	CN 7
Digastric	Trigeminal, facial	CN 5, 7
Infrahyoid group		
Sternohyoid	C1 to C3, hypoglossal	CN 12
Sternothyroid	C1 to C3, hypoglossal	CN 12
Thyrohyoid	C1, hypoglossal	CN 12
Omohyoid	C1 to C3, hypoglossal	CN 12

SUMMARY OF MUSCLE ACTION

The actions of the prime movers of the temporomandibular joint are summarized in Table 12–1.

SUMMARY OF MUSCLE INNERVATION

The innervation of the TMJ muscles comes from cranial nerve V, the trigeminal nerve. If the assisting muscles of the suprahyoid and infrahyoid group are included, innervation additionally comes from cranial nerves VII and XII (the facial and hypoglossal nerves, respectively). The hypoglossal nerve communicates with the first three cervical nerves as well. Innervation of all TMJ muscles is summarized in Table 12–2.

REVIEW QUESTIONS

1. The zygomatic arch is made up of which two bones?

2. Synonymous terms for TMJ motions are:
   a. opening the jaw
   b. closing the jaw
   c. moving the jaw posteriorly
   d. moving the jaw anteriorly
   e. moving the jaw toward the side

3. What two bones make up the temporomandibular joint?

4. What muscle can be palpated superior and anterior to the ear?

5. What muscle makes up the fullness of the posterior portion of the cheek?

6. What muscle works like a pulley?

7. The muscle in question #5 performs which pulley function?

8. If the 5th and 7th cranial nerves were damaged, which would impair function of the TMJ more?

9. Two motions occur during mandibular depression: (1) sliding the disk and condyle posteriorly and superiorly and (2) anterior rotation of the mandible on the disk. Which occurs first?

10. Lateral deviation of the mandible to the left involves both spinning and sliding motions. Describe how that happens.

11. What is another term for "Adam's apple"?

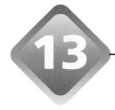

Neck and Trunk

The vertebral column establishes and maintains the longitudinal axis of the body. Because it is a multijointed rod, the vertebral column's motions occur as the result of the combined motions of individual vertebrae.

The spinal column provides a pivot point for motion and support of the head at the cervical region. The weight of the head, shoulder girdle, upper extremities, and trunk are transmitted through the vertebral column. Because it encases the spinal cord, the vertebral column is able to provide protection to the cord. Not only does this multijointed rod provide movement, but the arrangement of these segments also provides effective shock absorption and transmission.

Sitting on this long, multijointed rod (vertebral column) is the skull. The skull is the bony structure of the head and can be divided into the bones of the cranium, which contain and protect the brain and the facial bones. Because the sensory organs for sight, hearing, taste, and vestibular responses are located within the cranium, it is important that the head be able to move freely. This occurs through movements at various levels of the cervical spine.

Vertebral Curves

The vertebrae are arranged in such a way as to form anterior-posterior (concave-convex) curves in the vertebral column, which can be seen from the side (Fig. 13–1). These curves provide the vertebral column with much more strength and resilience, approximately 10 times more, than if it were a straight rod. The curves are summarized in Table 13–1.

Clarification of Terms

The term "spine" can be used in more than one way. The spinal cord, sometimes called the *spine,* is made of nervous tissue. The *spine, spinal column,* and *vertebral column* are synonymous terms referring to the bony components housing the spinal cord. This chapter discusses the spine as a bony structure.

Another term that needs clarifying is *facet.* A **facet** is a small, smooth, flat sur-

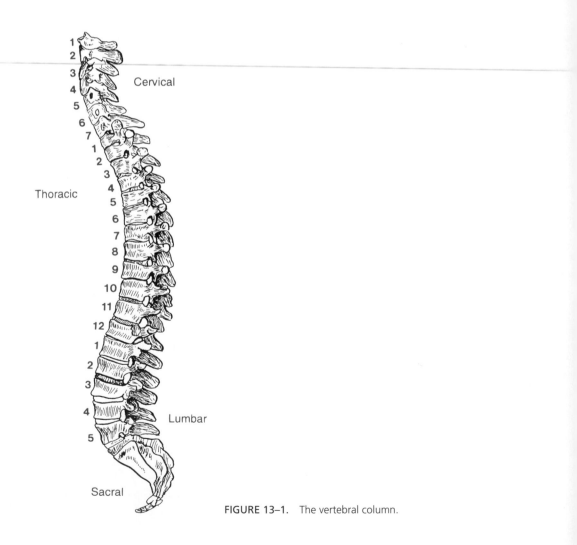

FIGURE 13–1. The vertebral column.

TABLE 13–1	**VERTEBRAL SEGMENTS**	
Segment	**Number**	**Anterior Curve**
Cervical	7	Convex
Thoracic	12	Concave
Lumbar	5	Convex
Sacral	5 (fused)	Concave

face on a bone. Facets, as will be discussed, are found on thoracic vertebrae at the point of contact with a rib. A **facet joint** is the articulation between the superior articular process of the vertebra below with the inferior articular process of the vertebra above.

Joint Motions

The vertebral column as a whole is considered to be triaxial. **Flexion, extension,** and **hyperextension** occur in the sagittal plane around a frontal axis (Fig. 13–2*A–C*). **Lateral bending,** also called *side bending* or *lateral flexion,* occurs in the frontal plane around a sagittal axis (Fig. 13–2*D*). **Rotation** occurs in the transverse plane around a vertical axis except between the skull and the atlas (C1) (Fig. 13–2*E*).

Although the spine has motion in the other two planes, it has no rotation. The alignment of the facet joints will greatly determine the amount of rotation and other motions possible. The cervical spine allows movement and positioning of the head. When describing motions of the cervical spine, motions of the head are also included.

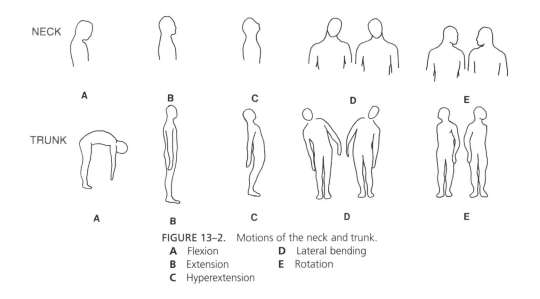

FIGURE 13–2.   Motions of the neck and trunk.
A Flexion   **D** Lateral bending
B Extension   **E** Rotation
C Hyperextension

Bones and Landmarks

The skull is made up of 21 separate bones and is considered the skeleton of the head (Fig. 13–3). Only those bones directly connected with the vertebral column will be discussed. They are as follows:

Occipital bone	Also called the occiput, it forms the posterior inferior part of the cranium.
Basilar area	Refers to the base, or inferior, portion of the occiput.
Foramen magnum	Opening in the occipital bone through which the spinal cord enters the cranium.
Occipital condyles	Located laterally to the foramen magnum on the occiput; provides articulation with the atlas (C1).
Temporal bone	Forms part of the base and lateral inferior sides of the cranium.
Mastoid process	Bony prominence behind the ear to which the sternocleidomastoid muscle attaches.

Vertebrae differ in size and shape but generally have the same layout (Figs. 13–4 and 13–5). The typical parts of a vertebra are as follows:

Body	Being primarily a cylindrical mass of cancellous bone, it is the anterior portion of the vertebra and the major weight-bearing structure. It is not present in the atlas (C1) and axis (C2).
	Between C3 and S1, bodies become progressively larger, bearing progressively more weight.
Neural arch	Also called the *vertebral arch;* it is the posterior portion of the vertebra with many different parts.
Vertebral foramen	Opening formed by the joining of the body and neural arch through which the spinal cord passes.
Pedicle	Portion of the neural arch just posterior to the body and anterior to the lamina.

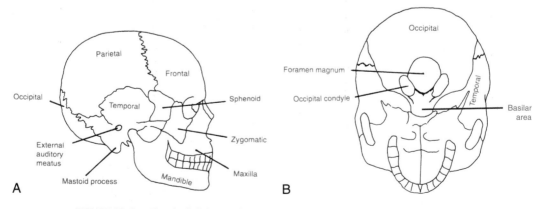

FIGURE 13–3.   The skull. (*A*) Lateral view. (*B*) The base of the skull, seen from below.

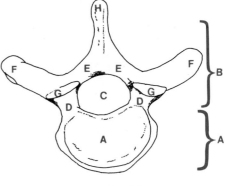

FIGURE 13–4. Typical vertebra.

A	Body	**E**	Lamina
B	Neural arch	**F**	Transverse process
C	Vertebral foramen	**G**	Articular process
D	Pedicle	**H**	Spinous process

SUPERIOR VIEW

Lamina	Posterior portion of the neural arch that unites from each side in the midline.
Transverse process	Formed at the union of the lamina and pedicle, the lateral projections of the arch to which muscles and ligaments attach.
Vertebral notches	Depressions located on the superior and inferior surfaces of the pedicle and that are so named.
Intervertebral foramen	Opening formed by the superior vertebral notch of the vertebra below and the inferior vertebral notch of the vertebra above.
Articular process	Projecting superiorly and inferiorly off the posterior surface of each lamina, and so named. Superior articular processes face posteriorly or medially while inferior processes face anteriorly or laterally.
Spinous process	The most posterior projection on the neural arch; located at the junction of the two lamina. It serves as a point of attachment for many muscles and ligaments, and can be palpated throughout the length of the vertebral column.

Between each vertebra is an **intervertebral disk** that articulates with adjacent bodies (Fig. 13–5 and 13–6). They are 23 in number, and their main function is to absorb and transmit shock and maintain flexibility of the vertebral column. The discs make up approximately 25 percent of the total length of the vertebral column.

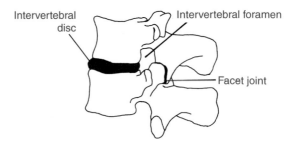

Intervertebral disc

Intervertebral foramen

Facet joint

FIGURE 13–5. Two vertebrae, seen from the side, with the intervertebral foramen, facet joint, and intervertebral disc.

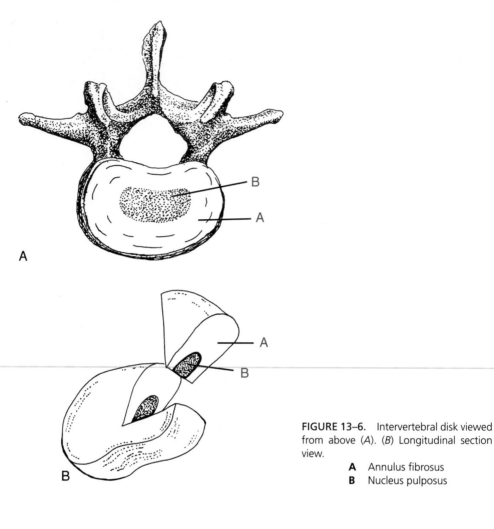

FIGURE 13–6.   Intervertebral disk viewed from above (*A*). (*B*) Longitudinal section view.

A   Annulus fibrosus
B   Nucleus pulposus

Annulus fibrosus	The outer portion, which consists of several concentrically arranged fibrocartilagenous rings that serve to contain the nucleus pulposus.
Nucleus pulposus	Pulpy gelatinous substance with a high water content in the center of the disk. At birth it is approximately 80 percent water, decreasing to less than 70 percent at 60 years of age. This is partially why an individual loses height with advanced age.

There are a few vertebrae with distinguishing characteristics that must be identified. They are as follows:

Atlas	The first cervical vertebra upon which the cranium rests (Fig. 13–7). It is named after the Titan in Greek mythology who held up the Earth because it supports the globe of the head. The atlas is ring-shaped and has no body or spinous process.
Anterior arch	The anterior portion of C1 (see Fig. 13–7*A*).

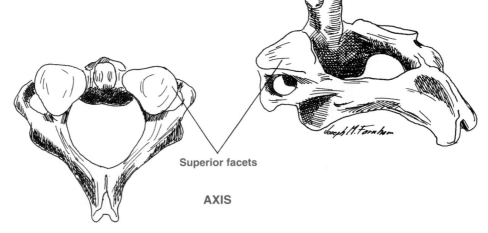

FIGURE 13–7. The atlas is the first cervical vertebra. This view is from above and behind.

A Anterior arch
B Articular process for the occipital bone
C Transverse foramen
D Posterior arch
E Transverse process
F Outline of odontoid process
G Vertebral foramen

Axis	The second cervical vertebra (Fig. 13–8) is so named because it forms the pivot upon which the atlas, supporting the head, rotates.
Dens	Also called the odontoid process; large vertical projection located anteriorly on the axis. Through its articulation with the atlas, cervical rotation occurs.
C7	Also known as vertebra prominens because of its long and prominent spinous process. It resembles a thoracic vertebra and can be easily palpated with the neck in flexion (see Fig. 13–8).
Transverse foramen	Holes or openings in the transverse process of the cervical vertebra through which the vertebral artery passes (see Fig. 13–7*C*).
Facet	Also called *costal facets,* they are located superiorly and inferiorly on the sides of the bodies and on the transverse processes of thoracic vertebrae (Fig. 13–9). It is here that the ribs articulate with the vertebrae.

Dens (odontoid process)

Superior facets

AXIS

FIGURE 13–8. The axis is the second cervical vertebra. (From Norkin, CC and Levangie, PK: Joint Structure and Function: A Comprehensive Analysis, ed 2. FA Davis, Philadelphia, 1992, p 146, with permission.)

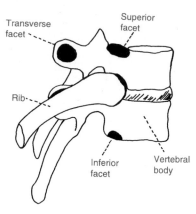

FIGURE 13–9.   Costal facets of thoracic vertebrae.

Demifacet	(In Latin *demi* means "half.") A partial, or half facet; located laterally on the superior and inferior edges of the vertebral body.

Although the three different vertebrae have all the same parts, there are differences. These differences are illustrated in Figure 13–10 and summarized in Table 13–2.

Joints and Ligaments

The cervical spine begins with two very different articulations. The **atlanto-occipital articulation** is formed by the condyles of the occiput articulating with the superior articular processes of the atlas. This union is strong and supports the weight of the head. The anterior atlanto-occipital membrane is an extension of the anterior longitudinal ligament, which is somewhat thin superiorly. The tectorial membrane is a continuation of the posterior longitudinal ligament. It serves as a sling to support the spinal cord as it enters the vertebral column. The posterior atlantoaxial ligament serves to secure the weight of the head on the neck. Each of the condyloid joints formed at the union of the occipital condyles and the superior articular processes of the atlas are synovial joints with a synovial membrane enclosed in an articular capsule.

The articulation between the atlas and the axis is known as the **atlantoaxial** articulation (Fig. 13–11). This consists of a synovial articulation between the odontoid process (dens) of the axis and the anterior arch of the atlas anteriorly and the transverse ligament posteriorly. There are two synovial cavities present, one on each side of the dens. Each is enclosed in an articular capsule. The anterior atlantoaxial ligament and the posterior atlantoaxial ligament are continuations of the anterior and posterior longitudinal ligaments, which traverse the length of the vertebral column.

The articulations between C2 through S1 are all basically the same. The strong, weight-bearing articulations occur anteriorly on the vertebra between vertebral bodies. The posterior portion of the vertebrae have two articulations (one on each side), called **facet joints** (also *apophyseal* or *zygapophyseal joints*) (see Fig. 13–5).

The facet joints are formed by the articulation between the superior articular process of the vertebra below with the inferior articular process of the vertebra above. Each facet joint is a synovial joint housing a synovial membrane and enclosed in an articular capsular ligament. Each vertebra has two superior articular processes and two inferior articular processes. Therefore, each vertebra is involved with two

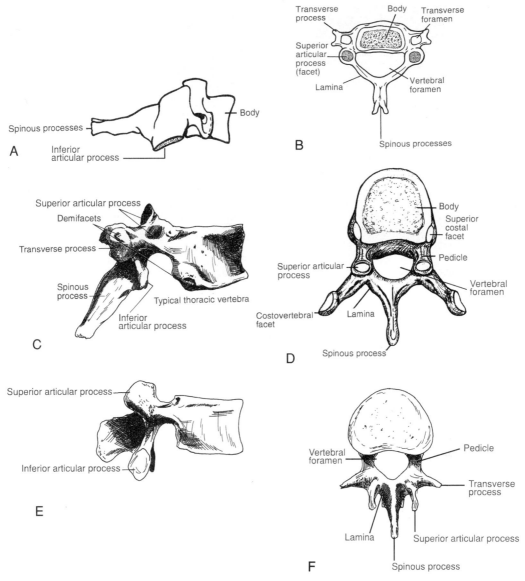

FIGURE 13–10.   Comparison of vertebrae. (Adapted from Norkin, CC and Levangie, PK: Joint Structure and Function: A Comprehensive Analysis, ed 2. FA Davis, Philadelphia, 1992, pp 131,144, 150, 152.)

A and **B**   Cervical
C and **D**   Thoracic
E and **F**   Lumbar

facet joints. These facet joints, by the direction they face, determine, to a great extent, the type and amount of motion possible (Fig. 13–12) at that part of the vertebral column.

In the lumbar area, the processes are located in the sagittal plane, whereas in the thoracic area they are in the frontal plane. Therefore, most flexion and extension of the vertebral column occurs in the lumbar spine, and most rotation and lateral bending occurs in the thoracic spine. Because the processes are located diagonally between the sagittal and frontal planes, the cervical spine has a great deal of all three

TABLE 13–2	**PARTS OF THE VERTEBRA**		
	Cervical	**Thoracic**	**Lumbar**
Size	Smallest	Intermediate	Largest
Body shape	Small oval	Heart shaped, with facets that connect with ribs	Large oval
Vertebral foramen	Large, triangular	Smallest	Intermediate
Transverse process	Foramen for vertebral artery; short, point laterally	Facets that connect with ribs; long, thick, point posteriorly and laterally	No foramen or articulation
Spinous process	Short, stout, bifid	Long, slender, point inferiorly	Thick, point posterioly
Superior articular process	Face posteriorly and laterally	Face posteriorly	Face medially
Vertebral notches	Equal depth	Deeper inferior notches	Deeper inferior notches

types of motion (Fig. 13–13). The attachment of ribs to the vertebra also contributes to the lack of flexion and extension in the thoracic spine.

Many ligaments hold these vertebrae together (Fig. 13–14). The **anterior longitudinal ligament** runs down the vertebral column on the anterior surface of the bodies and tends to prevent excessive hyperextension. It is thin superiorly and thick inferiorly to fuse to the sacrum. It is found in the thoracic and lumbar regions just deep to the aorta. The **posterior longitudinal ligament** runs along the vertebral bodies posteriorly inside the vertebral foramen. Its purpose is mainly to prevent excessive flexion. It is thick superiorly to help support the skull and thin inferiorly, which contributes to instability and increased disk injury in the lumbar region. The **supraspinal ligament** extends from the seventh cervical vertebra distally to the sacrum posteriorly along the tips of the spinous processes. The interspinous ligament

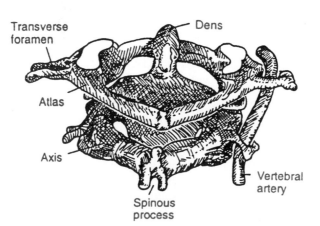

FIGURE 13–11. The relationship of the C1 and C2 vertebrae (atlas and axis). (Adapted from Norkin, CC and Levangie, PK: Joint Structure and Function: A Comprehensive Analysis, ed 2. FA Davis, Philadelphia, 1992, p 146.)

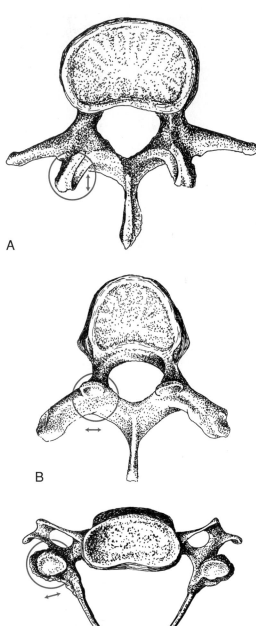

FIGURE 13–12. The positions of the superior articular processes on cervical, thoracic, and lumbar vertebrae.
A Lumbar orientation is in the sagittal plane
B Thoracic orientation is in the frontal plane
C Cervical orientation is triplanar

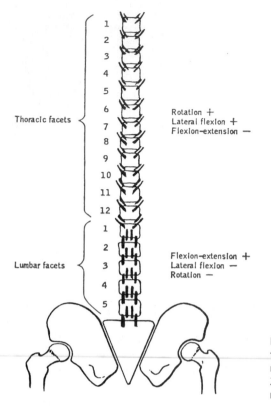

Thoracic facets

Rotation +
Lateral flexion +
Flexion–extension —

Lumbar facets

Flexion–extension +
Lateral flexion —
Rotation —

FIGURE 13–13. The planes of the articular facet joints determine the direction of spinal movement. (From Cailliet, R: Low Back Pain, ed 2. FA Davis, Philadelphia, 1968, p 9, with permission.)

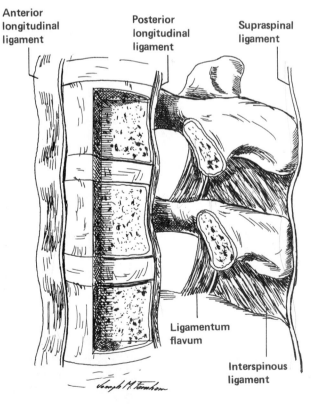

Anterior longitudinal ligament

Posterior longitudinal ligament

Supraspinal ligament

Ligamentum flavum

Interspinous ligament

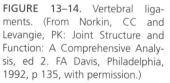

FIGURE 13–14. Vertebral ligaments. (From Norkin, CC and Levangie, PK: Joint Structure and Function: A Comprehensive Analysis, ed 2. FA Davis, Philadelphia, 1992, p 135, with permission.)

runs between successive spinous processes. The very thick ligamentum nuchae (nuchal ligament) takes the place of the supraspinal and **interspinal ligaments** in the cervical region (Fig. 13–15). The **ligamentum flavum** connect adjacent laminae anteriorly.

The lumbar spine is the region of the human body most often injured. It absorbs the majority of our body weight and any weight we carry. The center of gravity is located anterior to the second sacral vertebra. Most movement of the lumbar spine occurs between L4 and L5 and L5 and S1, and most disk herniations occur at these two levels.

The cervical spine is also freely movable. Unlike the lumbar spine, weight distribution is not its job. The cervical region supports the head, allows freedom of motion of the head on the neck, allows for the nervous tissue to enter the vertebral canal, and also allows for entrance and exit of the major blood vessels in the skull.

The thoracic spine has much less motion than the cervical and lumbar regions due to its attachments to the rib cage. The shape of the vertebral bodies and the length of the spinous processes also limit thoracic motion.

Muscles of the Neck and Trunk

Muscles of the neck and trunk are numerous and can be divided generally into anterior and posterior muscles as shown in Table 13–3. The quadratus lumborum muscle is the one exception. It is located in the middle of the frontal axis and is therefore neither an anterior nor posterior muscle. The clinical significance of the anterior or posterior location is function. As with most other joints, anterior muscles will have

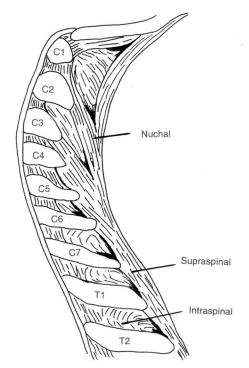

FIGURE 13–15. The nuchal ligament.

TABLE 13–3	**VERTEBRAL MUSCLES**	
	Neck	**Trunk**
Anterior	Sternocleidomastoid	Rectus abdominis
	Scalenes (3)	External oblique
	Prevertebra group (4)	Internal oblique
		Transverse abdominis
Posterior	Erector spinae group (3)	Erector spinae group (3)
	Splenius capitus	Transversospinalis group (3)
	Splenius cervicis	Interspinales
	Suboccipital group (4)	Intertransversarii
Lateral		Quadratus lumborum

a flexion function and posterior muscles will extend. Only those muscles that are clinically important from a physical therapy standpoint will be discussed here. Others will be summarized in charts and illustrations.

MUSCLES OF THE CERVICAL SPINE

Generally speaking, muscles located anterior to the vertebral column are neck flexors. The largest flexor, the sternocleidomastoid muscle, is a long, superficial, strap-like muscle originating as two heads from the medial aspect of the clavicle and superior end of the sternum (Fig. 13–16). It runs superiorly and posteriorly to insert on the mastoid process of the temporal bone. When it contracts bilaterally, it flexes the neck, and when it contracts unilaterally, it laterally bends and rotates the head to the opposite side. What "rotating to the opposite side" means is that, for example, when the right sternocleidomastoid muscle contracts, your neck would rotate so that you would be looking over your left shoulder.

Sternocleidomastoid Muscle

(O) Sternum and clavicle
(I) Mastoid process
(A) Bilaterally: flexes neck
   Unilaterally: laterally bends the neck; rotates head to the opposite side
(N) Accessory nerve (cranial nerve XI); second and third cervical nerves

---

Deep to the sternocleidomastoid muscle lie the three **scalene muscles** (Fig. 13–17). The **anterior scalene muscle** originates on the transverse processes of C3 through C6 and inserts into the superior surface of the first rib. The **middle scalene muscle** originates on the transverse processes of C2 through C7 and inserts into the superior surface of the first rib also. The **posterior scalene muscle,** the smallest and deepest, originates from C5 through C7, and inserts into the second rib. Because they all perform the same action and are located close to each other, it is not necessary to differentiate between them. Located laterally at the neck, they are very ef-

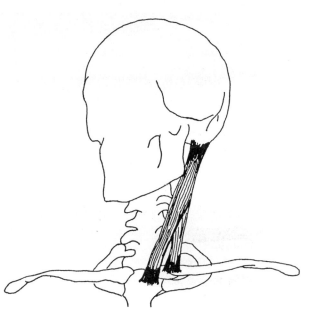

FIGURE 13–16. The sternocleidomastoid muscle.

fective in laterally bending the cervical spine. Because they are close to the axis, they
are only assistive in flexion.

Scalene Muscles	
(O)	Transverse processes of the cervical vertebrae
(I)	First and second ribs
(A)	Bilaterally: assists in neck flexion
	Unilaterally: neck lateral bending
(N)	Lower cervical nerve

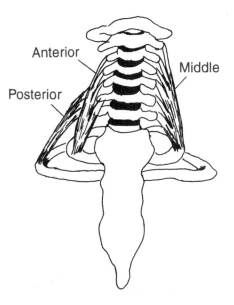

FIGURE 13–17. The scalene muscles.

There is an anterior group of muscles often referred to as the **prevertebral muscles**. They are located deep and run along the anterior portion of the cervical vertebrae (Fig. 13–18). These muscles have a role in flexing either the neck or head. Because of their small size in relation to other neck flexors, their greatest role, perhaps, is maintaining postural control. Table 13–4 summarizes their locations.

Several small muscles in the neck serve as anchors for the hyoid bone and the tongue. Except for the platysma, these muscles are illustrated in Figures 12–18 through 12–21. The hyoid bone is unique in that it has no bony articulation. It functions as a primary support for the tongue and its numerous muscles. The influence of these muscles on motions of the cervical spine is assistive at best. The muscles approach the base of the skull from all directions. Table 13–5 summarizes the actions of these muscles.

The **suboccipital muscles** are clustered together below the base of the skull and move only the head (Fig. 13–19). The muscles work together to either flex or extend the head with a rocking motion of the occipital condyles on the atlas, or to rotate by pivoting the skull and atlas around the odontoid process of the axis. These muscles are summarized in Table 13–6.

The postvertebral muscles are located posteriorly along the vertebral column and are considered the superior portions of the deep back muscles, known as the **erector spinae group**, which will be discussed later in more detail with the other trunk muscles. These muscles provide postural control over the gravitational pull of the head into flexion, and they act as extensors to bring the head back from the flexed position.

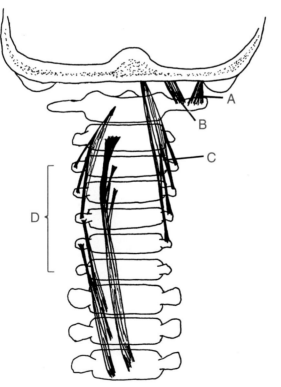

FIGURE 13–18. Prevertebral muscles.
    A Rectus capitis lateralis
    B Rectus capitis anterior
    C Longus capitis
    D Longus colli

TABLE 13–4	**PREVERTEBRAL MUSCLES**		
Muscle	**Origin**	**Insertion**	**Actions**
Longus colli	Bodies and transverse processes of C3–T2	Atlas and transverse processes and bodies of C2–C6	Flex neck
Longus capitis	Transverse processes of C3–C6	Occipital bone	Flex head
Rectus capitis anterior	Atlas	Occipital bone	Flex head
Rectus capitis lateralis	Transverse process of atlas	Occipital bone	Laterally bend head

Erector Spinae Muscles

See the section on the trunk for muscle summary.

The most superficial of the neck extensors are the **splenius capitis** and **splenius cervicis muscles.** As their names imply, they attach to the head and cervical spine with the splenius capitis muscle being the more superficial of the two. They both attach from the spinous processes of the lower cervical and upper thoracic vertebrae, and run superiorly and laterally to the lateral occiput (capitis) and transverse processes of the upper cervical vertebrae (cervicis) (Fig. 13–20). When the muscles on only one side contract, they rotate and laterally bend the head and neck to the same side. When both sides contract, however, they extend the head and neck.

Splenius Capitis Muscles

(O)	Lower half of nuchal ligament; spinous processes of C7 through T3
(I)	Lateral occipital bone; mastoid process
(A)	Bilaterally: extend head
	Unilaterally: rotate and laterally bend the head to same side
(N)	Middle and lower cervical nerves

TABLE 13–5	**MUSCLES OF THE MOUTH AND HYOID BONE**	
Group	**Muscle**	**Action**
Superficial cervical	Platysma	Draws lower lip down and out, tensing skin over neck
Suprahyoid	Digastric	Raises hyoid bone and/or tongue
	Stylohyoid	
	Mylohyoid	
	Genohyoid	
Infrahyoid	Sternohyoid	Lowers hyoid bone
	Sternohyoid	
	Sternohyoid	
	Thyrohyoid	
	Omohyoid	

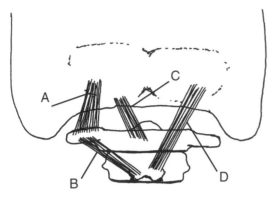

FIGURE 13–19.   Suboccipital muscles.
A   Obliquus capitis superior
B   Obliquus capitis inferior
C   Rectus capitis posterior minor
D   Rectus capitis posterior major

Splenius Cervicis Muscles

(O)	Spinous processes of T3 through T6
(I)	Transverse processes of C1 through C3
(A)	Bilaterally: extend head and neck
	Unilaterally: rotate and laterally bend the neck to same side
(N)	Middle and lower cervical nerves

It should be noted that the upper trapezius and levator scapula can assist the splenius capitis and cervicis under certain conditions. If the scapula is fixed, they can function in a reversal of muscle action. Instead of moving the scapula on the head and neck, the head and neck move on the scapula.

MUSCLES OF THE TRUNK

Spanning the anterior trunk in the midline is the **rectus abdominis muscle.** The two sides are separated from each other by the linea alba. The rectus abdominis muscle arises from the crest of the pubis and inserts into the costal cartilages of the fifth, sixth, and seventh ribs. There are several tendinous inscriptions dividing the muscle horizontally into several small units (Figs. 13–21 and 13–22). Located in the anterior midline, the rectus abdominis muscle is a strong trunk flexor and, along with the other anterior trunk muscles, compresses the abdominal contents.

Note that when doing a sit-up, the trunk is moving on the hips. The hip flexor

TABLE 13–6	SUBOCCIPITAL MUSCLES	
Muscle	**Location**	**Head Motion**
Obliquus capitis superior	Posterior	Extension
Obliquus capitis inferior	Posterior	Extension, lateral bending, rotation to the same side
Rectus capitis posterior minor	Posterior	Extension
Rectus capitis posterior major	Posterior	Extension, lateral bending, rotation to the same side

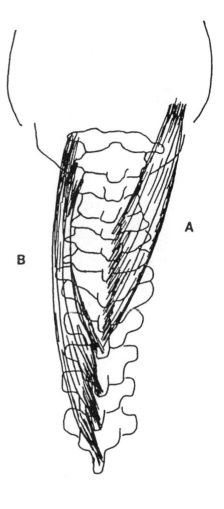

FIGURE 13–20. (*A*) The splenius capitis muscle. (*B*) The splenius cervicis muscle.

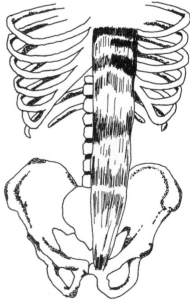

FIGURE 13–21. The rectus abdominis muscle.

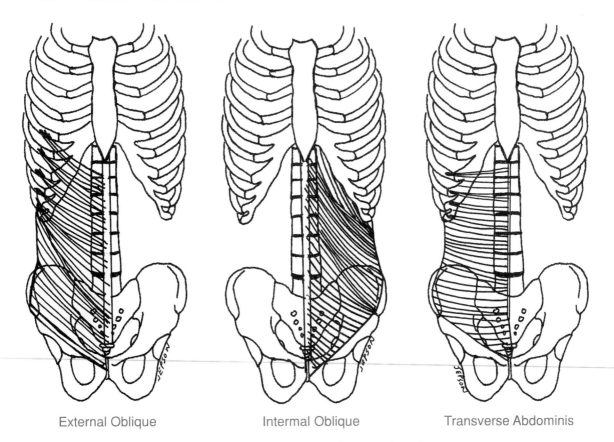

External Oblique   Intermal Oblique   Transverse Abdominis

FIGURE 13–22. The three layers of abdominal muscles.

muscles, in a reversal of muscle action, are also involved in performing a sit-up, expecially if the ankles are held down. Therefore, if the objective is to strengthen the abdominals (not the hip flexors), the hips and knees should be flexed and the ankles should not be held down. Flexing the hips and knees will shorten the hip flexors, making them less efficient. By not holding down the ankles, the hip flexors cannot work in a reversal of muscle action role.

Rectus Abdominis Muscles	
(O)	Pubis
(I)	Costal cartilages of fifth, sixth, and seventh ribs
(A)	Trunk flexion; compression of abdomen
(N)	Seventh through twelfth intercostal nerves

The **external oblique muscle** is a large, broad (see Fig. 13–22), flat muscle lying superficially on the anterolateral abdomen. It originates laterally on the lower eight ribs, runs inferiorly and medially to insert into the iliac crest and, via the abdominal aponeurosis, into the linea alba. The direction of the fibers on both sides form the shape of a "V." Bilaterally it flexes the trunk and compresses the abdominal contents, and unilaterally it laterally bends and rotates to the opposite side. This means that the right external oblique muscle would rotate the right shoulder toward the left.

Located deep to the external oblique muscle and running at right angles to the external oblique muscle is the **internal oblique muscle.** It originates from the inguinal ligament, iliac crest, and thoracolumbar fascia. It then runs superiorly and medially to insert into the last three ribs and, via the abdominal aponeurosis, into the linea alba (see Fig. 13–22). The direction of the fibers on both sides form the shape of an inverted "V." Like the external oblique muscle, when both sides contract, they flex and compress the abdominal contents. When one side contracts, it bends laterally. However, the internal oblique muscle has the opposite action in rotation by rotating the trunk to the same side. This means that the right internal oblique muscle would rotate the right shoulder toward the right.

External Oblique Muscle

(O)	Lower eight ribs laterally
(I)	Iliac crest and linea alba
(A)	Bilaterally: trunk flexion; compression of abdomen
	Unilaterally: lateral bending; rotation to opposite side
(N)	Eighth through twelfth intercostal, iliohypogastric, and ilioinguinal nerves

Internal Oblique Muscle

(O)	Inguinal ligament, iliac crest, thoracolumbar fascia
(I)	Tenth, eleventh, and twelfth ribs; abdominal aponeurosis
(A)	Bilaterally: trunk flexion; compression of abdomen
	Unilaterally: lateral bending; rotation to same side
(N)	Eighth through twelfth intercostal, iliohypogastric, and ilioinguinal nerves

The deepest of the abdominal muscles is the **transverse abdominis** muscle lying deep to the internal oblique muscle. It is named for the transverse, or horizontal, direction of its fibers. It originates from the lateral portion of the inguinal ligament, iliac crest, the thoracolumbar fascia, and the last six ribs. It spans the abdomen horizontally to insert into the abdominal aponeurosis and linea alba (see Fig. 13–22). Because of its horizontal line of pull, it plays no effective part in moving the trunk. However, it does work with the other abdominal muscles to compress and give support to the abdominal contents. This is important in such activities as coughing, sneezing, laughing, forced expiration, and "bearing down," such as during childbirth or while having a bowel movement.

Transverse Abdominis Muscle

(O)	Inguinal ligament, iliac crest, thoracolumbar fascia, and last six ribs
(I)	Abdominal aponeurosis and linea alba
(A)	Compression of abdomen
(N)	Seventh through twelfth intercostal, iliohypogastric, and ilioinguinal nerves

There are many groups of muscles that extend, and, as summarized in Table 13–7, some general statements can be made regarding attachments and actions. Generally speaking, muscles attaching from spinous process to spinous process have a vertical line of pull; thus, they extend. Because they are located in the mid-

TABLE 13–7	POSTERIOR TRUNK MUSCLES	
Attachments	**Action**	**Muscles**
Spinous processes	Extension	Spinalis (ES) Interspinales
Transverse processes	Extension, lateral bending	Longissimus (ES) Intertransversarii
Spinous to transverse process	Extension, rotation	Splenius cervicis
Transverse to spinous process	Extension, rotation	Semispinalis (T) Multifidus (T) Rotatores (T)
Transverse process to rib, or rib to rib	Extension, lateral bending	Iliocostalis (ES)

ES = erector spinae; T = transversospinalis.

line, there is only one set of them (Fig. 13–23*A*). Muscles that run from transverse process to transverse process have a vertical line of pull lateral to the midline; therefore, they laterally bend unilaterally and extend bilaterally (Fig. 13–23*B*). Muscles attaching from rib to rib have the same line of pull as those attaching between transverse processes. Being more lateral, muscles attaching to ribs are even more effective at lateral bending. Muscles attaching from spinous process to transverse process (Fig. 13–23*C*) or from transverse process to spinous process (Fig. 13–23*D*) have an oblique line and, therefore, extend bilaterally and rotate unilaterally. Of these, shorter muscles are more effective at rotation, and longer muscles are more effective at extension.

The intermediate layer of back extensors is a group of muscles called the **erector spinae muscles,** sometimes called the *sacrospinalis muscle group.* This muscle group can be subdivided into three groups that tend to run parallel to the vertebral column connecting spinous processes, transverse processes, and ribs (Fig. 13–24). The most medial group is the **spinalis muscle group** that primarily attaches the nuchal ligament and spinous processes of the cervical and thoracic vertebrae. The portion of this group that attaches to the occiput also attaches to the transverse processes of the cervical vertebrae. Located in the midline, these muscles are prime movers in trunk extension.

The intermediate muscles, the **longissimus muscle group,** are located lateral to the spinalis muscle group, attaching the transverse processes from the oc-

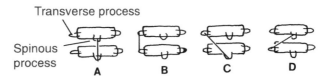

Transverse process

Spinous process

A   **B**   **C**   **D**

FIGURE 13–23.   Muscles that extend the spine mainly by:
A   Extension
B   Lateral bending
C and D   Extension and rotation (From Goldberg, S: Clinical Anatomy Made Ridiculously Simple. MedMaster, Miami, 1984, p 33, with permission.)

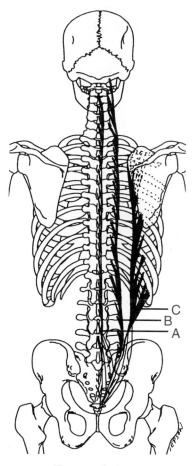

FIGURE 13–24. The erector spinae muscle.
A Spinalis
B Longissimus
C Iliocostalis

Erector Spine

ciput to the sacrum. These muscles have a vertical line of pull lateral to the midline and therefore, laterally bend when contracting unilaterally and extend when contracting bilaterally. The **iliocostalis muscles** are the most lateral group and primarily attach to the ribs posteriorly. Superiorly, they attach to transverse processes, and inferiorly they attach to the sacrum and ilium. Because of their lateral position, these muscles are excellent at lateral bending. Acting bilaterally, they are effective extensors. These three groups of muscles generally tend to be referred to as the erector spinae muscle group and, therefore, will be summarized as a group.

Erector Spinae Muscles

(O)   Spinous processes, transverse processes, and ribs from
            the occiput to the sacrum and ilium

(I)   Spinous processes, transverse processes, and ribs from
            the occiput to the sacrum and ilium

(A)   Bilaterally: extend
            Unilaterally: lateral bend

(N)   Spinal nerves

The deepest of the back extensor muscles is a group of three muscles called the **transversospinalis (transverse spinal) muscle group** (Fig. 13–25). They have an oblique line of pull essentially attaching from a transverse process to the spinous process of a vertebra above and, therefore, are very effective at rotation. The *semispinalis muscles* tend to span five or more vertebrae; the *multifidus* muscles tend to span two to four vertebrae; and the *rotatores* muscles, the shortest and deepest of this group, span only one vertebra. These muscles rotate to the opposite side and extend the spine.

Transversospinalis Muscles

(O)	Transverse processes
(I)	Spinous processes of vertebra above
(A)	Bilaterally: extend
	Unilaterally: rotate to opposite side
(N)	Spinal nerves

These next two muscles are located deep like the transversospinalis muscle group but have a vertical, not an oblique, line of pull and, therefore, must be considered separately. The names of the interspinales and intertransversarii muscles tell

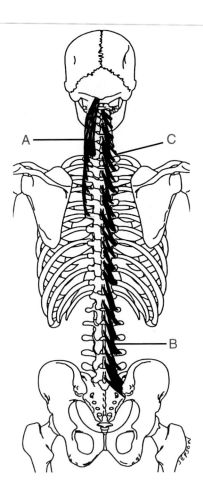

FIGURE 13–25. The transversospinalis muscle group.
A Semispinalis
B Multifidus
C Rotatores

you about their attachments. The **interspinales muscles** attach from the spinous process below to the spinous process above throughout most of the vertebral column (Fig. 13–26). With this vertical line of pull in the midline, they are effective extensors. The **intertransversarii muscles** attach from the transverse process below to the transverse process above, also throughout most of the vertebral column (Fig. 13–27). They are effective at lateral bending.

Inerspinales Muscles	
(O)	Spinous process below
(I)	Spinous process above
(A)	Trunk extension
(N)	Spinal nerves

Intertransversarii Muscles	
(O)	Transverse process below
(I)	Transverse process above
(A)	Trunk lateral bending
(N)	Spinal nerves

The **quadratus lumborum muscle** is a deep muscle that originates from the iliac crest and runs superiorly to insert into the last rib and transverse processes of the first four lumbar vertebrae (Fig. 13–28). Because it is located in the anterior-posterior midline, it does not have a function of flexion or extension; being vertical, it has no role in rotation. However, being lateral to the midline makes it effective at lateral bending. It has another function that occurs when its origin is pulled toward its insertion (reversal of muscle action). The action is called *hip hiking,* or *elevation,* of one side of the pelvis. This is an important function to anyone with a long leg cast or fused knee. It allows the foot to clear the floor without bending the knee.

Quadratus Lumborum Muscle	
(O)	Iliac crest
(I)	Twelfth rib, transverse processes of L2 to L5
(A)	Trunk lateral bending
(N)	Twelfth thoracic and first lumbar nerves

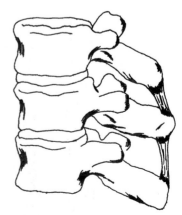

FIGURE 13–26.   Interspinales muscles.

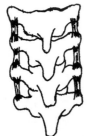

FIGURE 13–27. Intertransversarii muscles.

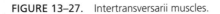

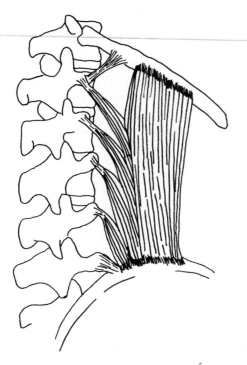

FIGURE 13–28. The quadratus lumborum muscle.

TABLE 13–8	PRIME MOVERS OF THE NECK AND TRUNK
Action	**Muscle**
	NECK
Flexion	Sterneocleidomastoid
Extension	Splenius capitis, splenius cervicis, erector spinae
Lateral bending	Sternocleidomastoid, splenius capitis, splenius cervicis, scalenes, erector spinae
Rotation (same side)	Splenius capitis, splenius cervicis
Rotation opposite side	Sternocleidomastoid
	TRUNK
Flexion	Rectus abdominis, external oblique, internal oblique
Extension	Erector spinae, transversospinalis, interspinales
Lateral bending	Quadratus lumborum, erector spinae, internal oblique, external oblique, intertransversarii
Rotation same side	Internal oblique
Rotation opposite side	External oblique, transversospinalis
Compression of abdomen	Rectus abdominis, external oblique, internal oblique, transverse abdominis

SUMMARY OF MUSCLE ACTIONS

Table 13–8 summarizes the muscle action of the prime movers of the neck and trunk.

SUMMARY OF MUSCLE INNERVATION

The muscles of the neck and trunk do not receive innervation from branches or terminal nerves of a plexus for the most part. Because they tend to be groups that span several vertebral levels, their innervation tends to reflect that. Generally speaking, they receive innervation from spinal nerves at various levels. For example, a spinal cord injury at T12 will not cause paralysis of all erector spinae muscles but will cause paralysis of those located below that level.

REVIEW QUESTIONS

1. Describe neck and trunk motions in:
   a. the frontal plane around the sagittal axis
   b. the transverse plane around the vertical axis
   c. the sagittal plane around the frontal axis

2. You are handed a cervical, thoracic, and lumbar vertebra. What identifying features help you distinguish among them?

3. What structural features allow the thoracic vertebrae to rotate but not to flex?

4. What structural features allow the lumbar vertebrae to flex but not to rotate?

5. Name the ligament that extends over the spinous processes from the occiput to C7 and from C7 to the sacrum.

6. What is the name of the series of ligaments that connect the lamina along the length of the vertebral column?

7. Name the ligaments that attach to the bodies of the vertebrae and run the length of the vertebral column.

8. Why does the quadratus lumborum muscle not play a role in trunk flexion or rotation?

9. Which posterior muscle groups are the most superficial?

10. You ask your patient, who is in the supine position, to raise her left shoulder toward her right knee. What joint motion(s) and prime movers are involved?

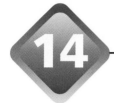

Respiration

The Thoracic Cavity

The thorax consists of the sternum, the ribs and costal cartilages, and the thoracic vertebrae (Fig. 14–1). It is bounded anteriorly by the sternum, posteriorly by the bodies of the 12 thoracic vertebrae, superiorly by the clavicle, and inferiorly by the diaphragm. The thorax is wider from side to side than it is from front to back.

The rib cage serves to attach the vertebral column posteriorly to the sternum anteriorly. Due to these attachments, movement within the thoracic spine is very limited. The internal organs (heart, lungs) are housed and protected within the rib cage. There are 12 ribs on each side, for a total of 24. The upper seven are called true ribs, attaching directly to the sternum anteriorly. Ribs eight through ten are called false ribs because they attach indirectly to the sternum via the costal cartilage of the seventh rib. The eleventh and twelfth ribs are called floating ribs because they have no anterior attachment. Each rib corresponds to the thoracic vertebral articulations above and below its number.

The **sternum** is the long, flat bone in the midline of the anterior chest wall. Its shape resembles a dagger and consists of three parts: manubrium, body, and xiphoid process (see Fig. 7–5). The *manubrium* (Latin, meaning "handle") is the superior part; the body is the middle and longest part; and the *xiphoid process* (Greek, meaning "sword") is the inferior tip portion. The ribs, sternum, and vertebral bodies form the thorax.

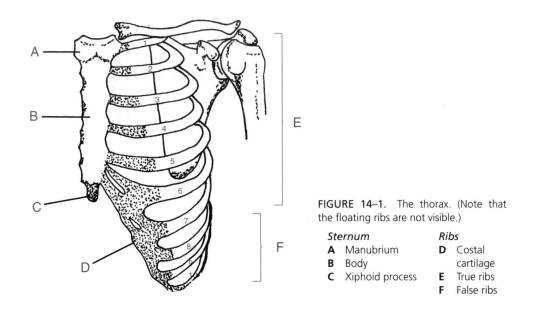

FIGURE 14-1. The thorax. (Note that the floating ribs are not visible.)

Sternum
A Manubrium
B Body
C Xiphoid process

Ribs
D Costal cartilage
E True ribs
F False ribs

JOINTS AND ARTICULATIONS

The ribs articulate with the vertebrae in mainly two areas: (1) the bodies of the vertebrae and (2) the transverse processes. These joints are called **costovertebral articulations** (Fig. 14–2). The articulating surface on the vertebral body is called the **facet** and is located laterally and posteriorly on the body near the beginning of the neural arch. Some ribs articulate partially with two bodies. These articulations are with the superior part of the vertebral body below and the inferior part of the vertebral body above. These facets are often called **demifacets** because they articulate with only about half of the rib. A facet that articulates with the tubercle and neck of the rib is located on the anterior tip of the transverse vertebra. These facets and demifacets are illustrated in Figure 14–3.

MOVEMENTS OF THE THORAX

Like the costovertebral articulations, the articulations of the ribs and the sternum, with the costal cartilage in between, are nonaxial, diarthrodial, gliding joints. Because most of the ribs attach anteriorly and posteriorly, there is little movement, but **ele-**

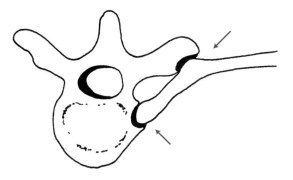

FIGURE 14–2. Costovertebral joints.

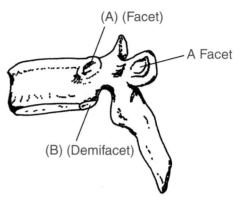

FIGURE 14–3. Thoracic vertebra, lateral view showing (*A*), facets which articulate with the rib and (*B*) demifacets (partial facets). Demifacets are not complete facets; therefore, the rib articulates with this one plus a demifacet on the vertebra below (or above).

vation and **depression** of the rib cage does occur. These movements are associated with inspiration and expiration of the lungs, respectively.

As you breathe in, the rib cage moves up and out; as you exhale, the rib cage moves down and in, returning to its starting position. This type of movement has been associated with the up and down movement of a bucket handle (Fig. 14–4). The handle (rib cage and sternum) is farthest from the bucket (vertebral column) in a horizontal position (inspiration). As the handle is lowered, it gets closer to the bucket. In comparison, as the sternum and ribs are lowered, the dimensions of the thorax decrease, resulting in expiration.

During inspiration, the thoracic cavity is made larger, causing the pressure within the thorax to decrease, forcing air into the lungs. Pulling apart the handles of a bellows (Fig. 14–5*A*) simulates this action. The reverse happens during expiration. The thoracic cavity returns to its smaller size, pressure in the thorax increases, and air is forced out of the lungs. This action is simulated by pushing the handles of the bellows together (Fig 14–5*B*).

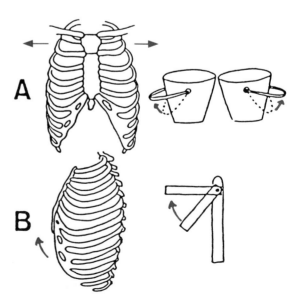

FIGURE 14–4. Bucket and pump handle models of inspiration. (*A*) As the bucket handle raises, there is an increased distance between the handle and the side of the bucket. Similarly, as the lateral aspect of the ribs elevate, it increases the mediolateral diameter of the chest cavity. (*B*) As the handle of the pump raises, there is an increased distance between the pump handle and the pump. Similarly, as the sternal end of the ribs elevate, the antero-posterior diameter of the chest cavity increases. (Adapted from Goldberg, S: Clinical Anatomy Made Ridiculously Simple. MedMaster, Miami, 1984, p 37, with permission.)

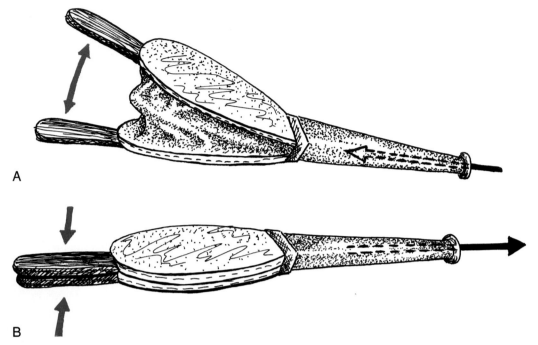

FIGURE 14–5. (A) Simulation of inspiration. As the handles of the bellows are pulled apart, air is brought into the bellows. As the ribs elevate and the diaphragm moves down, the thoracic cavity gets larger and air is pulled into the lungs. (B) Simulation of expiration. As the handles of the bellows are pushed together, air is pushed out of the bellows. Similarly, as the ribs move downward and the diaphragm moves upward, the thoracic cavity gets smaller and air is pushed out of the lungs.

Phases of Respiration

Inspiration is commonly broken down into three phases of increasing effort: quiet, deep, and forced. *Quiet inspiration* occurs when an individual is resting or sitting quietly. The diaphragm and external intercostal muscles are the prime movers. As *deep inspiration* occurs the actions of quiet inspiration are increased. A person needs more oxygen and is, therefore, breathing harder. Muscles that can pull the ribs up are being called into action. *Forced inspiration* occurs when an individual is working very hard, needs a great deal of oxygen, and is in a state of "air hunger." Not only are the muscles of quiet and deep inspiration working, but so are muscles that stabilize and/or elevate the shoulder girdle, thus directly, or indirectly, elevating the ribs.

Expiration is divided into two phases: quiet and forced. *Quiet expiration* is mostly a passive action. It occurs through relaxation of the external intercostal muscles, the elastic recoil of the thoracic wall and tissue of the lungs and bronchi, and gravity pulling the rib cage down from its elevated position. Essentially, no muscle action is occurring. *Forced expiration* brings in muscles that can pull down on the rib and muscles that can compress the abdomen, forcing the diaphragm upward.

Muscles of Respiration

The muscles of primary importance during respiration are the diaphragm and the intercostal muscles. The role of accessory muscles, which come into play during forced respiration, can be determined by noting whether a muscle's action will pull the ribs up (inspiration) or down (expiration). There has been a great deal of controversy over which muscles are active during which phases of respiration. In recent years, more refined electromyographic (EMG) instruments and techniques may have helped to clarify the roles of various muscles. Because there have been numerous studies conducted, many of which disagree, the waters are still cloudy.

DIAPHRAGM MUSCLE

The thoracic cavity is separated from the abdominal cavity by the diaphragm muscle, a large sheetlike, dome-shaped muscle (Fig. 14–6). It has a somewhat circular origin on the xiphoid process, the lower six ribs, and the upper lumbar vertebra. It inserts into itself at the broad central tendon. There are three openings in the diaphragm muscle to allow passage of the esophagus, the aorta, and the inferior vena cava. Because the insertion (central tendon) is located higher than the origin, the diaphragm muscle descends when it contracts (Fig. 14–7). This makes the thoracic cavity larger and the abdominal cavity smaller, causing inspiration.

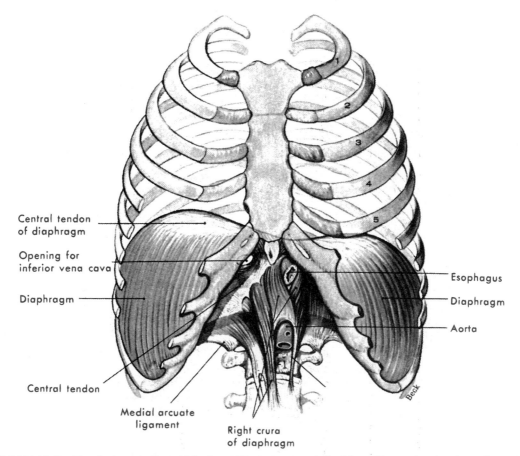

FIGURE 14–6. The diaphragm. (From Thibodeau, GA: Anatomy and Physiology. Times Mirror/Mosby College, St. Louis, 1987, p 263, with permission.)

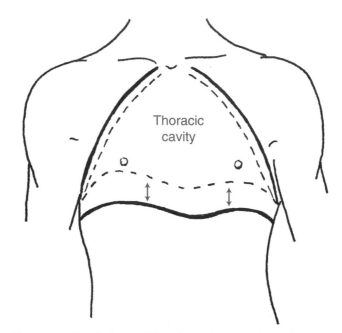

Thoracic cavity

FIGURE 14–7.   Movement of the diaphragm. When the diaphragm contracts, it descends, making the thoracic cavity larger. As in the bellows example, this allows air to be pulled into the lungs. When it relaxes, it moves upward, decreasing the size of the thoracic cavity and forcing air out of the lungs.

Diaphragm Muscle	
(O)	Xiphoid process, ribs, lumbar vertebrae
(I)	Central tendon
(A)	Inspiration
(N)	Phrenic nerve (C3, C4, C5)

INTERCOSTAL MUSCLES

The **intercostal muscles** are located between the ribs and run at right angles to each other (Fig. 14–8). The most superficial muscles are the **external intercostal muscles,** which run inferiorly and medially from the rib above to the rib below to elevate the ribs. *Anteriorly,* this is the same direction as the external oblique muscles, and the fibers are in the shape of a "V" (Fig. 14–9). The fibers of the internal intercostal muscles, deep and at a 90-degree angle to the external intercostals muscles, perform the opposite action. They run superiorly and medially from the rib below to the rib above and depress the ribs. *Anteriorly,* the fibers are in the shape of an inverted "V." If you view these muscles posteriorly, the direction of their fibers is just the opposite (Fig. 14–10).

To clearly understand how this change occurs, take a pencil and place it diagonally next to the sternum of a skeleton (or your partner). Next, move the pencil around the rib cage toward the vertebral column without changing the *direction* of the pencil. Notice that the pencil (muscle fibers) are in the opposite direction posteriorly, than when in front. Although the fibers have not changed direction, the ribs have curved 180 degrees.

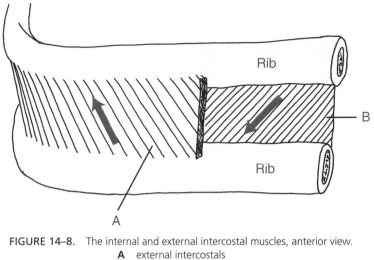

FIGURE 14–8.   The internal and external intercostal muscles, anterior view.
        A   external intercostals
        B   internal intercostals

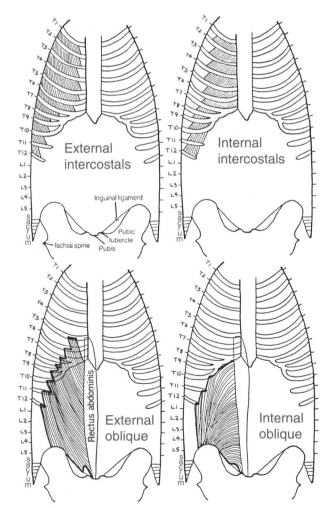

FIGURE 14–9. Comparison of the direction of muscle fibers in the intercostal muscles and the oblique muscles. (From Goldberg, S: Clinical Anatomy Made Ridiculously Simple. MedMaster, Miami, 1984, p 39, with permission.)

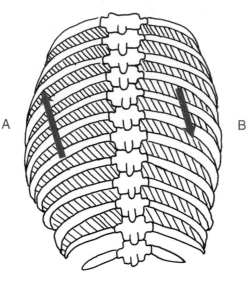

FIGURE 14–10.   Rib cage, posterior view showing the line of pull of the intercostals.
A   External intercostals—pulling up
B   Internal intercostals—pulling down

External Intercostal Muscles

(O)	Rib above
(I)	Rib below
(A)	Elevate ribs
(N)	Intercostal nerve (T2 through T6)

Internal Intercostal Muscles

(O)	Rib below
(I)	Rib above
(A)	Depress ribs
(N)	Intercostal nerve (T2 through T6)

Accessory muscles of inspiration assist the diaphragm and external intercostals in pulling up on the rib cage. These muscles are demonstrating reversal of muscle action by now pulling from origin toward insertion, instead of insertion toward origin. For example, the sternocleidomastoid usually pulls from its insertion on the skull toward the sternum, causing the head to move. When acting in inspiration, the head and neck are stabilized by other muscles and the sternocleidomastoid now pulls from origin on the sternum toward insertion on the head (Fig. 14–11). This muscle pull will elevate the rib cage.

It is common to see athletes who have just completed a sprint put their hands on their hips while trying to "catch their breath." What they are doing is making breathing a closed-chain activity. With the arms braced, the pectoralis major can now pull the sternum toward the humerus, thus increasing the diameter of the rib cage. Individuals with chronic obstructive pulmonary disease commonly brace their arms against the arms of the chair to accomplish the same thing (Fig. 14–12).

The scalenes usually move the head and neck. However, when they act as accessory breathing muscles, they elevate the first and second ribs assisting in inspiration.

Accessory expiratory muscles operate in much the same fashion, except that

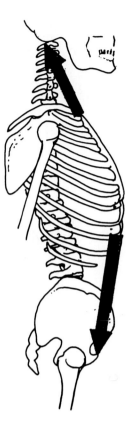

FIGURE 14–11.   Sternocleidomastoid muscle pulling up and Rectus Abdominis (RA) pulling down.

they pull down on the rib cage. For example, the rectus abdominis, which usually flexes the trunk, now pulls the sternum toward the pubis in a reversal of muscle action, which assists in expiration (see Fig. 14–10). The quadratus lumborum now pulls the lower ribs toward the iliac crest in the same fashion.

Many of the accessory breathing muscles have already been discussed with the vertebral column or shoulder girdle. Those that have not been discussed here or in previous chapters are illustrated in Figures 14–13 and 14–14. They are as follows:

ACCESSORY INSPIRATORY MUSCLES

DEEP INSPIRATION MUSCLES

Sternocleidomastoid
Pectoralis major
Scalenes
Levator costarum (Fig. 14–13)
Serratus posterior superior (Fig. 14–14a)

FORCED INSPIRATION MUSCLES

Levator scapulae
Upper trapezius
Rhomboids
Pectoralis minor

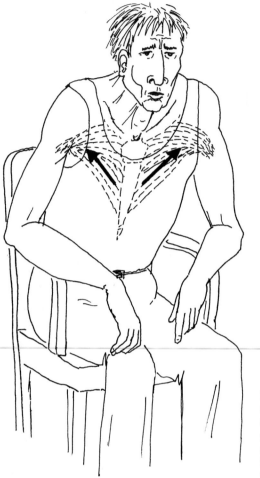

FIGURE 14–12. A person with chronic obstructive pulmonary disease (COPD) will often sit with the arms braced against the arms of the chair. This allows the pectoralis major, in a reversal of muscle action, to pull the sternum toward the humerus, thus increasing the diameter of the rib cage.

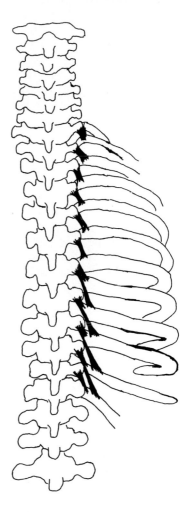

FIGURE 14–13.   The levator costarum muscles.

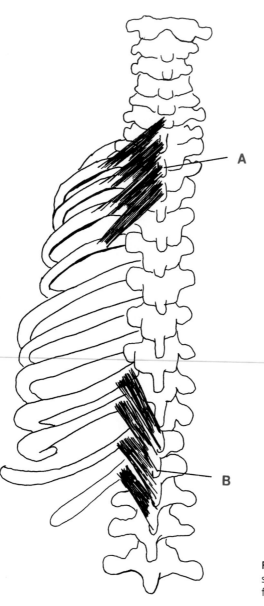

FIGURE 14–14. (*A*) The serratus posterior superior muscle. (*B*) The serratus posterior inferior muscle.

ACCESSORY EXPIRATORY MUSCLES

FORCED EXPIRATION MUSCLES

Rectus abdominis
External oblique
Internal oblique
Transverse abdominis
Quadratus lumborum
Serratus posterior inferior (see Fig. 14–14b)

Table 14–1 summarizes the activities of respiration.

TABLE 14–1	**ACTIVITIES OF RESPIRATION**
Action	**Muscles**

INSPIRATION: ELEVATION OF RIBS AND INCREASE IN SIZE OF THORACIC CAVITY VIA DESCENT OF THE DIAPHRAGM MUSCLE AND EXPANSION OF THE THORACIC WALL	
Quiet inspiration	Diaphragm
	External intercostals
Deep inspiration	Muscles of quiet inspiration *plus:*
	Sternocleidomastoid
	Scalenes
	Pectoralis major
	Levator costarum
	Serratus posterior superior
Forced inspiration	Muscles of quiet and deep inspiration *plus:*
	Levator scapula
	Upper trapezius
	Rhomboids
	Pectoralis minor
EXPIRATION: DEPRESSION (LOWERING) OF RIBS AND DECREASE IN SIZE OF THE THORACIC CAVITY	
Quiet expiration	Relaxation of external intercostals
	Elastic recoil of thoracic wall, lungs, and bronchi
	Gravity
	(Internal intercostals)
Forced expiration	Internal intercostals *plus:*
	Rectus abdominis
	External oblique
	Internal oblique
	Quadratus lumborum
	Transverse abdominis
	Serratus posterior inferior

SUMMARY OF MUSCLE INNERVATION

Muscles of respiration, like other trunk muscles, receive innervation from spinal nerves at various levels primarily in the thoracic region. The notable exception is the diaphragm muscle that receives its innervation from the phrenic nerve. The phrenic nerve arises from the third, fourth, and fifth cervical nerves. The functional significance of this is that an individual with a spinal cord injury at C3 or above will be dependent on a respirator. Individuals with a cervical spinal cord injury will have impaired respiration. Activities such as coughing, yelling, or taking deep breaths are limited. Not only are the intercostal muscles involved but other accessory breathing muscles as well. Activities requiring forced inspiration or expiration are affected to the degree that the accessory breathing muscles are involved.

REVIEW QUESTIONS

1. What bony structures make up the thorax?

2. Costovertebral articulations involve what bony structures?

3. What type of movement is allowed at the costovertebral articulations?

4. How do movements of the thorax affect inspiration and expiration? Of the diaphragm?

5. What is the muscle origin of all accessory inspiratory muscles in relation to the rib cage?

6. The external intercostal muscles form a "V" shape in front similar to the external obliques. Do the external intercostal muscles have this same shape in the back? If not, why?

7. Does the diaphragm have a bony attachment at each end of the muscle? If so, what are they? If not, how does the muscle work?

8. When you talk, are you doing so during inspiration, expiration, or both?

9. How do the accessory muscles assist with breathing?

10. Movement of the rib cage is often compared mechanically to what, while movement of the thoracic cavity (lung expansion/deflation) is often compared to what?

11. What is the functional significance between a person with a C3 spinal cord injury versus a person with a C5 level injury?

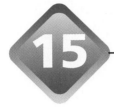

Pelvic Girdle

Structure and Function

Four bones make up the **pelvic girdle:** the sacrum, coccyx, and the two hip bones, comprised of the ilium, ischium, and pubis. The joints or articulations in the pelvic girdle include the right and left **sacroiliac joints** posterolaterally, the **symphysis pubis** anteriorly, and the **lumbosacral joint** superiorly (Fig. 15–1).

The pelvic girdle, also referred to as the **pelvis,** performs several functions. Perhaps most important to physical therapy is that it supports the weight of the body through the vertebral column and passes that force on to the hip bones. Conversely, it receives the ground forces generated when the foot contacts the ground, and transmits them upward toward the vertebral column. During walking, the pelvic girdle moves as a unit in all three planes to allow for relatively smooth motion. In addition, it supports and protects the pelvic viscera, provides attachment for muscles, and in females makes up the bony portion of the birth canal.

SACROILIAC JOINT

Joint Structure

The sacroiliac joint, commonly referred to as the **SI joint,** is a synovial, nonaxial joint between the sacrum and the ilium. It is described as a plane joint; however its articular surfaces are very irregular. It is this irregularity that helps to lock the two surfaces together.

The function of the sacroiliac joint is to transmit weight from the upper body through the vertebral column to the hip bones. It is designed for great stability and has very little mobility. Like other synovial joints, its articular surface is lined with hyaline cartilage. Synovial membrane lines the nonarticular portions of the joint. It

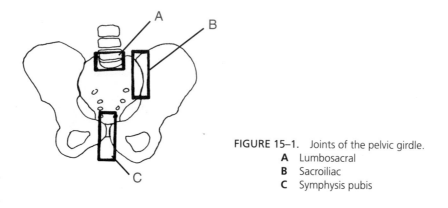

FIGURE 15–1. Joints of the pelvic girdle.
A Lumbosacral
B Sacroiliac
C Symphysis pubis

has a fibrous capsule reinforced by ligaments. This joint differs from other diarthrodial joints in that it has no voluntary motion.

Bones and Landmarks

The two bones of the SI joint are the sacrum and the superior portion of the hip bone, the ilium. The **sacrum** is wedge-shaped and consists of five fused sacral vertebrae. It is located between the two hip bones and makes up the posterior border of the bony pelvis. Its anterior surface, often called the pelvic surface, is concave (Fig. 15–2). Because it is tilted, the sacrum articulates with the fifth lumbar vertebra at an angle. This angle is referred to as the lumbosacral angle. The significant landmarks are as follows (Fig. 15–3):

Base	Superior surface of S1.
Promontory	Ridge projecting along the anterior edge of the body of S1.
Superior articular process	Located posteriorly on the base, it articulates with the inferior articular process of L5.
Ala	Lateral flared wings that are actually fused versions of transverse processes.
Foramina	Located on the anterior (pelvic) and dorsal surfaces are four pair of foramina. They serve as the exit for the anterior and posterior divisions of the sacral nerves. The anterior foramina are larger.
Auricular surface	Named (*auricula* is Latin for "earlike") because its shape is similar to the external ear. It is located on the lateral surface of the sacrum and articulates with the ilium. The irregular surface assists in locking the two surfaces together, providing greater stability.
Pelvic surface	Concave anterior surface.

The **ilium** will be described in more detail in Chapter 16. It makes up the superior part of the hip bone. Those landmarks relevant to the sacroiliac joint are as follows (Fig. 15–4):

Tuberosity	Large roughened area between the posterior portion of the iliac crest and the auricular surface. It serves as an attachment for the interosseous ligament.

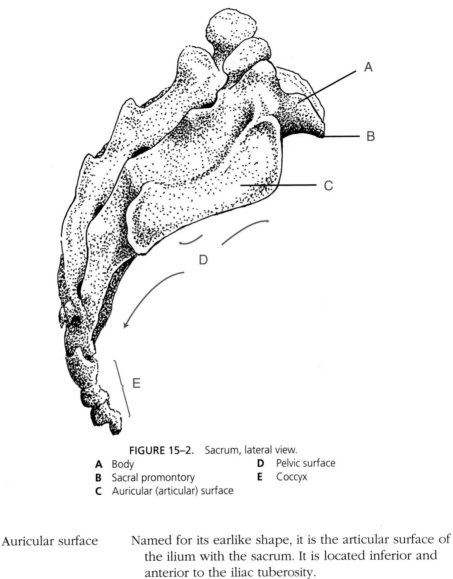

FIGURE 15–2.   Sacrum, lateral view.

A Body   **D** Pelvic surface
B Sacral promontory   **E** Coccyx
C Auricular (articular) surface

Auricular surface	Named for its earlike shape, it is the articular surface of the ilium with the sacrum. It is located inferior and anterior to the iliac tuberosity.
Iliac crest	Superior ridge of the ilium, the bony area felt when you place your hands on your hips.
Posterior superior iliac spine	Often abbreviated PSIS, it is the posterior projection of the iliac crest and serves as an attachment for the posterior sacroiliac ligaments.
Posterior inferior iliac spine	Often abbreviated PIIS; it lies inferior to the PSIS and serves as an attachment for the sacrotuberous ligament.
Greater sciatic notch	Formed by the ilium superiorly and the ilium and ischium inferiorly.
Greater sciatic foramen	Formed from the greater sciatic notch by ligamentous attachments. The sacrotuberous ligament forms the posterior medial border and the sacrospinous ligament forms the inferior border (see Figs. 15–5

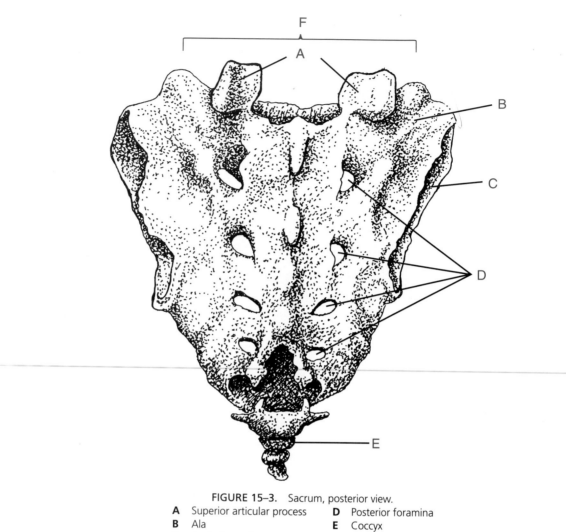

FIGURE 15–3. Sacrum, posterior view.

A	Superior articular process	**D**	Posterior foramina
B	Ala	**E**	Coccyx
C	Auricular surface	**F**	Base

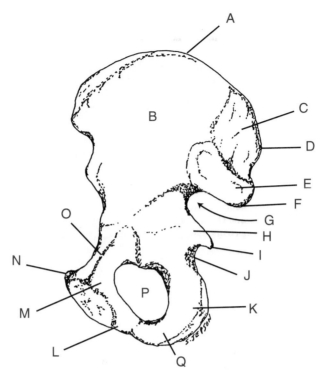

FIGURE 15–4. Right hip bone, medial view.

Ilium
A Iliac crest
B Iliac fossa
C Iliac tuberosity
D Posterior super-
     ior iliac spine
E Auricular surface
F Posterior inferior iliac spine
Combination of bones
G Greater sciatic notch (ilium and ischium)

Ischium
H Ischial body
I Ischial spine
J Lesser sciatic notch
K Ischial tuberosity
     ramus
Q Ischial Ramus

Pubis
L Inferior pubis ramus
M Pubic body
N Pubic tubercle
O Superior pubic
P Obturator foramen
     (ischium and pubis)

and 15–7). The sciatic nerve passes through this opening.

The **ischium** will also be described in more detail in the hip joint section. The portions of the ischium pertaining to the sacroiliac joint are (see Fig. 15–4):

Body — Makes up all of the ischium superior to the tuberosity.

Lesser sciatic notch — Smaller concavity located on the posterior body between the greater sciatic notch and the ischial tuberosity.

Spine — Located on the posterior portion of the body and inferior border of the greater sciatic notch superior to the lesser sciatic notch. It provides attachment for the sacrospinous ligament.

Tuberosity — The blunt, rough projection on the inferior part of the body. It is a weight-bearing surface when you are sitting.

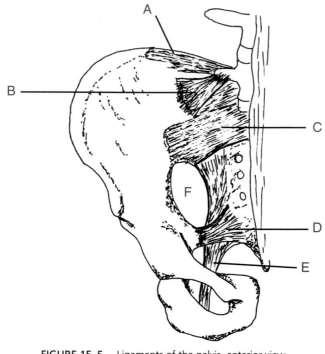

FIGURE 15–5. Ligaments of the pelvis, anterior view.

A	Iliolumbar ligament	**D**	Sacrospinous ligament
B	Lumbosacral ligament	**E**	Sacrotuberous ligament
C	Anterior sacroiliac ligament	**F**	Greater sciatic foramen

Ligaments

Because the sacroiliac joint is meant to take a great deal of stress while providing great stability, it is a joint heavily endowed with ligaments. The **anterior sacroiliac ligament** is a broad, flat ligament on the anterior (pelvic) surface connecting the ala and pelvic surface of the sacrum to the auricular surface of the ilium (Fig. 15–5). It holds the anterior portion of the joint together. The **interosseous sacroiliac ligament** is the deepest, shortest, and strongest of the sacroiliac ligaments (Fig. 15–6). It fills the roughened area immediately above and behind the auricular surfaces and anterior sacroiliac ligament. It connects the tuberosities of the ilium to the sacrum.

The posterior sacroiliac ligament is comprised of two parts (Fig. 15–7). The **short posterior sacroiliac ligament** runs more oblique between the ilium and the upper portion of the sacrum on the dorsal surface. It prevents forward movement of

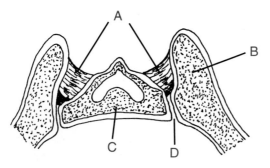

FIGURE 15–6. Cross section of the sacroiliac joints.

A	Interosseous sacroiliac ligament	**C**	Sacrum
B	Ilium	**D**	Sacroiliac joint

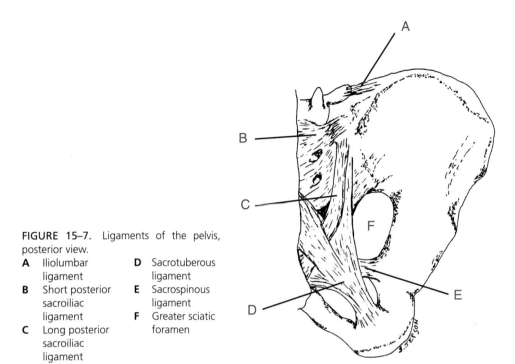

FIGURE 15–7. Ligaments of the pelvis, posterior view.

A	Iliolumbar ligament	**D**	Sacrotuberous ligament
B	Short posterior sacroiliac ligament	**E**	Sacrospinous ligament
C	Long posterior sacroiliac ligament	**F**	Greater sciatic foramen

the sacrum. The **long posterior sacroiliac ligament** runs more vertically between the posterior superior iliac spine and the lower portion of the sacrum. It prevents downward movement of the sacrum.

Three accessory ligaments further reinforce the sacroiliac joint. The **sacrotuberous ligament** is a very strong, triangular-shaped ligament running from between the PSIS and PIIS of the ilium, from the posterior and lateral side of the sacrum inferior to auricular surface, and from the coccyx (see Figs. 15–5*E* and 15–7*D*). These fibers come together to attach on the ischial tuberosity. It serves as an attachment for the gluteus maximus, and prevents forward rotation of the sacrum. The **sacrospinous ligament** is also triangular-shaped and lies deep to the sacrotuberous ligament. It has a broad attachment from the lower, lateral sacrum and coccyx on the posterior side (see Figs. 15–5*D* and 15–7*E*). It then narrows to attach to the spine of the ischium. These two ligaments convert the greater sciatic notch into a foramen through which passes the sciatic nerve. The **iliolumbar ligament** connects the transverse process of L5 with the ala of the sacrum (see Figs. 15–5*A* and 15–7*A*). It is described in more detail under the lumbosacral joint.

PUBIC SYMPHYSIS

The pubic symphysis joint is located in the midline of the body. The right and left pubic bones are joined anteriorly forming the pubic symphysis. A fibrocartilage disk lies between the two bones. Because it is an amphiarthrodial joint, there is little movement. However, in women during childbirth, it becomes much more moveable.

LIGAMENTS

The pubic symphysis is held together primarily by two ligaments (Fig. 15–8). The **superior pubic ligament** attaches to the pubic tubercles on each side of the body and strengthens the superior and anterior portions of the joint. The **inferior pubic ligament** attaches between the two inferior pubic rami. It strengthens the inferior portion of the joint.

Landmarks

The **pubis** will be described in greater detail under the hip joint. The landmarks relevant to the pubic symphysis are (see Fig. 15–4):

Body	Main portion of the pubic bone, it has a superior and inferior projection (ramus).
Superior ramus	Superior projection of the pubic body.
Inferior ramus	Inferior projection of the pubic body that provides attachment for the inferior pubic ligament.
Tubercle	Projects anteriorly on the superior ramus near the midline and provides attachment for superior pubic ligament.

LUMBOSACRAL JOINT

Joint Structure and Ligaments

The lumbosacral joint is made up of the fifth lumbar vertebra and the first sacral vertebra. The articulation between these vertebrae is the same as that for all other vertebrae. The bodies of these two bones are separated by an intervertebral disk and are held together at the bodies by the anterior and posterior longitudinal ligaments.

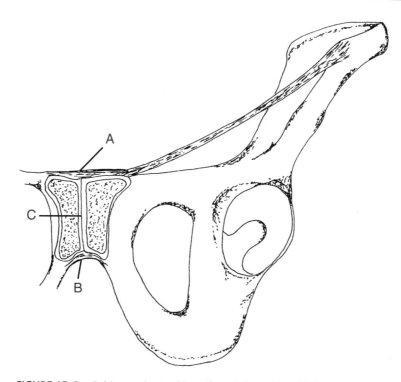

FIGURE 15–8. Pubic symphysis, oblique frontal view with pubic bone cut away.
A Superior pubic ligament
B Inferior pubic ligament
C Disk

The vertebrae articulate at the articular processes (inferior articular process of L5 and superior articular process of S1). The ligaments holding together this portion of the joint are the supraspinal, interspinal, and ligamentum flava. All of these ligaments are described in Chapter 13.

There are two additional ligaments that specifically hold the lumbosacral joint together (see Fig. 15–5). The **iliolumbar ligament** attaches on the transverse process of L5 and runs laterally to the inner lip of the posterior portion of the iliac crest. This ligament limits the rotation of L5 on S1, and assists the articular processes in preventing L5 from moving anteriorly on S1. The **lumbosacral ligament** also attaches on the transverse process of L5. It runs inferiorly and laterally to attach on the ala of the sacrum. Here its fibers intermingle with the fibers of the anterior sacroiliac ligament.

Lumbosacral Angle

Lumbosacral angle (Fig. 15–9) is determined by drawing one line parallel to the ground and another line along the base of the sacrum. This angle will increase as the pelvis tilts anteriorly and decrease as the pelvis tilts posteriorly. The optimal lumbosacral angle is approximately 30 degrees. As the lumbar lordosis increases, the an-

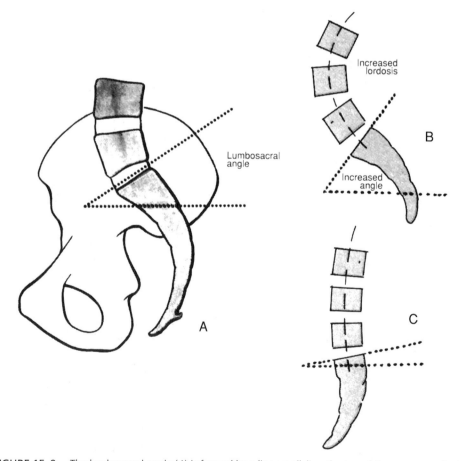

FIGURE 15–9. The lumbosacral angle (*A*) is formed by a line paralleling the top of the sacrum and a line drawn horizontally. The spine is balanced upon the sacrum. As the angle increases (*B*), the lordosis is greater. With a lesser angle (*C*), the lumbar lordosis is less. (From Soft Tissue Pain and Disability, Cailliet, R, ed 2, FA Davis, Philadelphia, 1988, p 52, with permission.)

gle increases. This causes the shearing stresses of L5 on S1 to increase. Forward movement of L5 on S1 is prevented by ligamentous support, the shape and fit of the inferior articular process of L5 inside, and behind the superior articular process of S1. Conversely, as the lumbar lordosis decreases, lumbosacral angle decreases.

Pelvic Girdle Motions

The joints directly involved in movement of the pelvic girdle include the two hip joints and the lumbar joints, particularly the lumbosacral articulation between L5 and S1. The pelvic motions occur in all three planes. When standing in the upright position, the pelvis should be level; in the sagittal plane, the anterior superior iliac spine (ASIS) and pubic symphysis should be in the same vertical plane. **Anterior tilt** occurs when the pelvis tilts forward, moving the ASIS anterior to the pubic symphysis. **Posterior tilt** occurs when the pelvis tilts backward moving the ASIS posterior to the pubic symphysis. These motions are shown in Figure 15–10.

For the body to remain upright when the pelvis tilts forward, movement in the opposite direction must occur in the joints above and below. Therefore, when the pelvis tilts anteriorly, the lumbar portion of the vertebral column goes into hyperextension while the hip joints flex. Thus, when a person with a hip flexion contracture stands in the upright position, the pelvis will tilt anteriorly while the lumbar region becomes hyperextended. Conversely, a person with tight hamstrings may stand with the pelvis tilted posteriorly and lumbar curve flattened.

In the frontal plane, the iliac crests should be level (Fig. 15–11). Placing your thumbs on the ASISs and determining if your thumbs are at the same level can assess this. **Lateral tilt** occurs when the two iliac crests are not level. Because the pelvis moves as a unit, one side moves up as the other side moves down (Fig. 15–12). Therefore, a point of reference must be used. *The side that is unsupported will be the point of reference.* During walking, the pelvis is level when both legs are in contact with the ground. However, when one leg leaves the ground (swing phase), it becomes unsupported and the pelvis on that side drops slightly. It is impossible to drop the pelvis on the weight-bearing side. Therefore, the point of reference for lateral tilt will be the unsupported, or less supported, side. Figure 15–13 illustrates a left lateral

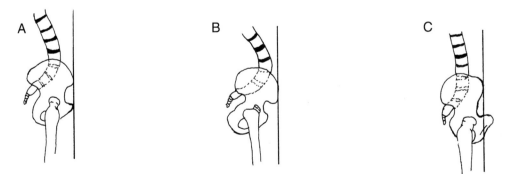

FIGURE 15–10.   Pelvic movement in the sagittal plane. In the neutral position (*A*), the anterior superior iliac spine and the pubic symphysis should be in the same vertical plane. Posterior tilt (*B*) occurs when the pelvis tilts backward, moving the ASIS posterior to the pubic symphysis. Anterior tilt (*C*) occurs when the pelvis tilts forward, moving the ASIS anterior to the pubic symphysis.

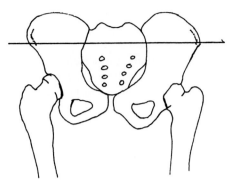

FIGURE 15–11. Pelvic movement in the frontal plane. When standing upright on both feet, the iliac crests should be level in the frontal plane and both anterior superior iliac spines should be level as well.

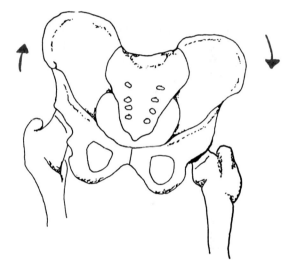

FIGURE 15–12. Lateral tilt.

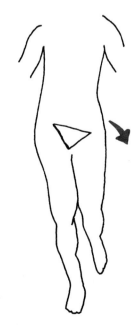

FIGURE 15–13. Left lateral tilt. When one leg leaves the ground, the pelvis on that side becomes unsupported. This causes the pelvis on that side to drop slightly. Therefore, lateral tilt is named by the unsupported side.

tilt. The person bears weight on the right leg while lifting the left leg from the ground. The left side of the pelvis becomes unsupported and drops, or laterally tilts to the left.

Some clinicians will identify the lateral tilt by the high side as is illustrated in *Kinesiology Laboratory Manual for Physical Therapist Assistants*. Therefore, the lateral tilt shown in Figure 15–12 would be a right lateral tilt. To avoid confusion, *unsupported side of the pelvis* will be used as the point of reference.

To keep the body balanced, joints directly above and below will shift in the opposite direction. Notice in Figure 15–14 that, as the pelvis tilts to the right, the vertebral column laterally bends to the left. While the weight-bearing hip joint (right) adducts, the unsupported hip (left) becomes more abducted.

Although this discussion has centered on one side of the pelvis dropping below the level of the other side, it is possible to raise the pelvis on the unsupported side. This is commonly called "hip hiking." When walking with a long leg cast or brace, this motion assists the foot in clearing the floor during the swing phase. Shifting from one ischial tuberosity to the other also involves raising the pelvis on one side. This is useful in allowing for some pressure relief during sitting.

Pelvic rotation occurs in the transverse plane around a vertical axis when one side of the pelvis moves forward or backward in relation to the other side. Looking down on the pelvis, as in Figure 15–15, the significant landmarks again are the ASISs. In the anatomical position, both ASISs should be in the same plane. In this example, the right leg is weight bearing and the left leg is swinging forward. Once again, *the unsupported side is the point of reference*. This causes the left side of the pelvis to rotate forward moving the left ASIS forward of the right ASIS. If the left leg were to swing backward, the pelvis would rotate backward. Stated another way, if you bear weight on your right leg and swing your left leg backward, the left side of your pelvis rotates backward.

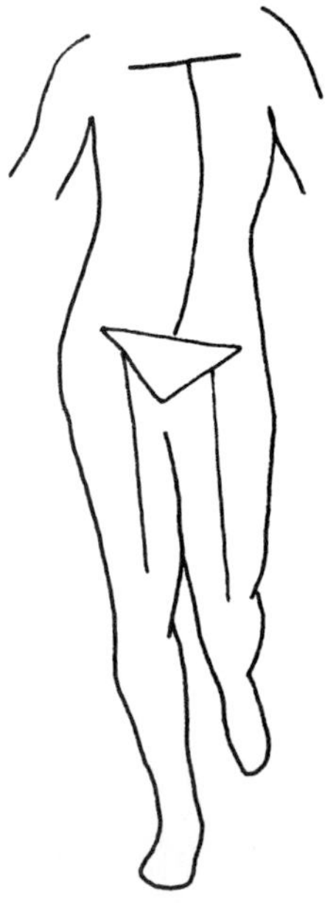

FIGURE 15–14. Associated motions. As the pelvis tilts to the left, the vertebral column laterally bends to the right. The right hip (weight-bearing side) adducts and the non-weight-bearing side abducts.

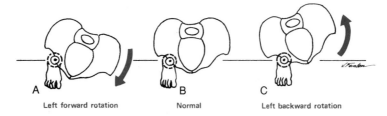

A — Left forward rotation   B — Normal   C — Left backward rotation

FIGURE 15–15. A superior view of rotation of the pelvis in the transverse plane. (*A*) Forward rotation of the pelvis around the right hip joint results in medial rotation of the right hip joint. (*B*) Neutral position of the pelvis and the right hip joint. (*C*) Backward rotation of the pelvis around the right hip joint results in lateral rotation of the right hip joint. (From Norkin, C and Levangie, P: Joint Structure and Function: A Comprehensive Analysis, ed 2, FA Davis, Philadelphia, p 314, with permission.)

This pelvic rotation is occurring because the pelvis is moving on the weight-bearing hip joint. As there is left forward rotation of the pelvis, there is medial rotation of the right hip. With left backward rotation of the pelvis, there is lateral rotation of the right hip. The combinations of joint motions occurring during walking will be described in greater detail in Chapter 6. However, a summary of some of the associated joint motions can be found in Table 15–1.

MUSCLE CONTROL

The pelvis is moved and controlled by groups of muscles acting as force couples. As the pelvis tilts in the anterior/posterior direction, it is opposing muscle groups that provide the movement and control (Fig. 15–16). To tilt the pelvis anteriorly, the lumbar trunk extensors, primarily the erector spinae, pull up posteriorly while the hip flexors pull down anteriorly. Conversely, to tilt the pelvis posteriorly, the abdominals pull up anteriorly while the gluteus maximus and hamstrings pull down posteriorly (Fig. 15–17). In both cases the opposite muscle groups are acting as a force couple causing the pelvis to tilt.

The force of gravity without any muscle action can tilt the pelvis laterally. However, to control or limit the amount of lateral tilting, opposite muscle groups work as a force couple as well. Using the example in Figure 15–18, in a reversal of muscle function action, the left trunk lateral benders, primarily the erector spinae and quadratus lumborum, pull up on the left while the right hip abductors pull down on the right side to keep the pelvis fairly level.

TABLE 15–1	ASSOCIATED MOTIONS OF THE PELVIC GIRDLE, VERTEBRAL COLUMN, AND HIP JOINTS	
Pelvic Girdle	**Vertebral Column**	**Hip**
Anterior tilt	Hyperextension	Flexion
Posterior tilt	Flexion	Extension
Lateral tilt (unsupported side)	Lateral bending to opposite side	Adduction—opposite side Abduction—same side
Rotation (forward)	Rotation—to opposite side	Medial rotation—weight-bearing side
Rotation (backward)	Rotation—to opposite side	Lateral rotation—weight-bearing side

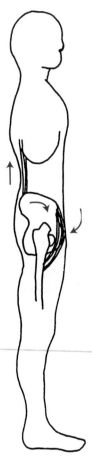

FIGURE 15–16.   Force couple causing anterior pelvic tilt. The posterior trunk extensors (erector spinae) pulling up and the anterior hip flexors pulling down cause the pelvis to tilt anteriorly.

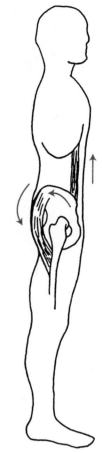

FIGURE 15–17. Force couple causing posterior pelvic tilt. The anterior trunk flexors pulling up and the posterior hip extensors cause the pelvis to tilt posteriorly.

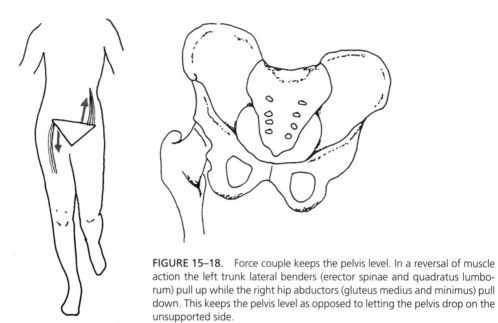

FIGURE 15–18.   Force couple keeps the pelvis level. In a reversal of muscle action the left trunk lateral benders (erector spinae and quadratus lumborum) pull up while the right hip abductors (gluteus medius and minimus) pull down. This keeps the pelvis level as opposed to letting the pelvis drop on the unsupported side.

All of these same muscle groups can work together to provide stability by preventing the pelvis from moving. Pelvic and trunk control is necessary to provide the stable foundation upon which the head and extremities can move.

REVIEW QUESTIONS

1. What pelvic girdle motions occur:

   a. In the sagittal plane around the frontal axis

   b. In the frontal plane around the sagittal axis

   c. In the transverse plane around the vertical axis

2. Concentric contraction of the right quadratus lumborum would cause the pelvis to laterally tilt to which side?

3. Motion occurs at the lumbosacral joint when the pelvis tilts anteriorly and posteriorly and at what other distal joint?

4. What associated hip motion occurs when the pelvis tilts:

   a. Anteriorly

   b. Posteriorly

   c. Laterally

5. What associated hip motion occurs when the left pelvis rotates:

   a. Forward

   b. Backward

6. What associated lumbar motion occurs when the pelvis tilts:

   a. Anteriorly

   b. Posteriorly

   c. Laterally

7. If a person maintained a posture in which the pelvis was tilted excessively in an anterior position, what muscle groups would tend to be tight?

Hip

Joint Structure and Motions

Bones and Landmarks

Ligaments and Other Structures

Muscles of the Hip

Summary of Muscle Action

Summary of Muscle Innervation

Review Questions

The lower extremity includes the pelvis, thigh, leg, and foot (Fig. 16–1). Bones of the pelvis are the two hip bones (os coxae bones), the sacrum, and coccyx. The hip bone consists of three bones (ilium, ischium, and pubis) fused together. The thigh contains the femur and patella. The leg includes the tibia and fibula, and the foot includes 7 tarsal bones, 5 metatarsals, and 14 phalanges. Table 16–1 summarizes these bones.

Joint Structure and Motions

The **hip** is the most proximal of the lower extremity joints. It is very important in weight-bearing and walking activities. Like the shoulder, it is a ball-and-socket joint. The rounded or convex-shaped femoral head fits into and articulates with the concave-shaped acetabulum (Fig. 16–2). Unlike the shoulder, the hip is a very stable joint and, therefore, sacrifices some range of motion. Conversely, the shoulder allows a great deal of motion but is not as stable.

Being a triaxial joint, the hip has motion in all three planes (Fig. 16–3). Flexion, extension, and hyperextension occur in the sagittal plane with approximately 120 degrees of flexion and 15 degrees of hyperextension. Extension is the return from flexion. Abduction and adduction occur in the frontal plane with about 45 degrees of abduction. Adduction is usually thought of as the return to anatomical position, although there is approximately an additional 25 degrees possible beyond the anatomical position. In the transverse plane, medial and lateral rotation are sometimes referred to as *internal* and *external rotation,* respectively. There are approximately 45 degrees of motion possible in each direction from the anatomical position.

The two hip bones are connected anteriorly to each other and to the sacrum posteriorly. The sacrum is also connected to the coccyx. These four bones (two hip bones, sacrum, and coccyx) are collectively known as the pelvis, or pelvic girdle (Fig. 16–4). Note that the pelvis does not include the femur.

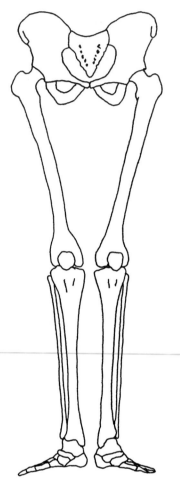

FIGURE 16–1. The lower extremities.

TABLE 16–1	**BONES OF THE LOWER EXTREMITY**	
Region	**Bones**	**Individual Bones**
Pelvis	Os coxae	Ilium, ischium, pubis
	Sacrum	
	Coccyx	
Thigh	Femur	
	Patella	
Leg	Tibia	
	Fibula	
Foot	Tarsals (7)	Calcaneus, talus, cuboid, navicular, cuneiform (3)
	Metatarsals (5)	First through fifth
	Phalanges (14)	Proximal (5), middle (4), distal (5)

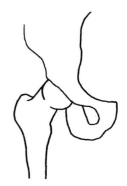

FIGURE 16–2. The hip joint.

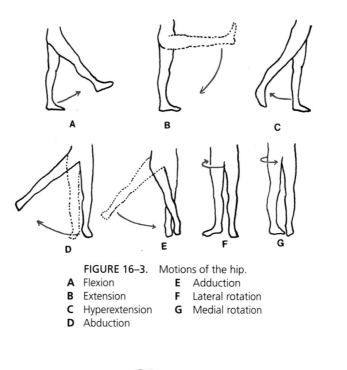

FIGURE 16–3. Motions of the hip.

A	Flexion	**E**	Adduction
B	Extension	**F**	Lateral rotation
C	Hyperextension	**G**	Medial rotation
D	Abduction		

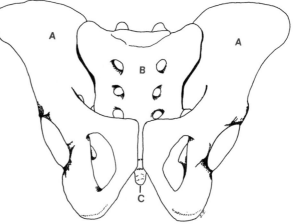

FIGURE 16–4. The bones of the pelvis. (*A*) Hip. (*B*) Sacrum. (*C*) Coccyx.

Bones and Landmarks

As mentioned, the hip joint is made up of the hip bone and the femur. The hip bone, also known as the *os coxae,* is irregularly shaped and actually made up of three bones (Fig. 16–5). These bones fuse together as one by adulthood. The three bones are the ilium, ischium, and pubis.

The fan-shaped **ilium** makes up the superior portion, and its significant landmarks are as follows (Fig. 16–6):

Iliac fossa	Large, smooth, concave area on the internal surface to which the iliac portion of the iliopsoas muscle attaches.
Iliac crest	Bony part that your hands rest on when you put your hands on your hips. Its

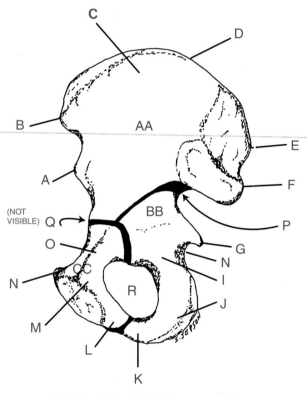

FIGURE 16–5. Right hip bone, medial view.

	Ilium		*Pubis*
A	Anterior inferior iliac spine	**K**	Inferior ramus
B	Anterior superior iliac spine	**L**	Body
C	Iliac fossa	**M**	Tubercle
D	Iliac crest	**N**	Superior ramus
E	Posterior superior iliac spine		
F	Posterior inferior iliac spine		*Combination*
		O	Greater sciatic notch
		P	Acetabulum (not visible)
	Ischium	**Q**	Obturator foramen
G	Ischial spine		
H	Body		*Bones*
I	Ischial tuberosity	**AA**	Ilium
J	Ramus	**BB**	Ischium
		CC	Pubis

borders are the anterior superior iliac spine (ASIS) anteriorly and the posterior superior iliac spine (PSIS) posteriorly.

Anterior Superior Iliac Spine	Abbreviated ASIS; the projection on the anterior end of the iliac crest. The tensor fascia lata, sartorius, and inguinal ligament attach here.
Anterior Inferior Iliac Spine	Abbreviated AIIS. The projection is just inferior to the ASIS to which the rectus femoris muscle attaches.
Posterior Superior Iliac Spine	Abbreviated PSIS. It is the posterior projection on the iliac crest.
Posterior Inferior Iliac Spine	Abbreviated PIIS; located just below the PSIS.

The **ischium** is the posterior inferior portion of the hip bone. Its significant landmarks are as follows (see Fig. 16–6):

Body	Makes up about two-fifths of the acetabulum.
Ramus	Extends medially from the body to connect with the inferior ramus of the pubis. The adductor magnus, obturator externus, and obturator internus muscles attach here.
Ischial tuberosity	Rough, blunt projection of the inferior part of the body which is weight bearing when you are sitting. It provides attachment for the hamstring and adductor magnus muscles.
Spine	Located on the posterior portion of the body and inferior border of the greater sciatic notch superior to the lesser sciatic notch. It provides attachment for the sacrospinous ligament.

The **pubis** forms the anterior inferior portion of the hip. It can be divided into three parts, the body and its two rami (see Fig. 16–5):

Body	Externally forms about one-fifth of the acetabulum and internally provides attachment for the obturator internus muscle.
Superior ramus	Lies superior between the acetabulum and the body and provides attachment for the pectineus muscle.
Inferior ramus	Lies posterior, inferior, and lateral to the body. Attachment for the adductor magnus and brevis and gracilis muscles.
Symphysis pubis	A cartilaginous joint connecting the bodies of the two pubic bones at the anterior midline.
Pubic tubercle	Projects anteriorly on the superior ramus near the symphysis pubis and provides attachment for the inguinal ligament.

The following are made up of combinations of the hip bones (see Fig. 16–5):

Acetabulum	A deep, cup-shaped cavity that articulates with the femur. It is made up of nearly equal portions of the ilium, ischium, and pubis.

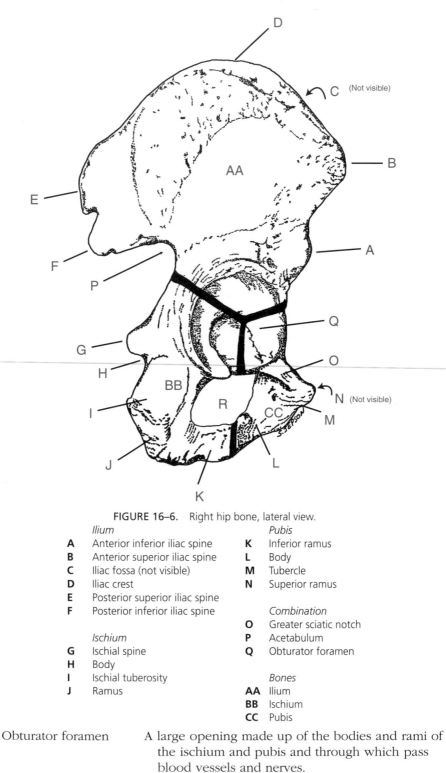

FIGURE 16–6. Right hip bone, lateral view.

Ilium
A Anterior inferior iliac spine
B Anterior superior iliac spine
C Iliac fossa (not visible)
D Iliac crest
E Posterior superior iliac spine
F Posterior inferior iliac spine

Ischium
G Ischial spine
H Body
I Ischial tuberosity
J Ramus

Pubis
K Inferior ramus
L Body
M Tubercle
N Superior ramus

Combination
O Greater sciatic notch
P Acetabulum
Q Obturator foramen

Bones
AA Ilium
BB Ischium
CC Pubis

Obturator foramen   A large opening made up of the bodies and rami of the ischium and pubis and through which pass blood vessels and nerves.

Greater sciatic notch   Large notch just below the PIIS that is actually made into a foramen by the sacrospinous ligament. The sciatic nerve, piriformis muscle, and other structures pass through this opening.

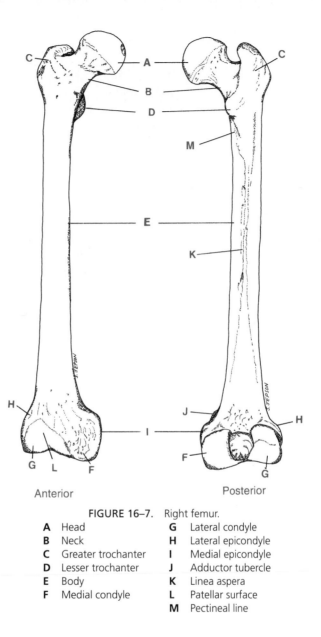

Anterior Posterior

FIGURE 16–7. Right femur.

A	Head	**G**	Lateral condyle
B	Neck	**H**	Lateral epicondyle
C	Greater trochanter	**I**	Medial epicondyle
D	Lesser trochanter	**J**	Adductor tubercle
E	Body	**K**	Linea aspera
F	Medial condyle	**L**	Patellar surface
		M	Pectineal line

The **femur** is the longest, strongest, and heaviest bone in the body. A person's height can roughly be estimated to be four times the length of the femur (Moore, p 403, 1985). It articulates with the hip bones to form the hip joint and has the following significant landmarks (Fig. 16–7):

Head	The rounded portion covered with articular cartilage articulating with the acetabulum.
Neck	The narrower portion located between the head and the trochanters.
Greater trochanter	Large projection located laterally between the neck and the body of the femur, providing attachment for the gluteus medius and minimus, and most deep rotator muscles.

Lesser trochanter	A smaller projection located medially and posteriorly just distal to the greater trochanter, providing attachment for the iliopsoas muscle.
Body	The long cylindrical portion between the bone ends; also called the *shaft*. It is bowed slightly anteriorly.
Medial condyle	Distal medial end.
Lateral condyle	Distal lateral end.
Lateral epicondyle	Projection proximal to the lateral condyle.
Medial epicondyle	Projection proximal to the medial condyle.
Adductor tubercle	Small projection proximal to the medial epicondyle to which a portion of the adductor magnus muscle attaches.
Linea aspera	Prominent longitudinal ridge or crest running most of the posterior length.
Pectineal line	Runs from below the lesser trochanter diagonally toward the linea aspera. It provides attachment for the adductor brevis.

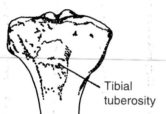

Tibial
tuberosity

Anterior

FIGURE 16–8. Right tibia, anterior view.

| Patellar surface | Between the medial and lateral condyle anteriorly. It articulates with the posterior surface of the patella. |

The **tibia** will be discussed in more detail in Chapter 17. It is important now, however, to identify one landmark (Fig. 16–8):

| Tibial tuberosity | Large projection at the proximal end in the midline. It provides attachment for the patellar tendon. |

Ligaments and Other Structures

Like all synovial joints, the hip has a fibrous **joint capsule.** It is strong and thick and covers the hip joint in a cylindrical fashion. It attaches proximally around the lip of the acetabulum and distally to the neck of the femur (Fig. 16–9). It forms a cylindrical sleeve that encloses the joint and most of the femoral neck.

Three ligaments reinforce the capsule. They are the iliofemoral, ischiofemoral, and pubofemoral ligaments (Fig. 16–10). The most important of these ligaments is the **iliofemoral ligament.** It reinforces the capsule anteriorly by attaching proximally to the anterior inferior iliac spine and crossing the joint anteriorly. It splits into two parts distally to attach to the intertrochanteric line of the femur. Because it resembles an inverted "Y," it is often referred to as the *Y ligament*. It is also known as the *ligament of Bigelow*. Its main function is to limit hyperextension.

The **pubofemoral ligament** spans the hip joint medially and inferiorly, attaching from the medial part of the acetabular rim and superior ramus of the pubis, running down and back to attach on the neck of the femur. Like the iliofemoral ligament, it also limits hyperextension. In addition, it limits abduction.

The **ischiofemoral ligament** covers the capsule posteriorly. It attaches on the ischial portion of the acetabulum, crosses the joint in a lateral and superior direc-

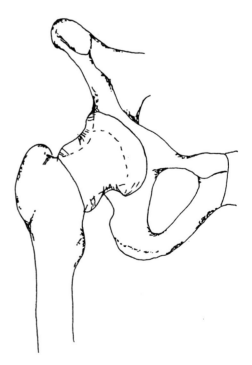

FIGURE 16–9. The hip joint capsule.

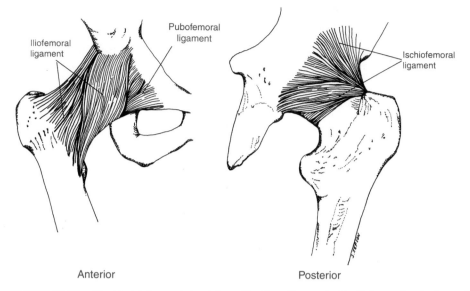

FIGURE 16–10.   The hip joint capsule is reinforced by three ligaments: the iliofemoral, pubofemoral, and ischiofemoral.

tion, and attaches on the femoral neck. Its fibers limit hyperextension and also medial rotation.

These three ligaments all attach along the rim of the acetabulum and cross the hip joint in a spiral fashion to attach on the femoral neck. The combined effect of this spiral attachment is to limit motion in one direction (hyperextension) while allowing full motion in the other (flexion). Therefore, these ligaments are slack in flexion and become taut as the hip moves into hyperextension. By thrusting the hips forward so that they are in front of the shoulders and knees, it is possible to stand in the upright position without using any muscles by, essentially, resting on the iliofemoral ligament. This is the basis for the standing posture of an individual with spinal cord paralysis (Fig. 16–11).

The **ligamentum teres** is a small intracapsular ligament of debatable importance (Fig. 16–12). It attaches proximally in the acetabulum and distally in the fovea of the femoral head. Some sources indicate that it becomes taut during adduction or

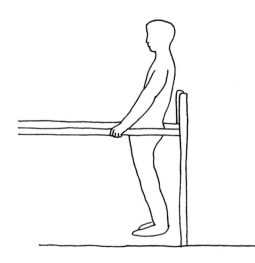

FIGURE 16–11.   The spiral attachment of the hip ligaments tends to limit hyperextension. A paraplegic individual can therefore stand in the upright position by thrusting the hips forward of the shoulders and knees.

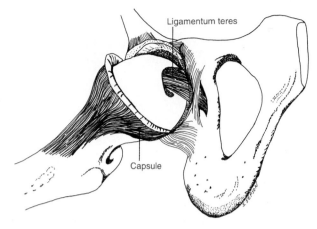

FIGURE 16–12. The ligamentum teres. Oblique view with femur laterally rotated and capsule cut away.

during lateral rotation, when the hip is semiflexed. However, given its size, it is doubtful that it adds significantly to the strength of the joint. Its other feature is that it contains a blood vessel that supplies the head of the femur. However, by itself, this vessel is unable to supply enough blood to the head to keep it viable.

The depth of the acetabulum is increased by the fibrocartilaginous **acetabular labrum,** which is located around the rim. The free end of the labrum surrounds the femoral head and assists in holding the head in the acetabulum.

Although the **inguinal ligament** has no function at the hip joint, it should be identified because of its presence. It runs from the anterior superior iliac spine to the pubic tubercle and is the landmark that separates the anterior abdominal wall from the thigh (Fig. 16–13). When the external iliac artery and vein pass under the inguinal ligament, their names change to the *femoral artery* and *vein*.

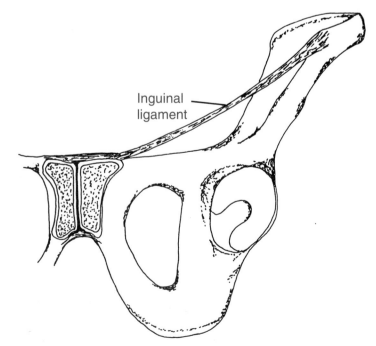

FIGURE 16–13. The inguinal ligament.

The **iliotibial band** or **tract** is the very long, tendinous portion of the tensor fascia latae muscle (see Fig. 16–25). It attaches to the anterior portion of the iliac crest and runs superficially down the lateral side of the thigh to attach to the tibia. Both the gluteus maximus and tensor fascia latae muscles have fibers attaching to it.

Muscles of the Hip

There are many similarities between the shoulder and hip joints. Like the shoulder, the hip has a group of one-joint muscles that provide most of the control and a group of longer, two-joint muscles that provide the range of motion. These muscles can also be grouped according to their location and somewhat by their function. For example, the anterior muscles tend to be flexors, lateral muscles tend to be abductors, posterior muscles tend to be extensors, and medial muscles tend to be adductors. Table 16–2 classifies the hip muscles by location and function.

The **iliopsoas muscle** is actually two muscles with separate proximal attachments and a common distal attachment (Fig. 16–14). The iliacus muscle portion arises from the iliac fossa, and the psoas major muscle portion comes from the transverse processes, bodies, and intervertebral disks of the T12 through L5 vertebrae. These muscles blend together to attach on the lesser trochanter of the femur. The iliopsoas muscle is a prime mover in hip flexion. The psoas muscle portion, because of its attachment on the vertebra, contributes to trunk flexion when the femur is stabilized.

Iliopsoas Muscle	
(O)	Iliac fossa, anterior and lateral surfaces of T12 through L5
(I)	Lesser trochanter
(A)	Hip flexion
(N)	Iliacus portion: Femoral nerve (L2, L3)
	Psoas major portion: L2 and L3

TABLE 16–2	**MUSCLES OF THE HIP**	
Muscle Group	**One-Joint Muscles**	**Two-Joint Muscles**
Anterior	Iliopsoas	Rectus femoris
		Sartorius
Medial	Pectineus	Gracilis
	Adductor magnus	
	Adductor longus	
	Adductor brevis	
Posterior	Gluteus maximus	Semimembranosus
	Deep rotators (6)	Semitendinosus
		Biceps femoris
Lateral	Gluteus medius	Tensor fascia latae
	Gluteus minimus	

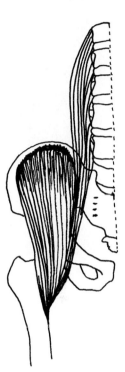

FIGURE 16–14. The iliopsoas muscle.

The **rectus femoris muscle** is part of the quadriceps muscle group and the only one of that group to cross the hip (Fig. 16–15). Its proximal attachment is on the AIIS. It runs almost straight down the thigh to be joined by the three vasti muscles to blend into the quadriceps muscle tendon. This tendon encases the patella, crosses the knee joint, and attaches to the tibial tuberosity. The rectus femoris muscle is a prime mover in hip flexion and knee extension.

Rectus Femoris Muscle

(O)	Anterior inferior iliac spine
(I)	Tibial tuberosity
(A)	Hip flexion, knee extension
(N)	Femoral nerve (L2, L3, L4)

The **sartorius muscle** is the longest muscle in the body (Fig. 16–16). This long, straplike muscle arises from the anterior superior iliac spine. It runs diagonally across the thigh from lateral to medial and proximal to distal to cross the medial knee joint posteriorly. Because of its line of pull, it is capable of flexing, abducting, and laterally rotating the hip and flexing the knee. However, it is not considered a prime mover in any one of these motions. It is most efficient when doing all four of these motions at the same time. An example of this motion is when you cross your legs by putting one foot on the opposite knee.

Sartorius Muscle

(O)	Anterior superior iliac spine
(I)	Proximal medial aspect of tibia
(A)	Combination of hip flexion abduction, lateral rotation
(N)	Femoral nerve (L2, L3)

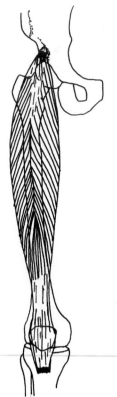

FIGURE 16–15.   The rectus femoris muscle.

Located medial to the iliopsoas muscle and lateral to the adductor longus muscle is the **pectineus muscle.** Its origin is on the superior ramus of the pubis, and its insertion is on the pectineal line of the femur (Fig. 16–17). Because it spans the hip anteriorly as well as medially, it provides hip flexion and adduction.

Pectineus Muscle

(O)	Superior ramus of pubis
(I)	Pectineal line of femur
(A)	Hip flexion and adduction
(N)	Femoral nerve (L2, L3, L4)

There are three other one-joint hip adductors, all with the same first name (Fig. 16–18). The **adductor longus muscle,** the most superficial of the three, originates from the anterior surface of the pubis near the tubercle and inserts on the middle third of the linea aspera of the femur. Because it is superficial, its tendon can easily be felt in the anterior-medial groin. Being able to palpate this tendon is important when checking for correct fit of the quadrilateral socket of the above-knee prosthesis. It is a prime mover in hip adduction.

Adductor Longus Muscle

(O)	Pubis
(I)	Middle third of the linea aspera
(A)	Hip adduction
(N)	Obturator nerve (L3, L4)

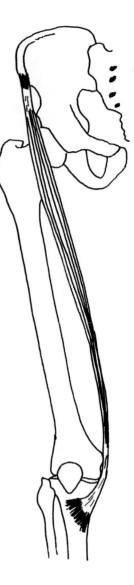

FIGURE 16–16.   The sartorius muscle.

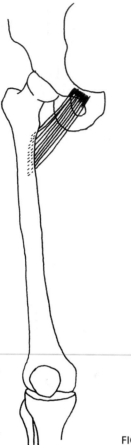

FIGURE 16–17. The pectineus muscle. Note that the distal attachment is on the posterior femur.

The **adductor brevis muscle** implies by its name that it is shorter. It lies deep to the adductor longus muscle, but superficial to the adductor magnus muscle. It arises from the inferior ramus of the pubis and inserts on the pectineal line and proximal linea aspera above the adductor longus muscle. It is a prime mover in hip adduction.

Adductor Brevis Muscle	
(O)	Pubis
(I)	Pectineal line and proximal linea aspera
(A)	Hip adduction
(N)	Obturator nerve (L3, L4)

The largest, most massive, and deepest of the adductors is the **adductor magnus muscle.** It arises from the ischial tuberosity and ramus of the ischium and inferior ramus of the pubis. It makes up most of the bulk on the medial thigh. It inserts along the entire linea aspera and adductor tubercle. There is an interruption, or hiatus, in the distal attachment between the linea aspera and adductor tubercle. The femoral artery and vein pass through this opening. After these structures have passed through to the posterior surface, their names become the *popliteal artery* and *vein*. Because of its size, the adductor magnus muscle is a very strong hip adductor.

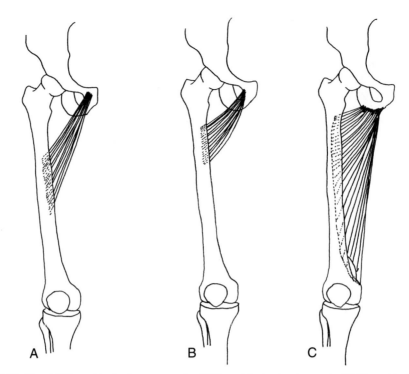

FIGURE 16–18. (A) The adductor longus muscle. (B) The adductor brevis muscle. (C) The adductor magnus muscle.

Adductor Magnus Muscle

(O)	Ischium and pubis
(I)	Entire linea aspera and adductor tubercle
(A)	Hip adduction
(N)	Obturator and sciatic nerve (L3, L4)

The only hip adductor that is a two-joint muscle is the **gracilis muscle** (Fig. 16–19). It arises from the symphysis and inferior ramus of the pubis and descends the thigh medially and superficially. It crosses the knee joint posteriorly and curves around the medial condyle to attach distally on the anteromedial surface of the proximal tibia.

Gracilis Muscle

(O)	Pubis
(I)	Anterior medial surface of proximal end of tibia
(A)	Hip adduction
(N)	Obturator nerve (L2, L3)

The **gluteus maximus muscle** can be described as a large, one-joint, quadrilateral-shaped, thick muscle located superficially on the posterior buttock (Fig. 16–20). It arises from the general area of the posterior sacrum, coccyx, and ilium, and runs in a diagonal direction distally and laterally to the posterior femur inferior to the greater trochanter. Some fibers also attach to the iliotibial band. Because it

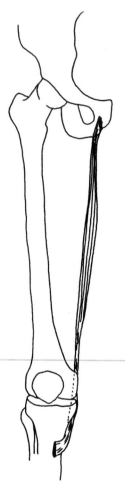
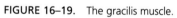

FIGURE 16–19.   The gracilis muscle.

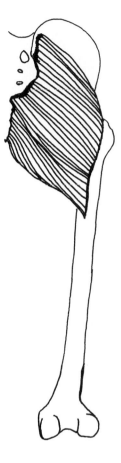

FIGURE 16–20.   The gluteus maximus muscle.

spans the hip posteriorly in this diagonal direction, it is very strong in hip extension, hyperextension, and lateral rotation.

Gluteus Maximus Muscle	
(O)	Posterior sacrum and ilium
(I)	Posterior femur distal to greater trochanter and to iliotibial band
(A)	Hip extension, hyperextension, lateral rotation
(N)	Inferior gluteal nerve (L5, S1, S2)

There are six small, deep, mostly posterior muscles that span the hip joint in a horizontal direction, and they all laterally rotate the hip. Because they all work together to produce the same motion, their individual attachments are not functionally important. Therefore, they can be grouped together as the **deep rotator muscles** (Fig. 16–21). The piriformis is, however, the best known of this group, perhaps, because of its close relationship to the sciatic nerve. Table 16–3 summarizes their attachments and innervation.

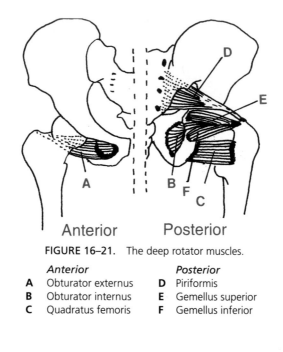

FIGURE 16–21.   The deep rotator muscles.

Anterior		*Posterior*	
A	Obturator externus	**D**	Piriformis
B	Obturator internus	**E**	Gemellus superior
C	Quadratus femoris	**F**	Gemellus inferior

Deep Rotator Muscles

(O)	Posterior sacrum, ischium, pubis
(I)	Greater trochanter area
(A)	Hip lateral rotation
(N)	Numerous, see Table 16–3

Three muscles that are known collectively as the **hamstring muscles** cover the posterior thigh. They consist of the semitendinosus, the semimembranosus, and the biceps femoris muscles (Fig. 16–22). They have a common site of origin on the ischial tuberosity.

TABLE 16–3	DEEP ROTATOR MUSCLES		
Muscle	**Proximal Attachment**	**Distal Attachment**	**Innervation**
Obturator externus	Rami of pubis and ischium	Trochanteric fossa	Obturator nerve
Obturator internus	Rami of pubis and ischium	Greater trochanter	Nerve to obturator internus
Quadratus femoris	Ischial tuberosity	Intertrochanteric crest	Nerve to quadratus femoris
Piriformis	Sacrum	Greater trochanter	S1, S2 segments
Gemellus superior	Ischium	Greater trochanter	Nerve to obturator internus
Gemellus inferior	Ischial tuberosity	Greater trochanter	Nerve to quadratus femoris

The **semimembranosus muscle** runs down the medial side of the thigh deep to the semitendinosus muscle and inserts on the posterior surface of the medial condyle of the tibia. The **semitendinosus muscle** has a much longer and narrower distal tendon that, after spanning the knee joint posteriorly, moves anteriorly to attach to the anteromedial surface of the tibia with the gracilis and sartorius muscles. The **biceps femoris muscle** has two heads and runs down the thigh laterally on the posterior side. The long head arises with the other two muscles on the ischial tuberosity, but the short head arises from the lateral lip of the linea aspera. Both heads join together spanning the knee posteriorly to attach laterally on the head of the fibula and by a small slip to the lateral condyle of the tibia. Because they span the knee posteriorly, they flex the knee. The long head, because it spans the hip posteriorly, also extends the hip.

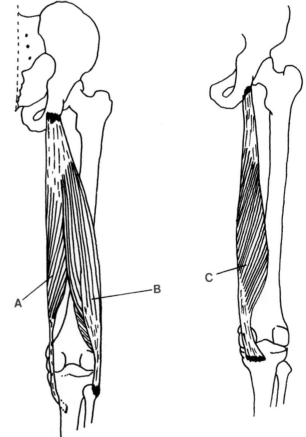

FIGURE 16–22. The hamstring muscles: (*A*) Semitendinosus. (*B*) Biceps femoris. (*C*) Semimembranosus.

Semimembranosus Muscle

(O)	Ischial tuberosity
(I)	Posterior surface of medial condyle of tibia
(A)	Extend hip and flex knee
(N)	Sciatic nerve (L5, S1, S2)

Semitendinosus Muscle

(O)	Ischial tuberosity
(I)	Anteromedial surface of proximal tibia
(A)	Extend hip and flex knee
(N)	Sciatic nerve (L5, S1, S2)

Biceps Femoris Muscle

(O)	Long head: ischial tuberosity
	Short head: lateral lip of linea aspera
(I)	Fibular head
(A)	Long head: extend hip and flex knee
	Short head: flex knee
(N)	Long head: sciatic nerve (S1, S2, S3)
	Short head: common peroneal nerve (L5, S1, S2)

The other two gluteal muscles are more laterally located. The **gluteus medius muscle** is triangular shaped, much like the deltoid muscle of the shoulder (Fig. 16–23). It attaches proximally to the outer surface of the ilium and distally to the lateral surface of the greater trochanter. Because it spans the hip laterally, it is able to abduct the hip. Its anterior fibers are able to assist the gluteus minimus muscle in medially rotating the hip.

Gluteus Medius Muscle

(O)	Outer surface of the ilium
(I)	Lateral surface of the greater trochanter
(A)	Hip abduction
(N)	Superior gluteal nerve (L4, L5, S1)

Proximally the **gluteus minimus muscle** lies deep and inferior to the gluteus medius muscle on the lateral ilium (Fig. 16–24). The distal attachment is on the anterior aspect of the greater trochanter. This gives the gluteus minimus muscle a somewhat diagonal line of pull, making it able to medially rotate the hip. Because it spans the hip laterally, it also abducts the hip.

Gluteus Minimus Muscle

(O)	Lateral ilium
(I)	Anterior surface of the greater trochanter
(A)	Hip abduction, medial rotation
(N)	Superior gluteal nerve (L4, L5, S1)

Attaching to the ilium and the femur and spanning the hip laterally, these two gluteal muscles have another very important function. When you stand on one

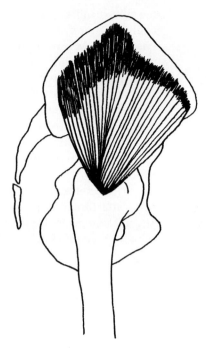

FIGURE 16–23. The gluteus medius muscle.

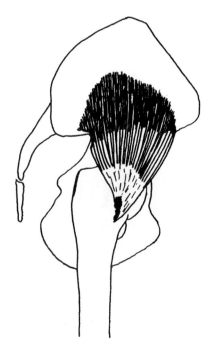

FIGURE 16–24. The gluteus minimus muscle.

leg, the distal segment (femur) becomes more stable than the proximal segment (pelvis); therefore, the origin moves toward the insertion. Another term for this change is **reversal of muscle function.** If these muscles did not contract when you stood on one leg, the opposite side of your pelvis would drop (Fig. 16–25). Therefore, the gluteus medius and minimus muscles contract to keep the pelvis fairly level and prevent the opposite side of the pelvis from dropping very much when you stand on one leg. This occurs every time you pick up one leg, as when walking. Weakness or loss of these muscles results in a "Trendelenberg gait." For example, if your right hip abductors are weak, your left pelvis will drop significantly when you stand on your right leg and lift your left leg off the ground.

The **tensor fascia latae muscle** is a very short muscle with a very long tendinous attachment (Fig. 16–26). It arises from the ASIS, crosses the hip laterally and slightly anteriorly, then attaches to the long fascial band called the *iliotibial band,* which proceeds down the lateral thigh and attaches into the tibia. It is a hip abductor, but because of its slight anterior position, it is perhaps strongest when performing a combination of flexion and abduction. Stated another way, it is most efficient when abducting in a slightly anterior direction.

Tensor Fascia Latae Muscle	
(O)	Anterior superior iliac spine
(I)	Lateral condyle of tibia
(A)	Combined hip flexion and abduction
(N)	Superior gluteal nerve (L4, L5)

SUMMARY OF MUSCLE ACTION

Table 16–4 summarizes the actions of the prime movers of the hip joint.

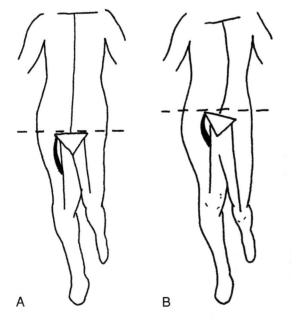

FIGURE 16–25. (*A*) In reversal of muscle function, the right hip abductors contract to keep the pelvis steady when the left leg is lifted. (*B*) When right hip abductors are weak, the left side of the pelvis drops.

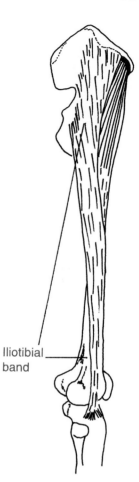

Iliotibial band

FIGURE 16–26. The tensor fascia latae muscle. The very long, tendinous portion of this muscle is known as the iliotibial band.

TABLE 16–4	**PRIME MOVERS OF THE HIP JOINT**
Action	**Muscle**
Combination of flexion and abduction	Tensor fascia latae
Combination of flexion, abduction, and lateral rotation	Sartorius
Flexion	Rectus femoris, iliopsoas, pectineus
Extension	Gluteus maximus, semitendinosus, semimembranosus, biceps femoris (long head)
Hyperextension	Gluteus maximus
Abduction	Gluteus medius, gluteus minimus
Adduction	Pectineus, adductor longus, adductor brevis, adductor magnus, gracilis
Medial rotation	Gluteus minimis
Lateral rotation	Gluteus maximus, deep rotators

TABLE 16–5	INNERVATION OF THE MUSCLES OF THE HIP	
Muscle	**Nerve**	**Spinal Segment**
Iliopsoas: psoas part	Anterior rami	L2, L3
Iliacus part	Femoral	L2, L3
Rectus femoris	Femoral	L2, L3, L4
Sartorius	Femoral	L2, L3
Pectineus	Femoral	L2, L3
Gracilis	Obturator	L2, L3
Adductor longus	Obturator	L2, L3, L4
Adductor brevis	Obturator	L2, L3, L4
Adductor magnus	Obturator	L3, L4
Gluteus maximus	Inferior gluteal	L5, S1, S2
Gluteus medius	Superior gluteal	L5, S1, S2
Gluteus minimis	Superior gluteal	L5, S1, S2
Tensor fascia latae	Superior gluteal	L4, L5
Semitendinosus	Sciatic	L5, S1, S2
Semimembranosus	Sciatic	L5, S1, S2
Biceps femoris		
Long	Sciatic	L5, S1, S2
Short	Common peroneal	L5, S1, S2
Obturator externus	Obturator	L3, L4
Obturator internus	Nerve to the obturator internus	L5, S1
Gemellus superior	Nerve to the obturator internus	L5, S1
Quadratus femoris	Nerve to the quadratus femoris	L5, S1
Gemellus inferior	Nerve to the quadratus femoris	L5, S1
Piriformis	Anterior rami	S1, S2

TABLE 16–6	SEGMENTAL INNERVATION OF HIP MUSCLES						
Spinal Cord Level	**L2**	**L3**	**L4**	**L5**	**S1**	**S2**	**S3**
Iliopsoas	X	X					
Sartorius	X	X					
Gracilis	X	X					
Rectus femoris	X	X	X				
Pectineus	X	X	X				
Adductor longus		X	X				
Adductor brevis		X	X				
Adductor magnus		X	X				
Tensor fascia latae			X	X			
Gluteus medius			X	X	X		
Gluteus minimus			X	X	X		
Semitendinosus				X	X	X	
Semimembranosus				X	X	X	
Biceps femoris				X	X	X	X
Deep rotators		X	X	X	X	X	

SUMMARY OF MUSCLE INNERVATION

Generally speaking, the femoral nerve innervates muscles on the anterior surface of the hip and thigh region (hip flexors). The obturator nerve innervates hip adductors, on the medial side. The hip abductors on the lateral side are supplied by the superior gluteal nerve. The hamstring muscles, which are hip extensors and located posteriorly, receive innervation from the sciatic nerve.

There are, of course, exceptions to all generalizations. The gluteus maximus, a posterior muscle, receives innervation from the inferior gluteal nerve. The deep rotators do not fit neatly into any sort of generalization; therefore, they are included in the summary of hip joint muscle innervation in Table 16–5 individually instead of as a group. Table 16–6 summarizes the segmental innervation. As has been stated in previous chapters, there is variation among sources regarding some segmental innervation. The deep rotators are included here as a group.

REVIEW QUESTIONS

1. List the bones that make up the:
   a. Pelvis
   b. Hip bone
   c. Hip joint
   d. Acetabulum
   e. Obturator foramen
   f. Greater sciatic notch

2. If you were handed an unattached hip bone, what landmarks would you use to determine if it was a right or left hip bone?

3. How would you determine if an unattached femur is a right or left one?

4. Describe the hip joint:
   a. Number of axes:
   b. Shape of joint:
   c. Type of motion allowed:

5. What hip motions occur in:
   a. the transverse plane around the vertical axis?
   b. the sagittal plane around the frontal axis?
   c. the frontal plane around the sagittal axis?

6. What is referred to as the *Y ligament?* Why?

7. Why is the hip joint not prone to dislocation?

8. What is the direction of the line of attachment of the ligaments of the hip—vertical, horizontal, or spiral? What does this line of attachment allow for?

9. Which hip joint muscles are two-joint muscles that attach below the knee?

10. Which hip joint muscles are not prime movers in any single action but are effective in a combination of movements? List the movements.

11. What muscle(s) keeps your pelvis from dropping on one side when you lift one foot off the floor? Describe what happens.

Knee

Joint Structure and Motions

At first glance the knee joint appears to be a relatively simple joint; however, it is one of the more complex joints in the body. Because it is supported and maintained entirely by muscles and ligaments with no bony stability, and because it is frequently exposed to severe stresses and strains, it should be no surprise that it is one of the most frequently injured joints in the body.

The knee joint is the largest joint in the body and it is classified as a synovial hinge joint (Fig. 17–1). The motions possible at the knee are flexion and extension (Fig. 17–2). From 0 degrees of extension there are approximately 120 to 135 degrees of flexion. However, unlike the elbow, the knee joint is not a true hinge because it has a rotational component. This rotation is not a free motion but an accessory motion that accompanies flexion and extension.

This rotation occurs because the articular surface of the femoral medial condyle is longer than that of the lateral condyle. As extension occurs, the articular surface of the lateral condyle is used up while some articular surface remains medially. Therefore, the medial condyle of the femur must also glide posteriorly to use all of its articular surface. It is this posterior gliding of the medial condyle during the last few degrees of weight-bearing extension (closed chain action) that causes the femur to rotate medially (spin) on the tibia (Fig. 17–3). In non-weight-bearing extension (open chain action), the tibia rotates laterally on the femur. These last few degrees of motion lock the knee in extension, which is sometimes referred to as the *screw-home mechanism* of the knee (Fig. 17–4). With the knee fully extended, an individual can stand for a long time without using muscles. The knee must be "*un*locked"

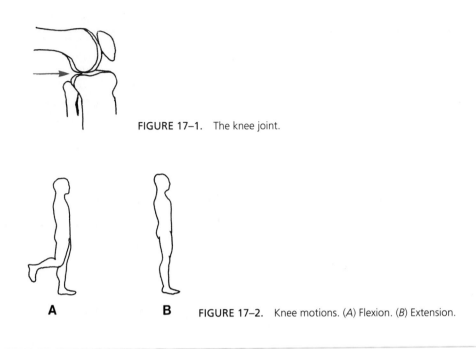

FIGURE 17–1. The knee joint.

A **B** **FIGURE 17–2.** Knee motions. (*A*) Flexion. (*B*) Extension.

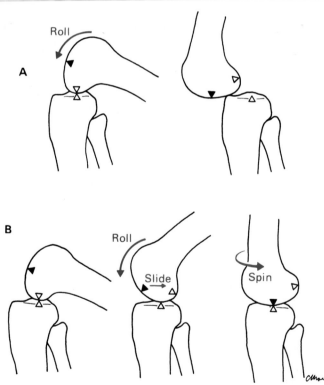

FIGURE 17–3. Arthrokinematic movements of the joint surfaces. (*A*) Pure rolling or hinge motion of the femur or the tibia would cause joint dislocation. (*B*) Normal motion of the knee demonstrates a combination of rolling, sliding, and spinning in the last 20 degrees of extension (terminal rotation of the knee). (Adapted from Smith, LK, Weiss, EL, and Lehmkuhl, LD: Brunnstrom's Clinical Kinesiology, ed 5. FA Davis, Philadelphia, 1996, p 13.)

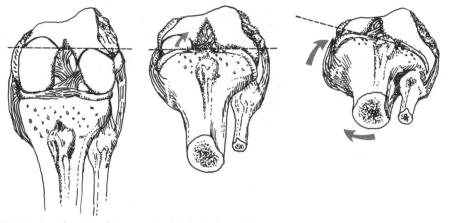

FIGURE 17–4. The screw-home motion of the knee. In the non-weight-bearing position, the tibia laterally rotates on the femur as the knee moves into the last few degrees of extension.

by the femur rotating laterally on the tibia for knee flexion to occur. It is this small amount of rotation of the femur on the tibia, or vice versa, that keeps the knee from being a true hinge joint. Because this rotation is not an independent motion, it will not be considered a knee motion.

The articulation between the femur and patella is referred to as the **patellofemoral joint** (Fig. 17–5). The posterior surface of the patella is smooth and glides over the patellar surface of the femur. The patella's main functions are to increase the mechanical advantage of the quadriceps muscle and to protect the knee joint. An increased mechanical advantage is achieved by lengthening the moment arm. As discussed in Chapter 6 on torque, moment arm is the perpendicular distance between the muscle's line of action and the center of the joint (axis). By placing the patella between the quadriceps tendon and the femur, the action line of the quadriceps muscles is further away (Fig. 17–6). Hence the moment arm is lengthened, which allows the muscle to have greater angular force. Without the patella, the moment arm would be smaller and much of the force of the muscle would be directed back into the joint (stabilizing force).

The **Q angle,** or *patellofemoral angle,* is the angle between the quadriceps muscle, primarily the rectus femoris muscle, and the patellar tendon. It is determined by drawing a line from the anterior superior iliac spine (ASIS) to the midpoint of the patella and from the tibial tuberosity to the midpoint of the patella. The angle formed by the intersecting of these lines represents the Q angle (Fig. 17–7). Sources vary, but in knee extension in normal individuals, this angle ranges from 13 to 18 degrees and tends to be greater in females (Magee, p 296). Many different knee problems are associated with Q angles being greater or less than this range.

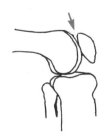

FIGURE 17–5. The patellofemoral joint.

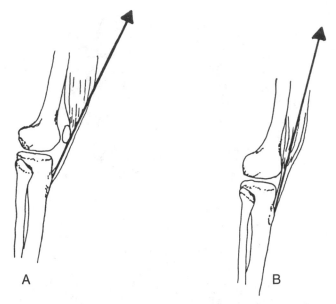

FIGURE 17–6. Moment arm of the quadriceps muscles is greater with a patella (*A*), than without a patella (*B*).

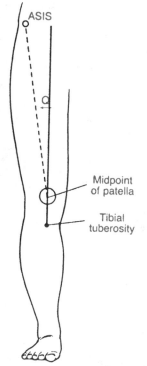

FIGURE 17–7. Measurement of the Q angle. (From Gould, JA and Davies, GJ: Orthopaedic and Sports Physical Therapy, ed 2. Mosby-Year Book, St. Louis, 1989, p 186, with permission.)

Bones and Landmarks

The knee is composed of the distal end of the femur articulating with the proximal end of the tibia. The significant landmarks for the femur were discussed in the previous chapter. The landmarks of the tibia significant to the knee are as follows (Fig. 17–8):

Intercondylar eminence	A double-pointed prominence on the proximal surface at about the midpoint, which extends up into the intercondylar fossa of the femur.
Medial condyle	The proximal medial end.
Lateral condyle	The proximal lateral end.

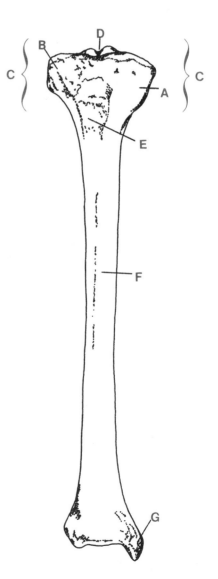

FIGURE 17–8. Right tibia, anterior view.

A	Medial condyle	**E**	Tibial tuberosity
B	Lateral condyle	**F**	Crest
C	Tibial plateau	**G**	Medial malleolus
D	Intercondylar eminence		

Plateau — The enlarged proximal end including the medial and lateral condyles and the intercondylar eminence.

Tibial tuberosity — Large projection at the proximal end on the anterior surface in the midline.

The **fibula** is lateral to, and smaller than, the tibia. It is set back from the anterior surface of the tibia, allowing a large space for muscle attachment (Fig. 17–9). This feature gives the lower leg its rounded circumference. The fibula is not part of the knee joint because it does not articulate with the femur. Although it does provide a point of attachment for some of the knee structures, it has a larger role at the ankle.

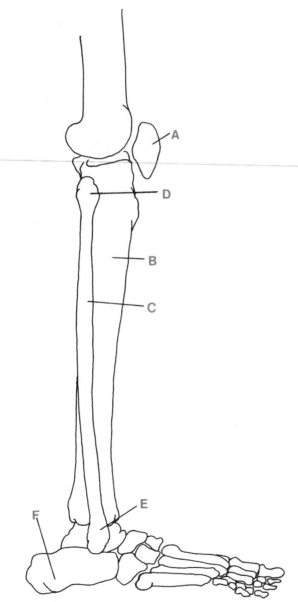

FIGURE 17–9. Right leg, lateral view.

A Patella	**D** Fibular head
B Tibia	**E** Lateral malleolus
C Fibula	**F** Calcaneus

The **patella** is a triangular-shaped sesamoid bone within the quadriceps muscle tendon (Fig. 17–10). It has a broad superior border and a somewhat pointed distal portion.

The **calcaneus** (see Fig. 17–9F) is the most posterior of the tarsal bones and is commonly known as the *heel*. It is identified here because it provides attachment for the gastrocnemius muscle.

Ligaments and Other Structures

As earlier, the knee is held together not by its bony structure but by ligaments and muscles. The cruciate and collateral ligaments are the two main sets of ligaments for this task (Fig. 17–11). The cruciates are located within the joint capsule and are therefore called **intracapsular ligaments.** Located between the medial and lateral condyles, the cruciates cross each other obliquely (*cruciate means* "resembling a cross" in Latin). They are named by their attachment on the *tibia* (Fig. 17–12). The **anterior cruciate ligament** attaches to the anterior surface of the tibia in the intercondylar area just medial to the medial meniscus. It spans the knee laterally to the posterior cruciate ligament and runs in a superior and posterior direction to attach posteriorly on the lateral condyle of the femur. The **posterior cruciate ligament** attaches to the posterior tibia in the intercondylar area and runs in a superior and anterior direction on the medial side of the anterior cruciate ligament. It attaches to the anterior femur on the medial condyle. To summarize these attachments, the anterior cruciate runs from anterior tibia to posterior femur, and the posterior cruciate runs from posterior tibia to anterior femur.

The cruciates provide stability in the sagittal plane. The anterior cruciate ligament keeps the femur from being displaced posteriorly on the tibia or, conversely, the tibia from being displaced anteriorly on the femur. It tightens during extension, preventing excessive hyperextension of the knee. When the knee is partly flexed, the anterior cruciate keeps the tibia from being moved anteriorly. Conversely, the posterior cruciate ligament keeps the femur from being displaced anteriorly on the tibia or the tibia from being displaced posteriorly on the femur. It tightens during flexion and is injured much less frequently than is the anterior cruciate ligament.

Located on the sides of the knee are the collateral ligaments. The **medial collateral,** or **tibial collateral, ligament** is a flat, broad ligament attaching to the medial condyles of the femur and tibia. Fibers of the medial meniscus are attached to this ligament, which contributes to frequent tearing of the medial meniscus when there is excessive stress to the medial collateral ligament. On the lateral side is the **lateral collateral,** or **fibular collateral, ligament.** It is a round, cordlike ligament

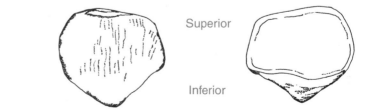

Superior

Inferior

FIGURE 17–10. The patella.   Anterior surface   Posterior surface

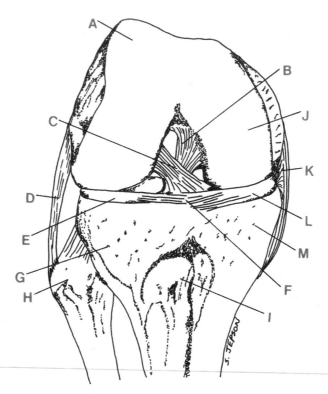

FIGURE 17–11. The right knee in flexion, anterior view.

Lateral Side

A Lateral condyle of the femur
B Posterior cruciate ligament
C Anterior cruciate ligament
D Lateral collateral ligament
E Lateral meniscus
F Transverse ligament
G Lateral condyle of the tibia

H Head of the fibula
I Tibial tuberosity

Medial Side

J Medial condyle of the femur
K Medial collateral ligament
L Medial meniscus
M Medial condyle of the tibia

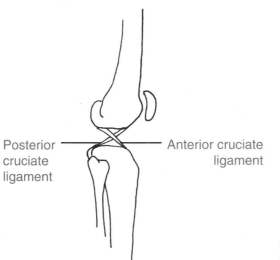

Posterior cruciate ligament

Anterior cruciate ligament

FIGURE 17–12. Cruciate ligaments are named for their attachment on the tibia.

that attaches to the lateral condyle of the femur and runs down to the head of the fibula, independent of any attachment to the lateral meniscus. It protects the joint from stresses to the medial side of the knee. It is quite strong and not commonly injured.

The collateral ligaments provide stability in the frontal plane. The medial collateral ligament, providing medial stability, prevents excessive motion from a blow to the lateral side of the knee. The lateral collateral ligament provides just the opposite stability. Because their attachments are offset posteriorly and superiorly to the axis of flexion, the collateral ligaments become tight during extension, contributing to the stability of the knee, and slack during flexion.

The **medial** and **lateral meniscus** are two half moon, wedge-shaped fibrocartilage disks located on the superior surface of the tibia and are designed to absorb shock (Fig. 17–13). Because they are thicker laterally and the proximal surfaces are concave, the menisci deepen the relatively flat joint surface. The medial meniscus, perhaps because of its attachment to the medial collateral ligament, is more frequently torn. Shock absorption is another function of the menisci.

The purpose of a bursa is to reduce friction, and approximately 13 are located at the knee joint. They are needed because the many tendons located around the knee have a relatively vertical line of pull against bony areas or other tendons. Figure 17–14 illustrates most of the bursae around the knee. Table 17–1 summarizes the most commonly discussed bursae.

The **popliteal space** is the area behind the knee, and it contains important nerves (tibial and common peroneal) and blood vessels (popliteal artery). This diamond-shaped fossa is bound superiorly on the medial side by the semitendinosus and semimembranosus muscles and by the biceps femoris muscle on the lateral side (Fig. 17–15). The inferior boundaries are the medial and lateral heads of the gastrocnemius muscle.

The **pes anserine** (Latin, meaning "goose foot") **muscle group** is made up of the sartorius, gracilis, and the semitendinosus (Fig. 17–16) muscles. Each has a different proximal attachment. The sartorius muscle arises anteriorly from the iliac spine, the gracilis muscle medially from the pubis, and the semitendionosus muscle posteriorly from the ischial tuberosity. They all cross the knee posteriorly and medially, then join together to have a common distal attachment on the anteromedial surface of the proximal tibia. Orthopedic surgeons sometimes alter this common attachment to provide for medial stability to the knee.

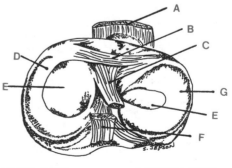

FIGURE 17–13. Right knee, superior view.

A Quadriceps tendon	**E** Articular surface of the tibia
B Transverse ligament	
C Anterior cruciate ligament	**F** Posterior cruciate ligament
D Medial meniscus	**G** Lateral meniscus

MEDIAL SIDE   LATERAL SIDE

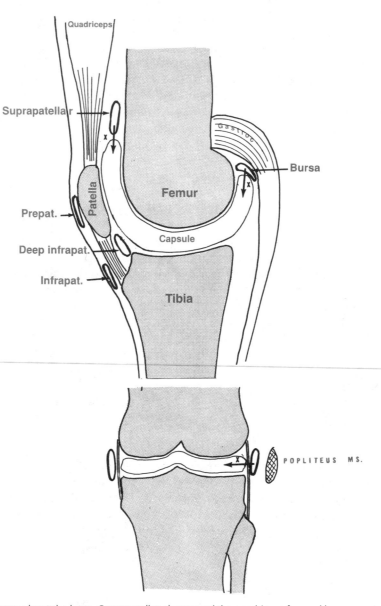

FIGURE 17–14. Bursae about the knee. *Suprapatellar,* also termed the quadriceps femoral bursa, may communicate with the knee capsule. *Prepatellar,* between the skin and the patella; *Infrapatellar* (superficial), between skin and patellar tendon. *Deep Infrapatellar,* between patellar tendon and tibia; and bursae between the lateral head of the gastrocnemius and the joint capsule, the fibular collateral ligament and the biceps or popliteal tendon, and the popliteal tendon and the lateral femoral condyle. *X* indicates possible communication with the joint capsule. (Adapted from Cailliet, R: Knee Pain and Disability. FA Davis, Philadelphia, 1973, p 31, with permission.)

TABLE 17–1	BURSAE OF THE KNEE

Name	Location
ANTERIOR	
Subcutaneous prepatellar	Between the patella and skin
Deep infrapatellar	Between proximal tibia and patellar ligament
Subcutaneous infrapatellar	Between tibial tuberosity and skin
Suprapatellar*	Between distal femur and quadriceps tendon
POSTERIOR	
Gastrocnemius*	Between lateral head of gastrocnemius muscle and capsule
Biceps	Between fibular collateral ligament and biceps tendon
Popliteal*	Between popliteus tendon and lateral femoral condyle
Gastrocnemius*	Between medial head of gastrocnemius muscle and capsule
Semimembranosus	Between tendon of semimembranosus muscle and head of tibia

*Communicates with knee joint

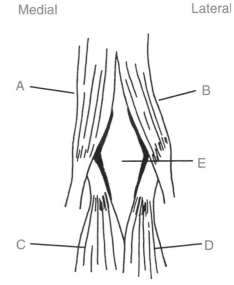

FIGURE 17–15. Boundaries of the right popliteal space.

A Semimembranosus and semitendinosus muscles
B Biceps femoris muscle
C Gastrocnemius muscle (medial)
D Gastrocnemius muscle (lateral)
E Popliteal space

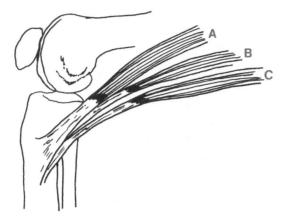

FIGURE 17–16. The pes anserine. (*A*) Sartorius muscle. (*B*) Gracilis muscle. (*C*) Semitendinosus muscle.

Muscles of the Knee

Many of the two-joint muscles of the knee were discussed with the hip. Further clarification of these muscles, however, does need to be made. Table 17–2 shows the muscles that cross the knee, although not all have a major function.

ANTERIOR MUSCLES

The quadriceps muscles comprise four muscles that cross the anterior surface of the knee (Fig. 17–17). The **rectus femoris muscle** was described in Chapter 16 as originating from the anterior inferior iliac spine (**AIIS**) and superficially descending the thigh in the midline. The **vastus lateralis muscle** is located lateral to the rectus femoris muscle. It originates from the linea aspera of the femur, and spans the thigh laterally to join the other quadriceps muscles at the patella. The **vastus medialis muscle** also comes from the linea aspera, but spans the thigh medially. Located deep

TABLE 17–2	MUSCLES OF THE KNEE	
Area	**One-Joint Muscle**	**Two-Joint Muscle**
Anterior	Vastus lateralis	Rectus femoris
	Vastus medialis	
	Vastus intermedialis	
Posterior	Biceps femoris (short)	Biceps femoris (long)
	Popliteus	Semimembranosus
		Semitendinosus
		Sartorius
		Gracilis
		Gastrocnemius
Lateral		Tensor fascia latae

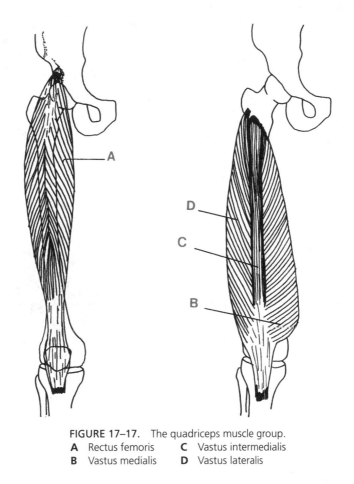

FIGURE 17–17. The quadriceps muscle group.
A Rectus femoris   **C** Vastus intermedialis
B Vastus medialis   **D** Vastus lateralis

to the rectus femoris muscle is the **vastus intermedialis muscle.** It arises from the anterior surface of the femur and spans the thigh anteriorly. It blends together with the other vasti muscles along its length. All four quadriceps muscles attach to the base of the patella and the tibial tuberosity via the patellar tendon. Because all four muscles span the knee anteriorly, they all extend the knee. Because the rectus femoris muscle also spans the hip anteriorly, it flexes the hip.

Rectus Femoris Muscle

(O)	AIIS
(I)	Tibial tuberosity via patellar tendon
(A)	Hip flexion, knee extension
(N)	Femoral nerve (L2, L3, L4)

Vastus Lateralis Muscle

(O)	Linea aspera
(I)	Tibial tuberosity via patellar tendon
(A)	Knee extension
(N)	Femoral nerve (L2, L3, L4)

Vastus Medialis Muscle

(O)	Linea aspera
(I)	Tibial tuberosity via patellar tendon
(A)	Knee extension
(N)	Femoral nerve (L2, L3, L4)

Vastus Intermedialis Muscle

(O)	Anterior femur
(I)	Tibial tuberosity via patellar tendon
(A)	Knee extension
(N)	Femoral nerve (L2, L3, L4)

POSTERIOR MUSCLES

Three muscles that are known collectively as the hamstring muscles cover the posterior thigh. They consist of the semitendinosus, the semimembranosus, and the biceps femoris muscles (Fig. 17–18). Because they were described in Chapter 16, they will only be summarized here.

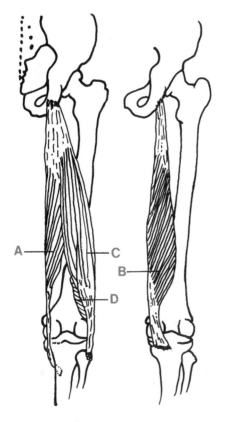

FIGURE 17–18. The hamstring muscle group.
A Semitendinosus
B Semimembranosus
C Biceps femoris, long head
D Biceps femoris, short head

Semimembranosus Muscle

(O)   Ischial tuberosity
(I)   Posterior surface of medial condyle of tibia
(A)   Extend hip and flex knee
(N)   Sciatic nerve (L5, S1, S2)

Semitendinosus Muscle

(O)   Ischial tuberosity
(I)   Anteromedial surface of proximal tibia
(A)   Extend hip and flex knee
(N)   Sciatic nerve (L5, S1, S2)

Biceps Femoris Muscle

(O)   Long head: ischial tuberosity
Short head: lateral lip of linea aspera
(I)   Fibular head
(A)   Long head: extend hip and flex knee
Short head: flex knee
(N)   Long head: sciatic nerve (L5, S1, S2)
Short head: common peroneal nerve (L5, S1, S2)

The **popliteus muscle** is a one-joint muscle located posteriorly at the knee in the popliteal space deep to the two heads of the gastrocnemius muscles (Fig. 17–19). It originates on the lateral side of the lateral condyle of the femur and crosses the knee posteriorly at an oblique angle to insert medially on the posterior proximal tibia. Because it spans the knee posteriorly, it flexes the knee. It is credited with "unlocking" the knee, or initiating knee flexion.

Popliteus Muscle

(O)   Lateral condyle of femur
(I)   Posterior medial condyle of tibia
(A)   Initiates knee flexion
(N)   Tibial nerve (L4, L5, S1)

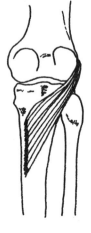

FIGURE 17–19. The popliteus muscle.

The **gastrocnemius muscle** is a two-joint muscle that crosses the knee and the ankle (Fig. 17–20). It is an extremely strong ankle plantar flexor but also has a significant role at the knee. It attaches by two heads to the posterior surface of the medial and lateral condyles of the femur. After descending the posterior calf superficially, it forms a common tendon with the soleus muscle and attaches to the posterior surface of the calcaneus. Although its major function is at the ankle, it does span the knee posteriorly, has a good angle of pull, and is a large muscle. Therefore, its contribution as a knee flexor cannot be overlooked. Its unusual contribution to knee *extension* has been demonstrated in individuals with no quadriceps muscle function (Fig. 17–21). In a closed kinetic chain action with the foot planted on the ground so that the distal segment (leg) is stationary, the proximal segment (thigh) becomes the movable part. This is also a reversal of muscle action, in which the femur is pulled posteriorly, or into knee extension. This feature of the gastrocnemius muscle makes it possible for a person to stand upright without the use of quadriceps muscles.

Gastrocnemius Muscle

(O)	Medial and lateral condyles of femur
(I)	Posterior calcaneus
(A)	Knee flexion, ankle plantar flexion
(N)	Tibial nerve (S1, S2)

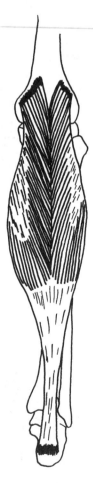

FIGURE 17–20. The gastrocnemius muscle.

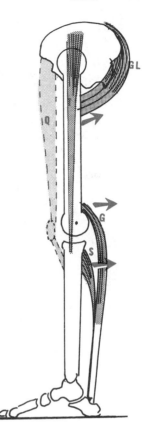

FIGURE 17–21. The gastrocnemius muscle as a knee extensor. With a nonfunctioning quadriceps, stance is possible by gluteus maximus and gastrocnemius action. In the weight-bearing position, the two muscles contract, pulling the knee into extension. The soleus assist the gastrocnemius. (Adapted from Cailliet, R: Knee Pain and Disability. FA Davis, Philadelphia, 1973, p 30, with permission.)

Q	Quadriceps	**G**	Gastrocnemius
T	Tensor fascia latae	**S**	Soleus
GL	Gluteus maximus		

The gracilis, sartorius, and tensor fascia latae muscles span the knee joint posteriorly, but because of their angle of pull, size in relation to other muscles, and other such factors, they do not have a prime-mover function. They do, however, provide stability to the joint.

The **tensor fascia latae muscle** spans the knee laterally essentially in the middle of the joint axis for flexion and extension. It contributes greatly to lateral stability. The **gracilis** and **sartorius muscles** span the knee medially, contributing greatly to medial stability. The gastrocnemius and hamstring muscles provide posterior stability both medially and laterally, and the quadriceps muscles provide anterior stability.

SUMMARY OF MUSCLE ACTION

The actions of the prime movers of the knee are summarized in Table 17–3.

SUMMARY OF MUSCLE INNERVATION

The femoral and sciatic nerves play a major part in the innervation of the knee joint. The femoral nerve innervates the quadriceps muscle group, and the sciatic nerve innervates the hamstring muscle group. The only exception to this is the short head of the biceps femoris muscle, which receives innervation from the common peroneal nerve.

TABLE 17–3	PRIME MOVERS OF THE KNEE
Action	**Muscle**
Extension	Quadriceps group
	Rectus femoris
	Vastus medialis
	Vastus intermedialis
	Vastus lateralis
Flexion	Hamstring group
	Semimembranosus
	Semitendinosus
	Biceps femoris
	Popliteus
	Gastrocnemius

TABLE 17–4	INNERVATION OF THE MUSCLES OF THE KNEE	
Muscle	**Nerve**	**Spinal Segment**
	QUADRICEPS	
Rectus femoris	Femoral	L2, L3, L4
Vastus lateralis	Femoral	L2, L3, L4
Vastus intermedialis	Femoral	L2, L3, L4
Vastus medialis	Femoral	L2, L3, L4
	HAMSTRINGS	
Semimembranosus	Sciatic	L5, S1, S2
Semitendinosus	Sciatic	L5, S1, S2
Biceps femoris		
Long head	Sciatic	L5, S1, S2
Short head	Common peroneal	L5, S1, S2
	OTHERS	
Popliteus	Tibial	L4, L5, S1
Gastrocnemius	Tibial	S1, S2

TABLE 17–5	SEGMENTAL INNERVATION OF THE KNEE					
Spinal Cord Level	**L2**	**L3**	**L4**	**L5**	**S1**	**S2**
Knee extensors						
Rectus femoris	X	X	X			
Vastus lateralis	X	X	X			
Vastus intermedialis	X	X	X			
Vastus medialis	X	X	X			
Knee flexors						
Popliteus			X	X	X	
Semitendinosus				X	X	X
Semimembranosus				X	X	X
Biceps femoris				X	X	X
Gastrocnemius					X	X

The other two knee flexors, the popliteus and gastrocnemius muscles, receive innervation from the tibial nerve. Not included in this discussion or in Table 17–4 are those two-joint hip muscles that span the knee but do not act as prime movers at the knee. As you can see, the knee extensors receive innervation from the femoral nerve, which comes off the spinal cord at a higher level than the knee flexors. This is significant when dealing with individuals with spinal cord injuries. Tables 17–4 and 17–5 summarize the innervation to the knee. It should be noted that there is some discrepancy among various sources regarding spinal cord level of innervation.

REVIEW QUESTIONS

1. Describe the knee joints:

	Knee	*Patellofemoral*
a. Number of axes:	_____	_____
b. Shape of joint:	_____	_____
c. Type of motion allowed:	_____	_____

2. Describe knee joint motion in terms of planes and axes.

3. What is the "*Q* angle"? Why is it important?

4. Identify the ligaments that provide anterior/posterior stability to the knee.

5. Identify the ligaments that provide medial/lateral stability to the knee.

6. Which bones make up the knee joint?

7. List the muscles that cross the knee anteriorly.

8. List the muscles that cross the knee posteriorly.

9. Why is the action of the popliteus muscle often described as "unlocking" the joint?

10. Which muscles extend the hip and flex the knee?

11. Which muscles flex the hip and extend the knee?

12. Which muscles extend the hip and extend the knee?

13. What is the pes anserine?

14. An individual with a spinal cord injury at L3 would be expected to have what knee motion?

15. What type of kinetic chain activity is demonstrated in Figure 17–21?

16. In Figure 17–21, is either the gastrocnemius or gluteus maximus muscle working in a reversal of muscle action role?

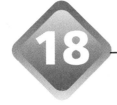

Ankle Joint and Foot

The leg, that portion of the lower extremity extending from the knee to the ankle, is composed of the tibia and fibula. A strong interosseous membrane keeps the two bones together and also provides a greater surface for muscle attachment (Fig. 18–1).

Bones and Landmarks

The tibia, the larger of the two bones is the only true weight-bearing bone of the leg. Triangular in shape, the tibia's apex (crest) is located anteriorly. The long, thin fibula is set back in line with the posterior surface of the tibia (Fig. 18–2). Laterally, this forms a gully, with the interosseous membrane as the floor, permitting attachment of several muscles without distorting the shape of the leg. Tibial landmarks in addition to those discussed in Chapter 17 are as follows:

Crest   Anterior and most prominent of the three borders
Medial malleolus   The enlarged distal medial surface

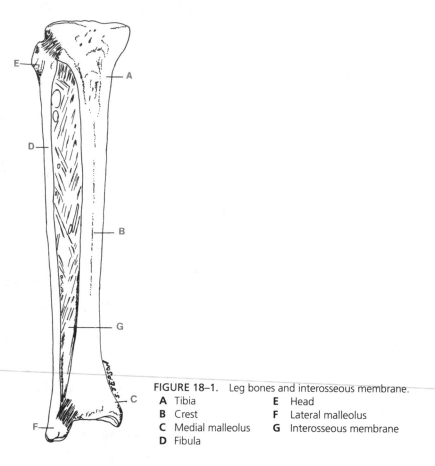

FIGURE 18–1. Leg bones and interosseous membrane.

A	Tibia	**E**	Head
B	Crest	**F**	Lateral malleolus
C	Medial malleolus	**G**	Interosseous membrane
D	Fibula		

The landmarks of the fibula are as follows:

Head	Enlarged proximal end of the bone
Lateral malleolus	Enlarged distal end

The bones of the foot include the tarsals, metatarsals, and phalanges. The seven **tarsal bones** and their landmarks consist of the following (Fig. 18–3):

Calcaneus	Largest and most posterior tarsal bone.
Tuberosity	Projection on the posterior inferior surface of the calcaneus.
Sustentaculum tali	Medial superior part projecting out from the rest of the bone, supporting the medial side of the talus. Three tendons loop around this projection, changing directions from the posterior leg to the plantar foot.
Talus	Sitting on the calcaneus, it is the second largest tarsal.
Navicular	On the medial side in front of the talus and proximal to the three cuneiforms.
Tuberosity	Projection on the navicular; easily seen on the medial border of the foot.
Cuboid	On the lateral side of the foot proximal (superior) to the fourth and fifth metatarsals and distal (inferior) to the calcaneus.

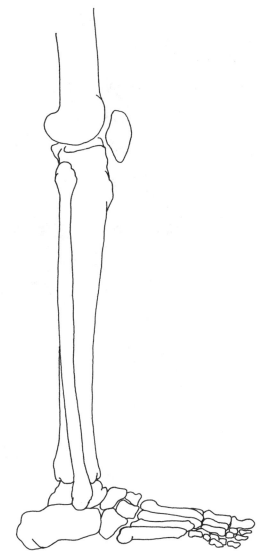

FIGURE 18–2.   Right leg, lateral view. Note the posterior position of the fibula.

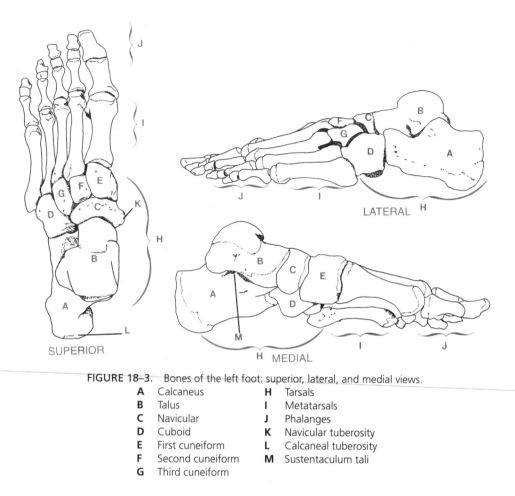

FIGURE 18–3. Bones of the left foot: superior, lateral, and medial views.

A	Calcaneus	**H**	Tarsals
B	Talus	**I**	Metatarsals
C	Navicular	**J**	Phalanges
D	Cuboid	**K**	Navicular tuberosity
E	First cuneiform	**L**	Calcaneal tuberosity
F	Second cuneiform	**M**	Sustentaculum tali
G	Third cuneiform		

Cuneiforms	Three in number; named the first through third, going from the medial toward the lateral side in line with the metatarsals. The first is the largest of the three.

The **metatarsals** are numbered 1 through 5, starting medially (see Fig. 18–3). Normally, the first and fifth metatarsals are weight-bearing bones and the second, third, and fourth are not. We tend to stand on a triangle. Weight is borne from the base of the calcaneus to the heads of the first and fifth metatarsals. The significant features and landmarks of the metatarsals are as follows:

Base	Proximal end of each metatarsal
Head	Distal end of each bone
First	Thickest and shortest metatarsal; located on the medial side of the foot
Second	The longest; articulates with the second cuneiform
Third	Articulates with the third cuneiform
Fourth	With the fifth metatarsal, articulates with the cuboid
Fifth	Has prominent tuberosity located on the lateral side of its base

The **phalanges** of the foot have the same composition as those of the hand (see Fig. 18–3). The first digit, the **great toe,** has a proximal and distal phalanx but no middle phalanx. The second through fifth digits, also called the four lesser toes, each have a proximal, middle, and distal phalanx.

FUNCTIONAL ASPECTS OF THE FOOT

The foot can be divided into three parts (Fig. 18–4). The **hindfoot** is made up of the talus and calcaneus. In the gait cycle, the hindfoot is the first part of the foot that makes contact with the ground, thus influencing the function and movement of the other two parts. The **midfoot** is made up of the navicular and cuboid bones. The mechanics of this part provide stability and mobility to the foot as it transmits movement from the hindfoot to the forefoot. The **forefoot** is made up of the three cuneiforms, five metatarsals, and all of the phalanges. This part of the foot adapts to the level of the ground. It is also the last part of the foot to be in contact with the ground during stance phase.

The ankle joint and foot perform three main functions: acting as a shock absorber as the heel strikes the ground at the beginning of stance phase; adapting to the level (or unevenness) of the ground; and providing a stable base of support from which to propel the body forward.

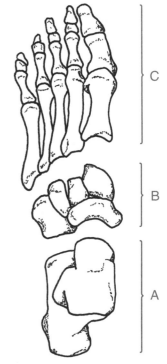

FIGURE 18–4.   Functional areas of the foot.
    A   Hindfoot
    B   Midfoot
    C   Forefoot

Joints and Motions

ANKLE MOTIONS

Motions of the ankle joint and foot need to be defined because there is variation among authors. **Plantar flexion** is movement toward the plantar surface of the foot, whereas **dorsiflexion** is movement toward the dorsal surface of the foot. These motions occur in the sagittal plane. The terms **flexion** and **extension** should not be used because of conflicting definitions. Functionally speaking, *plantar flexion* is the same as extension, part of the general extension movement of the hip, knee, and ankle. However, anatomically speaking, *dorsiflexion* is the same as extension, meaning movement toward the extensor side of the foot.

Movement in the frontal plane is called inversion and eversion. **Inversion** is the raising of the medial border of the foot, or rotation at the tarsal joints turning the forefoot inward. **Eversion,** the opposite motion, is the raising of the lateral border of the foot, or rotation of the tarsal joints turning the forefoot outward. Movement in the transverse plane is called **adduction** and **abduction.** These motions occur in the forefoot (Fig. 18–5), and accompany inversion and eversion, respectively.

In recent years, clinicians have begun using supination and pronation to describe ankle joint and foot motion. **Supination** describes a combination of plantar flexion, inversion and adduction, and **pronation** describes a combination of dorsiflexion, ever-

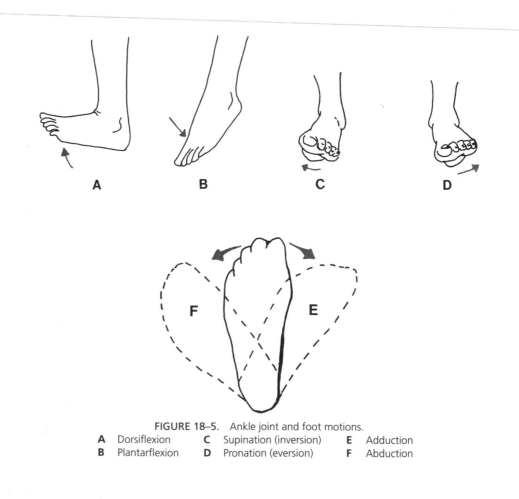

FIGURE 18–5. Ankle joint and foot motions.

A Dorsiflexion	**C** Supination (inversion)	**E** Adduction
B Plantarflexion	**D** Pronation (eversion)	**F** Abduction

sion, and abduction. To avoid further confusion of terms, valgus and varus must be defined. These terms are more commonly used to describe a *position,* usually an abnormal one. **Valgus** refers to a position in which the distal segment is positioned away from the midline. Conversely, **varus** refers to a position in which the distal segment is positioned toward the midline. Therefore, a calcaneal valgus is a position in which the distal (inferior) part of the calcaneus is angled away from the midline (Fig. 18–6). These terms will not be used here because *motion,* not *position,* is the emphasis.

In summary, the terminology commonly used by clinicians to describe ankle and foot motions are: dorsiflexion, plantar flexion, supination (combination of plantar flexion, inversion, and forefoot adduction), and pronation (combination of dorsiflexion, eversion, and forefoot abduction). These motions are illustrated in Figure 18–5. However, when describing muscle action, inversion and eversion are used in place of supination and pronation, respectively.

Two joints with little motion that are not part of the true ankle joint but play a small role in the proper function of the ankle are the tibiofibular joints (Fig. 18–7). The **superior tibiofibular joint** is the articulation between the head of the fibula and the posterior lateral aspect of the proximal tibia. It is a uniaxial plane joint. Being a synovial joint, it has a joint capsule. Ligaments reinforce the capsule. The gliding motion present is relatively small. The **inferior tibiofibular joint** is a syndesmosis (fibrous union) between the distal tibia, which is concave, and the distal fibula, which is convex. Because it is not a synovial joint, there is no joint capsule. However, there is fibrous tissue separating the bones and several ligaments holding the joint together. Much of the strength of the ankle joint is dependent upon a strong union at this joint.

ANKLE JOINTS

The true **ankle joint** (*talocrural joint* or *talotibial joint*) is made up of the distal tibia sitting on the talus with the medial malleolus of the tibia fitting down around the medial aspect of the talus, and the lateral malleolus of the fibula fitting down around the lateral aspect. This type of joint often is described using a carpentry term as a *tenon and mortise joint.* A mortise is a notch cut in a piece of wood to receive a projecting piece (tenon) shaped to fit. Therefore, the tibia and fibula would be the mortise, and the talus would be the tenon (Fig. 18–8).

To summarize, the ankle is a uniaxial hinge joint consisting of articulation between the distal end and medial malleolus of the tibia and the lateral malleolus of the fibula with the talus. The ankle joint allows approximately 30 to 50 degrees of plantar flexion and 20 degrees of dorsiflexion. In the anatomical position, the ankle is in a neutral position. Because the axis of rotation is at an angle, it is considered **triplanar,** a term used to describe motion around an obliquely oriented axis that passes through all three planes.

The **subtalar,** or **talocalcaneal, joint** consists of the inferior surface of the talus articulating with the superior surface of the calcaneus. This joint has a primarily gliding motion (Fig. 18–9). The anterior surfaces of the talus and calcaneus articulating with the posterior surfaces of the navicular and the cuboid, respectively, make up the **transverse tarsal joint** (midtarsal joint) (Fig. 18–10). However, very little movement occurs between the navicular and the cuboid. Pronation and supination, which are motions between the hindfoot and forefoot, occur here and are triplanar motions.

Functionally, the subtalar and transverse tarsal joints cannot be separated. Therefore, supination and pronation are actually combinations of motions. Supina-

Medial   Lateral

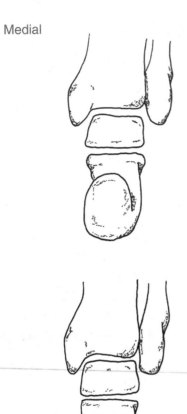

A

B

C

FIGURE 18–6.   Calcaneal positions.
    A   Neutral
    B   Calcaneal valgus
    C   Calcaneal varus

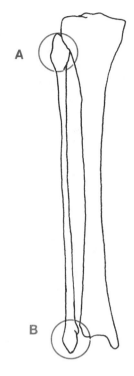

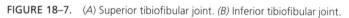

FIGURE 18–7.   (*A*) Superior tibiofibular joint. (*B*) Inferior tibiofibular joint.

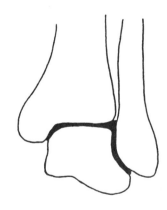

FIGURE 18–8.   Ankle joint.

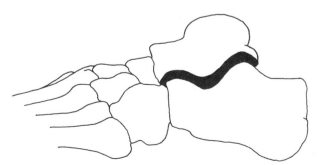

FIGURE 18–9.   Subtalar joint.

tion, is a combination of inversion, adduction, and plantar flexion. Pronation is the reverse combination of eversion, abduction, and dorsiflexion.

Therefore, when the ankle is described as moving in plantar flexion and dorsiflexion, these motions are occurring at the talocrural joint. When the ankle moves in inversion and eversion, these motions are occurring at the subtalar and transverse tarsal joints.

FOOT JOINTS

The **metatarsophalangeal (MTP) joints** consist of the metatarsal heads articulating with the proximal phalanges (Fig. 18–11). Like the metacarpophalangeal joints of the hand, there are five joints allowing flexion, extension, hyperextension, abduction, and adduction (Fig. 18–12). The first MTP joint is much more mobile. It allows approximately 45 degrees flexion and extension, and 90 degrees of hyperextension. The second through fifth MTP joints allow about 40 degrees of flexion and extension, and only about 45 degrees of hyperextension. This hyperextension is very important during the toe-off phase of walking. The point of reference for abduction and adduction is the second toe. Like the middle finger of the hand, the second toe abducts in both directions but adducts only as a return motion from abduction.

Also like the hand, there is a **proximal interphalangeal (PIP)** and **distal interphalangeal (DIP) joint** on each of the lesser toes (two through five). Because there is less dexterity required of the foot, these joints individually are not as significant as in the hand. The great toe has a proximal and distal phalanx but no middle phalange. Therefore, it has only one joint, the **interphalangeal (IP) joint** (see Fig. 18–11).

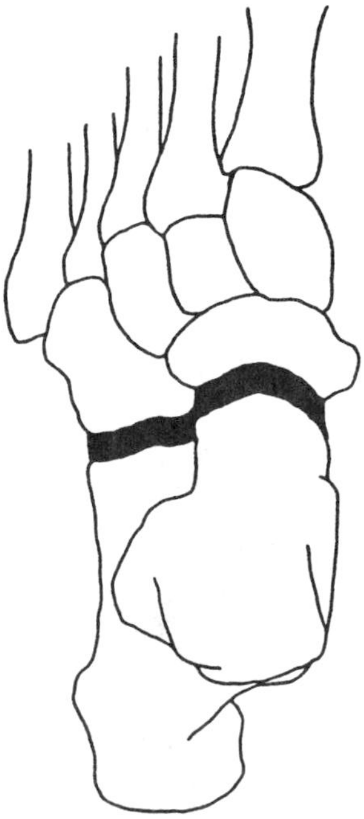

FIGURE 18–10. Transverse tarsal joint.

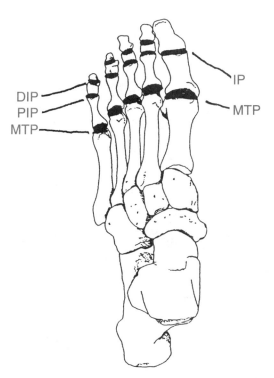

FIGURE 18–11. Joints of the phalanges of the foot. (DIP = distal interphalangeal; PIP = proximal interphalangeal; MTP = metatarsophalangeal; IP = interphalangeal.)

Ligaments and Other Structures

The ankle joint, a synovial joint, has a **joint capsule.** This capsule is rather thin anteriorly and posteriorly but is reinforced by collateral ligaments on the sides. These collateral ligaments are actually groups of several ligaments. On the medial side is a triangular-shaped **deltoid ligament** whose apex is located along the tip of the medial malleolus with a broad base spreading out to attach to the talus, navicular, and calcaneus in four parts (Figs. 18–13 and 18–14). The most anterior fibers attach to the navicular (tibionavicular ligament). The middle fibers (tibiocalcaneal ligament) descend directly to the sustentaculum tali of the calcaneus. The posterior fibers (posterior tibiotalar ligament) run backward to the talus. The deep fibers (anterior tibio-

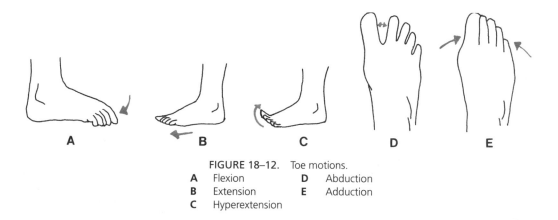

FIGURE 18–12. Toe motions.

A Flexion	**D** Abduction
B Extension	**E** Adduction
C Hyperextension	

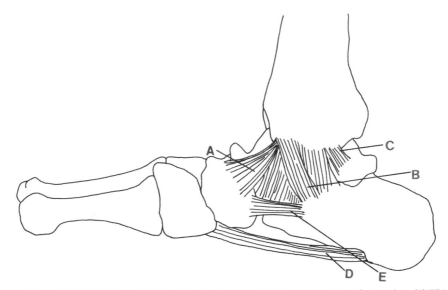

FIGURE 18–13. Ligaments of the medial ankle. Deltoid ligament: (*A*) Tibionavicular portion. (*B*) Tibiocalcaneal portion. (*C*) Posterior tibiotalaris portion. Note: The anterior tibiotalar portion of the deltoid ligament lies deep and is not visible in this view. Other ligaments: (*D*) long plantar ligaments; (*E*) spring ligament. (Adapted from Kessler, RM and Hurtling, D: Management of Common Musculoskeletal Disorders. Lippincott, Philadelphia, 1983, p 457.)

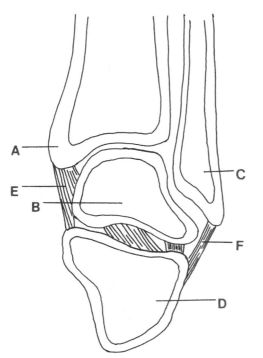

FIGURE 18–14. Frontal section through the ankle and subtalar joints. (Adapted from Kessler, RM and Hertling, D: Management of Common Musculoskeletal Disorders. Lippincott, Philadelphia, 1983, p 456.)

A Medial malleolus	**D**	Calcaneus
B Talus	**E**	Deltoid ligament
C Fibula	**F**	Calcaneofibular ligament

talar ligament) cannot be seen from the medial side because they are deep to the tibiocalcaneal portion. The deltoid ligament strengthens the medial side of the ankle joint, holds the calcaneus and navicular against the talus, and helps to maintain the medial longitudinal arch.

On the lateral side of the ankle joint is a group of three ligaments commonly referred to as the **lateral ligament** (Fig. 18–15). This ligament consists of three parts connecting the lateral malleolus to the talus and calcaneus. The rather weak anterior talofibular ligament attaches the lateral malleolus to the talus. Posteriorly, the fairly strong posterior talofibular ligament runs almost horizontally to connect the lateral malleolus to the talus. In the middle is the long and fairly vertical calcaneofibular ligament that attaches the malleolus to the calcaneus. The ankle is considered the most frequently injured joint in the body and the lateral ligament is the most frequently injured ligament. One or more of its three parts may be stretched or torn.

Numerous other ligaments attach the various tarsals to each other, to the metatarsals, and so on. They tend to be named for the bones to which they attach. Their individual names and locations will not be discussed here.

ARCHES

Because the foot is the usual point of impact with the ground, it must be able to absorb a great deal of shock, adjust to changes in terrain, and propel the body forward during movement. To allow these things to occur, the bones of the foot are arranged in arches. We tend to stand on a triangle with weight bearing borne from the base of the calcaneus to the heads of the first and fifth metatarsals (Fig. 18–16). Between these three points we have two arches (medial and lateral longitudinal) (Fig. 18–17) at right angles to the third (transverse) arch (Fig. 18–18).

The **medial longitudinal arch** makes up the medial border of the foot running from the calcaneus posteriorly through the talus, navicular, and three cuneiforms anteriorly to the first three metatarsals. The talus is at the top of the arch and often referred to as the *keystone* because it receives the weight of the body. A keystone is

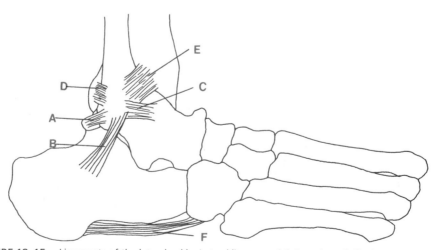

FIGURE 18–15. Ligaments of the lateral ankle. Lateral ligament: (*A*) Posterior talofibular portion. (*B*) Calcaneofibular portion. (*C*) Anterior talofibular portion. Other ligaments: (*D*) posterior tibiofibular ligament; (*E*) anterior tibiofibular ligament; (*F*) long plantar ligament. (Adapted from Kessler, RM and Hertling, D: Management of Common Musculoskeletal Disorders. Lippincott, Philadelphia, 1983, p 455.)

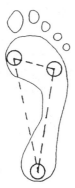

FIGURE 18–16.   The main weight-bearing surfaces of the foot.

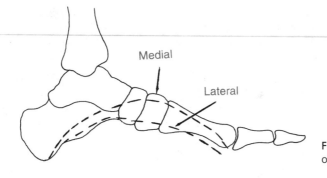

FIGURE 18–17.   Longitudinal arches of the foot.

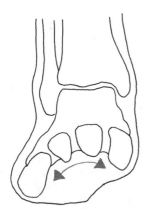

FIGURE 18–18.   Transverse arch of the foot.

an essential part of an arch, usually the central or topmost, part. This arch depresses somewhat during weight bearing and then recoils when the weight is removed. Normally it never touches the ground.

The **lateral longitudinal arch** runs from the calcaneus anteriorly through the cuboid to the fourth and fifth metatarsals. It normally rests on the ground during weight bearing. The **transverse arch** runs from side to side through the three cuneiforms to the cuboid. The second cuneiform is the keystone of this arch.

These three arches are maintained by (1) the shape of the bones and their relation to each other, (2) the plantar ligaments and aponeurosis (Figs. 18–19 and 18–20), and (3) muscles. The ligaments and aponeurosis are perhaps the most important features. The **spring ligament** (plantar calcaneonavicular) attaches to the calcaneus and runs forward to the navicular. It is short, wide, and most important because it supports the medial side of the longitudinal arch.

The **long plantar ligament,** the longest of the tarsal ligaments, is more superficial than the spring ligament. It attaches posteriorly to the calcaneus and runs forward to attach on the cuboid and bases of the third, fourth, and fifth metatarsals. It is the primary support of the lateral longitudinal arch. The long plantar ligament is assisted by the **short plantar ligament,** which also attaches the calcaneus to the cuboid. The longitudinal arch is further supported by the **plantar aponeurosis,** which runs from the calcaneus forward to the proximal phalanges. It acts as a tie rod, keeping the posterior segments (calcaneus and talus) from separating from the anterior portion (anterior tarsals and metatarsal heads).

The arches also are supported by muscles, mainly the invertors and evertors of the foot. The tibialis posterior, flexor hallucis longus, and flexor digitorum longus muscles all span the ankle posteriorly on the medial side, passing under the sustentaculum tali of the calcaneus. Thus, they give some support to the medial side of the foot. The flexor hallucis longus and flexor digitorum longus muscles span the medial longitudinal arch and help support it. The peroneus longus muscle spans the foot from the lateral to the medial side providing support to the transverse and lateral longitudinal arches. However, the total muscular support to the arches has been estimated to bear only about 15 to 20 percent of the total stress to the arches.

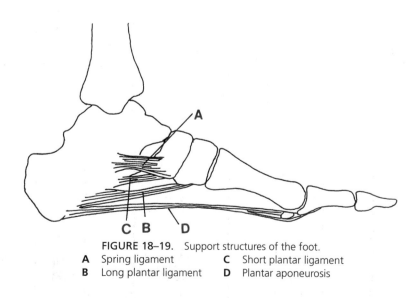

FIGURE 18–19.   Support structures of the foot.
A   Spring ligament   **C**   Short plantar ligament
B   Long plantar ligament   **D**   Plantar aponeurosis

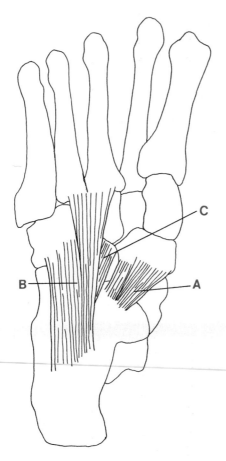

FIGURE 18–20. Inferior view of the foot. (*A*) Spring ligaments. (*B*) Long plantar ligament. (*C*) Short plantar ligament. (Adapted from Kessler, RM and Hertling, D: Management of Common Musculoskeletal Disorders. Lippincott, Philadelphia, 1983, p 454.)

Muscles of the Ankle and Foot

EXTRINSIC MUSCLES

As with the wrist and hand, there are extrinsic and intrinsic muscles in the ankle and foot. The extrinsic muscles originate on the leg, and the intrinsic muscles originate on the tarsal bones. The extrinsic muscles of the leg are found in groups of three or combinations of three and are located in three anatomical areas. All have proximal attachments on the femur, tibia, or fibula, and all cross the ankle joint. Table 18–1 summarizes these muscles.

Superior Posterior Group

The superficial posterior group includes the gastrocnemius, soleus, and plantaris muscles. Because the gastrocnemius muscle was described in Chapter 17, it will only be summarized here (Fig. 18–21). Its proximal attachment is posterior on the condyles of the femur, and its distal attachment is via the large Achilles' tendon to the posterior calcaneus.

TABLE 18–1	**EXTRINSIC MUSCLES OF THE ANKLE AND FOOT**	
Muscle	**Joint Crossing**	**Possible Actions**
Posterior Superficial Group		
Gastrocnemius	Posterior	Plantar flexion
Soleus	Posterior	Plantar flexion
Plantaris	Posterior	Plantar flexion
Posterior Deep Group		
Tibialis posterior	Posterior, medial	Plantar flexion, inversion
Flexor digitorum longus	Posterior, medial	Plantar flexion, inversion, toe flexion
Flexor hallucis longus	Posterior, medial	Plantar flexion, inversion, toe flexion
Anterior Group		
Tibialis anterior	Anterior, medial	Dorsiflexion, inversion
Extensor hallucis longus	Anterior, medial	Dorsiflexion, inversion, great toe extension
Extensor digitorum longus	Anterior	Dorsiflexion, lesser toe extension
Lateral Group		
Peroneus longus	Posterior, lateral	Plantar flexion, eversion
Peroneus brevis	Posterior, lateral	Plantar flexion, eversion
Peroneus tertius	Anterior	Dorsiflexion, eversion

Gastrocnemius Muscle

(O)   Medial head: medial condyle of femur
Lateral head: lateral condyle of femur
(I)   Posterior calcaneus
(A)   Knee flexion; ankle plantar flexion
(N)   Tibial nerve (S1, S2)

The **soleus** muscle is a large, one-joint muscle located deep to the gastrocnemius muscle (Fig. 18–22). Originating on the posterior tibia and fibula, it spans the posterior leg blending with the gastrocnemius muscle to form the large, strong Achilles' tendon that inserts on the posterior calcaneus. Because the soleus muscle spans the ankle in the midline, its only function is to plantar flex the ankle. The two heads of the gastrocnemius and soleus muscles make up what is sometimes referred to as the triceps surae muscle, meaning "three-headed calf muscle."

Soleus Muscle

(O)   Posterior tibia and fibula
(I)   Posterior calcaneus
(A)   Ankle plantar flexion
(N)   Tibial nerve (S1, S2)

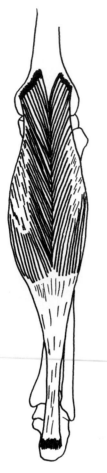

FIGURE 18–21. The gastrocnemius muscle.

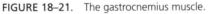

The **plantaris** muscle is a long, thin, two-joint muscle with no significant function (see Fig. 18–22). It originates on the posterior surface of the lateral epicondyle of the femur, spans the posterior leg medially, and blends with the gastrocnemius and soleus muscles in the Achilles' tendon. Theoretically, it should flex the knee and plantar flex the ankle. However, because of its size in relation to the prime movers of those actions, it is assistive at best.

Plantaris Muscle	
(O)	Posterior lateral condyle of femur
(I)	Posterior calcaneus
(A)	Very weak assist in knee flexion; ankle plantar flexion
(N)	Tibial nerve (L4, L5, S1)

Deep Posterior Group

The deep posterior group is made up of the tibialis posterior, flexor hallucis longus, and flexor digitorum longus muscles. They all attach to the posterior tibia and/or fibula, and all terminate in the foot. Because they all cross the ankle posteriorly, they all plantar flex it. However, because of their size in relation to the soleus and gastrocnemius muscles, they are only assistive.

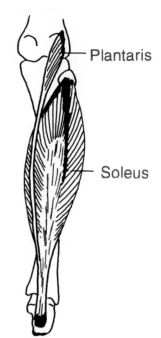

FIGURE 18–22. The soleus and plantaris muscles.

The **tibialis posterior** muscle is the deepest lying posterior muscle with its proximal attachment on the interosseous membrane and adjacent portions of the tibia and fibula (Fig. 18–23). It descends on the posterior aspect of the leg, looping around the medial malleolus to attach on the navicular with fibrous expansions to the cuboid, the three cuneiforms, sustentaculum tali of the calcaneus, and the bases of the second through fourth metatarsals. Because the tibialis posterior muscle crosses the ankle medially and posteriorly, it can plantar flex and invert. Because of its size in relation to the other plantar flexors, it is assistive in this action.

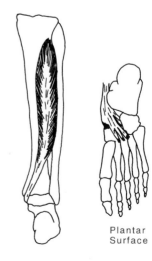

Plantar
Surface

FIGURE 18–23. The tibialis posterior muscle.

Tibialis Posterior Muscle

(O)	Interosseous membrane, adjacent tibia and fibula
(I)	Navicular and most tarsals and metatarsals
(A)	Ankle inversion; assists in plantar flexion
(N)	Tibial nerve (L5, S1)

Situated mostly on the lateral side of the leg, the **flexor hallucis longus** muscle arises from the posterior fibula and interosseous membrane. It descends the leg posteriorly, loops around the medial malleolus through a groove in the posterior talus, and goes under the sustentaculum tali of the calcaneus. This muscle travels down the foot through the two heads of the flexor hallucis brevis muscle to attach at the base of the distal phalanx of the great toe (Fig. 18–24). This distal attachment is similar to the flexor digitorum profundus and superficialis muscles in the hand. The flexor hallucis longus muscle flexes the great toe and assists in inversion and, to a lesser degree, assists in plantar flexion of the ankle.

Flexor Hallucis Longus Muscle

(O)	Posterior fibula and interosseous membrane
(I)	Distal phalanx of the great toe
(A)	Flexes great toe; assists in inversion and plantar flexion of the ankle
(N)	Tibial nerve (L5, S1, S2)

Situated mostly on the medial side of the leg, the **flexor digitorum longus** muscle arises from the posterior tibia (Fig. 18–25). It descends the leg posteriorly, loops around the medial malleolus, and runs down the foot, splitting into four tendons to insert into the distal phalanx of the second through fifth toes. This muscle passes through the split in the flexor digitorum brevis tendon in a similar fashion to the flexor digitorum profundus muscle, which goes through the split in the flexor digitorum superficialis muscle in the hand. It flexes the four lesser toes and assists in inversion and plantar flexion of the ankle.

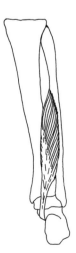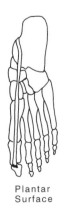

Plantar
Surface

FIGURE 18–24.   The flexor hallucis longus muscle.

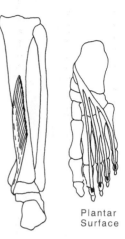

Plantar
Surface

FIGURE 18–25.   The flexor digitorum longus muscle.

Flexor Digitorum Longus Muscle	
(O)	Posterior tibia
(I)	Distal phalanx of four lesser toes
(A)	Flexes the four lesser toes; assists in ankle inversion and plantar flexion of the ankle
(N)	Tibial nerve (L5, S1)

The relationships among the deep posterior muscles are interesting, crossing and intertwining with one another from their proximal to distal attachments. This feature provides added strength, much like a braided rope, which is stronger than one whose individual fibers run parallel to one another. Table 18–2 summarizes this changing relationship.

Anterior Group

The anterior muscle group is made up of the tibialis anterior, extensor hallucis longus, and the extensor digitorum longus muscles. They all attach proximally on the anterolateral leg and cross the ankle anteriorly.

The **tibialis anterior** muscle originates on the lateral side of the tibia and interosseous membrane, descends the leg to insert medially on the first cuneiform and base of the first metatarsal (Fig. 18–26). It makes up most of the bulk of the anterolateral leg. Because the tibialis anterior muscle spans the ankle anteriorly and medially, it dorsiflexes and inverts the ankle.

TABLE 18–2	**DEEP POSTERIOR GROUP**				
Location				**Relationship**	
Origin (medial to lateral)		FDL	TP		FHL
Medial malleolus (superior to inferior)		TP	FDL		FHL
Insertion (medial to lateral)		FHL	TP		FDL

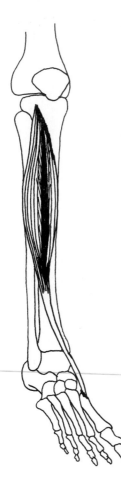

FIGURE 18–26. The tibialis anterior muscle.

Tibialis Anterior Muscle

(O)   Lateral tibia and interosseous membrane
(I)   First cuneiform and metatarsal
(A)   Ankle inversion and dorsiflexion
(N)   Deep peroneal nerve (L4, L5, S1)

The **extensor hallucis longus** muscle, a thin muscle lying deep to and between the tibialis anterior and the extensor digitorum longus muscles, originates on the fibula and interosseous membrane and inserts into the base of the distal phalanx of the great toe (Fig. 18–27). Its primary function is to extend the great toe, but this muscle also assists in dorsiflexing and inverting the ankle.

Extensor Hallucis Longus Muscle

(O)   Fibula and interosseous membrane
(I)   Distal phalanx of great toe
(A)   Extends first toe; assists in ankle inversion and dorsiflexion
(N)   Deep peroneal nerve (L4, L5, S1)

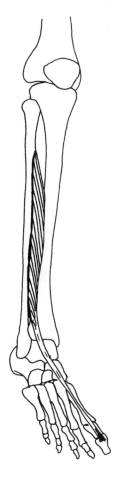

FIGURE 18–27.   The extensor hallucis longus muscle.

The most lateral of the anterior muscles, the **extensor digitorum longus** muscle attaches to most of the anterior fibula, interosseous membrane, and the lateral condyle of the tibia. It descends the leg to attach to the distal phalanx of the four lesser toes (Fig. 18–28). The extensor digitorum longus muscle functions primarily to extend the second through fifth toes, but it also assists in dorsiflexing the ankle.

Extensor Digitorum Longus Muscle	
(O)	Fibula, interosseous membrane, tibia
(I)	Distal phalanx of four lesser toes
(A)	Extends four lesser toes, assists in ankle dorsiflexion
(N)	Deep peroneal nerve (L4, L5, S1)

Lateral Group

The lateral group of muscles consists of the peroneus longus, peroneus brevis, and peroneus tertius muscles. They all originate proximally on the fibula and run distally to the foot. Two cross the ankle joint posteriorly, and one crosses the ankle anteriorly.

The **peroneus longus** muscle is the more superficial of the peroneal muscles. Arising from the proximal end of the fibula and interosseous membrane, it descends

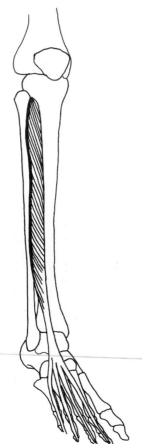

FIGURE 18–28. The extensor digitorum longus muscle.

the lateral leg and loops behind the lateral malleolus with the peroneus brevis muscle. Then the peroneus longus muscle goes deep to cross the foot obliquely from the lateral to the medial side of the foot inserting into the plantar surface of the first metatarsal and first cuneiform (Fig. 18–29). This distal attachment is very close to the attachment of the tibialis anterior muscle. Together, the peroneus longus and tibialis anterior muscles are sometimes referred to as the **stirrup of the foot** because the peroneus longus muscle vertically descends the leg laterally before crossing the foot medially to join the tibialis anterior muscle. The tibialis anterior muscle vertically descends the leg medially to meet the peroneus longus muscle, forming a U or stirrup. Crossing the foot as it does, the peroneus longus muscle provides some support to the lateral longitudinal and transverse arches of the foot. Its prime function is to evert the ankle, although this muscle is able to assist somewhat in ankle plantar flexion.

Peroneus Longus Muscle	
(O)	Lateral proximal fibula and interosseous membrane
(I)	Plantar surface of first cuneiform and metatarsal
(A)	Ankle eversion; assists in ankle plantar flexion
(N)	Superficial peroneal nerve (L4, L5, S1)

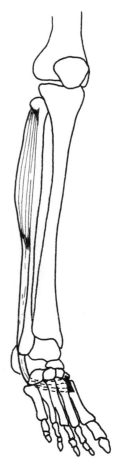

FIGURE 18–29. The peroneus longus muscle (dotted lines indicate location on plantar surface).

Deep to the peroneus longus muscle is the smaller, shorter **peroneus brevis** muscle. It attaches laterally on the distal fibula, descends the leg, and loops behind the lateral malleolus before coming forward to attach on the base of the fifth metatarsal (Fig. 18–30). The peroneus brevis muscle is superficial from the lateral malleolus forward. Like the peroneus longus muscle, this muscle's prime function is to evert the ankle, although it is able to assist somewhat in plantar flexion.

Peroneus Brevis Muscle

(O)	Lateral distal fibula
(I)	Base of fifth metatarsal
(A)	Ankle eversion; assists in plantar flexion
(N)	Superficial peroneal nerve (L4, L5, S1)

The **peroneus tertius** muscle, not present in all people, is difficult to identify and often is confused as part of the extensor digitorum longus muscle. The muscle arises from the distal medial fibula and interosseous membrane, and crosses the ankle anteriorly to insert on the dorsal surface of the base of the fifth metatarsal, near the peroneus brevis muscle (see Fig. 18–30). Theoretically, this muscle should dorsiflex and evert the ankle, but due to its size, it is assistive at best.

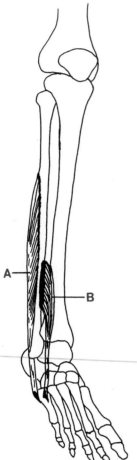

FIGURE 18–30. (*A*) Peroneus brevis muscle. (*B*) Peroneus tertius muscle.

Peroneus Tertius Muscle	
(O)	Distal medial fibula
(I)	Base of fifth metatarsal
(A)	Assists in ankle eversion and dorsiflexion
(N)	Deep peroneal nerve (L4, L5, S1)

Table 18–3 summarizes the actions of the prime movers of the ankle.

INTRINSIC MUSCLES

Intrinsic muscles have both attachments distal to the ankle joint. Because we do not use these muscles to perform intricate actions, they do not tend to be as well developed as their counterparts in the hand. Their names tell a great deal about their location and action. All intrinsic muscles are located on the plantar surface, essentially in layers, except the extensor digitorum brevis muscle, which is on the dorsal surface. Table 18–4 summarizes the intrinsic muscles according to surface location, depth location, function, and similar structure in the hand. Table 18–5 summarizes the innervation of these muscles.

TABLE 18–3	PRIME MOVERS OF THE FOOT AND ANKLE

Action	Muscle
Plantar flexion	Gastrocnemius
Plantar flexion	Soleus
No significant action	Plantaris
Inversion	Tibialis posterior
Flexion of second through fifth toes	Flexor digitorum longus
Flexion of first toe	Flexor hallucis longus
Eversion	Peroneus longus
Eversion	Peroneus brevis
No significant action	Peroneus tertius
Extension of second through fifth toes	Extensor digitorum longus
Extension of first toe	Extensor hallucis longus
Dorsiflexion, inversion	Tibialis anterior

TABLE 18–4	INTRINSIC MUSCLES OF THE FOOT

Muscle	Action	Comparable Hand Muscle
	DORSAL SURFACE	
Extensor digitorum brevis	Extends PIP joints of digits 2–5	None
	PLANTAR SURFACE	
First layer		
Abductor hallucis	Abducts; flexes IP of first toe	Abductor pollicis brevis
Flexor digitorum brevis	Flexes PIP of digits 2–5	Flexor digitorum superficialis
Abductor digiti minimi	Flexes; abducts fifth digit	Same name
Second layer		
Quadratus plantae	Straightens diagonal line of pull of flexor digitorum longus	None
Lumbricales	Flexes MPs; extends PIPs and DIPs	Same name
Third layer		
Flexor hallucis brevis	Flexes MP of first digit	Flexor pollicis brevis
Adductor hallucis	Adducts; flexes first digit	Adductor pollicis
Flexor digiti minimi	Flexes PIP of fifth digit	Same name
	DORSAL SURFACE	
Fourth Layer		
Dorsal interossei	Abducts second through fourth digits	Same name
Plantar interossei	Adducts second through fourth digits	Palmar interossei

TABLE 18–5	INNERVATION OF THE INTRINSIC MUSCLES OF THE FOOT

Muscle	Nerve
DORSAL SURFACE	
Extensor digitorum brevis	Deep peroneal
PLANTAR SURFACE	
Abductor hallucis	Tibial
Flexor digitorum brevis	Tibial
Abductor digiti minimi	Tibial
Quadratus plantae	Tibial
Lumbricales	Tibial
Flexor hallucis brevis	Tibial
Adductor hallucis	Tibial
Flexor digiti minimi	Tibial
Dorsal interossei	Tibial
Plantar interossei	Tibial

TABLE 18–6	INNERVATION OF THE MUSCLES OF THE LEG AND FOOT

Muscle	Nerve	Spinal Segment
Gastrocnemius	Tibial	S1, S2
Soleus	Tibial	S1, S2
Plantaris	Tibial	L4, L5, S1
Tibialis posterior	Tibial	L5, S1
Flexor digitorum longus	Tibial	L5, S1
Flexor hallucis longus	Tibial	L5, S1, S2
Peroneus longus	Superficial peroneal	L4, L5, S1
Peroneus brevis	Superficial peroneal	L4, L5, S1
Peroneus tertius	Deep peroneal	L4, L5, S1
Extensor digitorum longus	Deep peroneal	L4, L5, S1
Extensor digitorum brevis	Deep peroneal	L5, S1
Extensor hallucis longus	Deep peroneal	L4, L5, S1
Tibialis anterior	Deep peroneal	L4, L5, S1
Abductor hallucis	Medial plantar (tibial)	L4, L5
Flexor hallucis brevis	Medial plantar (tibial)	L4, L5, S1
Flexor digitorum brevis	Medial plantar (tibial)	L4, L5
Lumbricales (medial 1)	Medial plantar (tibial)	L4, L5
Lumbricales (lateral 3)	Lateral plantar (tibial)	S1, S2
Abductor digiti minimi	Lateral plantar (tibial)	S1, S2
Quadratus plantae	Lateral plantar (tibial)	S1, S2
Adductor hallucis	Lateral plantar (tibial)	S1, S2
Flexor digiti minimi	Lateral plantar (tibial)	S1, S2
Dorsal interossei	Lateral plantar (tibial)	S1, S2
Plantar interossei	Lateral plantar (tibial)	S1, S2

TABLE 18–7	SEGMENTAL INNERVATION OF THE ANKLE JOINT AND FOOT			
Spinal Cord Level	**L4**	**L5**	**S1**	**S2**
Gastrocnemius			X	X
Soleus			X	X
Plantaris	X	X	X	
Tibialis posterior		X	X	
Flexor digitorum longus		X	X	
Flexor hallucis longus		X	X	X
Peroneus longus	X	X	X	
Peroneus brevis	X	X	X	
Peroneus tertius	X	X	X	
Extensor digitorum longus	X	X	X	
Extensor digitorum brevis		X	X	
Extensor hallucis longus	X	X	X	
Tibialis anterior	X	X		
Abductor hallucis	X	X		
Flexor hallucis brevis	X	X	X	
Flexor digitorum brevis	X	X		
Lumbricales	X	X	X	X
Abductor digiti minimi			X	X
Quadratus plantae			X	X
Adductor hallucis			X	X
Flexor digiti minimi			X	X
Dorsal interossei			X	X
Plantar interossei			X	X

SUMMARY OF MUSCLE INNERVATION

The ankle and foot muscles fall into relatively tidy groupings according to innervation. Those muscles located on the posterior leg and plantar surface of the foot receive innervation from the tibial nerve. The plantar foot divides into two groups similar to the hand. The lateral plantar branch of the tibial nerve innervates muscles located on the lateral side, and the medial plantar branch innervates those on the medial side.

The superficial peroneal nerve innervates muscles on the lateral side of the leg (peroneals). The peroneus tertius muscle is the exception, because it crosses the ankle anteriorly to receive innervation with the other anterior muscles from the deep peroneal nerve.

Tables 18–6 and 18–7 summarize ankle and foot innervation. As has been noted in the previous chapters, there is some variation among sources regarding spinal cord level. When discrepancy occurred, *Gray's Anatomy,* 29th edition, was used as the reference source.

REVIEW QUESTIONS

1. Describe the ankle (talotibial) joint:
   a. Number of axes:
   b. Shape of joint:
   c. Type of action allowed:
   d. Bones involved:

2. What bones are involved in the subtalar joint? In the transverse tarsal joint?

3. What is (are) the function(s) of the interosseous membrane?

4. What ligament(s) provides medial stability to the ankle?

5. What ligament(s) provides lateral stability to the ankle?

6. List the bones involved in the medial longitudinal arch. What is the function of each?

7. List the bones involved in the transverse arch. What is the function of each?

8. Which muscle(s) passes behind the medial malleolus?

9. Which muscle(s) attaches on the medial side of the foot?

10. Which muscle(s) passes behind the lateral malleolus?

11. Which muscle(s) attaches on the lateral side of the foot?

12. Which muscles form the "stirrup" of the foot? Describe how the stirrup is formed.

13. If an individual had a L4 spinal cord level injury, would you expect to see any ankle plantar flexion?

Posture

In general, posture is the position of your body parts in relationship to each other at any given time. Posture can be static, as in a stationary position such as standing, sitting, or lying. It can be dynamic as the body moves from one position to another. Posture deals with alignment of the various body segments. These body segments can be compared to blocks. If you start stacking blocks, one directly on top of the other, the column would remain relatively stable. However, if you stack them off center from each other, the column will remain upright only if the block, or blocks, above counter the block or blocks below, and remain within the base of support. In the human body, each joint involved with weight bearing can be considered a postural segment.

Vertebral Alignment

The vertebral column can be compared to the column of blocks. It is not completely straight, but has a series of counter-balancing anterior-posterior curves. These curves, which must be maintained during rest and activity, act as shock absorbers and reduce the amount of injury. The thoracic and sacral curves counter the cervical and lumbar curves (Fig. 19–1). The thoracic and sacral curves are concave anteriorly and convex posteriorly. Conversely, the lumbar and cervical curves are convex anteriorly and concave posteriorly. When one or more of these vertebral curves either increases or decreases significantly from what is considered good posture, poor posture re-

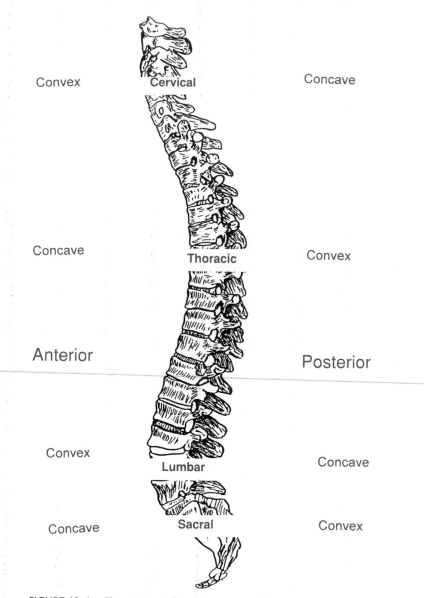

Convex   **Cervical**   Concave

Concave   **Thoracic**   Convex

Anterior   Posterior

Convex   **Lumbar**   Concave

Concave   **Sacral**   Convex

FIGURE 19–1. The convex and concave curves of the vertebral column.

sults. For example, a "sway back" is an increased lumbar curve, whereas a "flat back" is a decreased thoracic curve. In most cases, if there is an increased lumbar curve, there is also an increased thoracic curve. No lateral curves should exist. Any lateral curvature of the spine is a pathologic condition called scoliosis.

DEVELOPMENT OF POSTURAL CURVES

At birth, the entire vertebral column is concave anteriorly. This concave curve is called a **primary curve.** The thoracic and sacral curves are considered primary curves for this reason. As the child grows, **secondary curves** develop. These are the anteriorly convex curves of the cervical and lumbar regions. Figure 19–2 shows the development of the vertebral curves and the postural changes that occur with age.

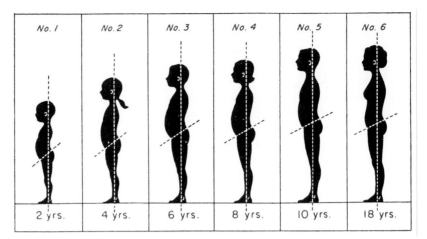

No. 1	No. 2	No. 3	No. 4	No. 5	No. 6
2 yrs.	4 yrs.	6 yrs.	8 yrs.	10 yrs.	18 yrs.

FIGURE 19–2. Postural changes with age. Apparent kyphosis at ages 6 and 8 is due to scapular winging. (From Magee, DJ: Orthopedic Physical Assessment. WB Saunders, Philadelphia, 1987, p 378, with permission; original source, McMorris, RO: Pediatr Clin North Am 8:214, 1961.)

The position of the pelvis has great influence on the vertebral column, especially the lumbar region. The pelvis should be in a neutral position. This position is defined as (1) when the anterior superior iliac spine (ASIS) and posterior superior iliac spine (PSIS) are level with each other in a transverse plane; and (2) when the ASIS is in the same vertical plane as the symphysis pubis. When the pelvis is in a neutral position, the lumbar curve has the desired amount of curvature. When the pelvis is tilted anteriorly, there is an increased amount of lumbar curvature, or lordosis. When the pelvis is tilted posteriorly, there is a decreased amount of curve, or flat back. These positions are illustrated in Figure 15–10.

With weight evenly distributed on both legs, the pelvis should remain level from side to side, with both ASISs being at the same level. During walking, however, the pelvis dips from side to side as weight is shifted from stance to swing phase. This **lateral pelvic tilt** is controlled by the hip abductors, mainly the gluteus medius and gluteus minimus, and the trunk lateral benders, mainly the erector spinae and quadratus lumborum. If you bend your right knee and lift your foot off the ground, your pelvis on the right side becomes unsupported and will drop. Force couple action of the hip abductors and trunk lateral benders hold the pelvis level. The left hip abductors (opposite side) contract to pull the pelvis down on the left side while trunk lateral benders on the right (same side) contract to pull the pelvis up on the right side. These motions are illustrated in Figures 15–16 and 15–17. A lateral pelvic tilt can also occur if both legs are not of equal length. This will result in a lateral curvature, or scoliosis.

In the upright position, both static and dynamic posture depends primarily upon muscle contractions to remain upright. The muscles most involved are called **antigravity muscles.** These muscles are the hip and knee extensors, and the trunk and neck extensors. Other muscles, perhaps less involved, but also important in maintaining the upright position are the trunk and neck flexors and lateral benders, hip abductors and adductors, and the ankle pronators and supinators. If all of these muscles were to relax, the body would collapse.

The ankle plantar flexors and dorsiflexors are important in controlling postural sway. **Postural sway** is anterior-posterior motion of the upright body caused by motion occurring primarily at the ankles. This sway is the result of constant displacement and correction of the center of gravity within the base of support. Therefore, a high center of gravity and small base of support tends to increase the amount of postural sway. To demonstrate this, stand upright with your feet slightly apart. Notice how much your body tends to move back and forth. Next, observe the amount of sway when you stand on your toes in the upright position with your feet close together. You should notice much more motion in the latter position, because you have raised your center of gravity and made your base of support smaller.

Good posture, which means good alignment, is important because it decreases the amount of stress placed on ligaments, muscles, and tendons. Good alignment also improves function and decreases the amount of muscle energy needed to keep the body upright. For example, if the knee is in full extension, little muscle contraction is needed to keep the knee from buckling. However, when the knee is partially flexed, the muscles at that joint (knee extensors) must contract to keep the knee from collapsing. Because standing is a closed chain activity, muscles at the hip and ankle must also contract to keep the body's center of gravity over its base of support.

Standing Posture

Posture is easier to describe in a static standing position because, except for a slight amount of sway when standing, the body is not moving. However, many of the guidelines for static posture can be applied to dynamic posture. Assessing a person's posture can be done most accurately with the use of a plumb line suspended from the ceiling or a posture grid behind the person as a point of reference. A plumb line is a string or cord with a weight attached to the lower end. Because the string is weighted, it makes a perfectly straight vertical line of gravity.

LATERAL VIEW

In the standing position and viewed from the **lateral position,** the plumb line should be aligned so that it passes slightly in front of the lateral malleolus (Fig. 19–3). For ideal posture, the body segments should be aligned so that the plumb line passes through the landmarks listed below as follows:

Head:	through the ear lobe
Shoulder:	through tip of the acromion process
Thoracic spine:	anterior to the vertebral bodies
Lumbar spine:	through the vertebral bodies
Pelvis:	level with an anterior or posterior tilt
Hip:	through the greater trochanter (slightly posterior to the hip joint axis)
Knee:	slightly posterior to the patella (slightly anterior to the knee joint axis) with the knees in extension
Ankle:	slightly anterior to the lateral malleolus with the ankle joint in a neutral position between dorsiflexion and plantar flexion

Common postural deviations that can be detected from the side view are summarized in Table 19–1. Because standing is a closed kinetic chain activity, the position or motion of one joint will effect the position or motions of other joints.

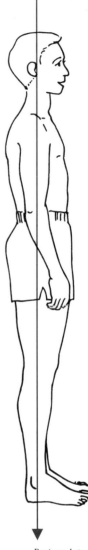

FIGURE 19–3. Posture, lateral view. (From Minor, MA and Lippert, LS: Kinesiology Laboratory Manual for Physical Therapist Assistants. FA Davis, Philadelphia, 1998, p 280, with permission.)

Posture, lateral view.

ANTERIOR VIEW

In the standing position and viewed from the **anterior position,** the plumb line should be aligned to pass through the midsagittal plane of the body, thus dividing the body into two equal halves (Fig 19–4). The following body segments listed below should be aligned as follows:

Head:	extended and level, not flexed or hyperextended
Shoulders:	level and not elevated or depressed
Sternum:	centered in the midline
Hips:	level with both ASISs in the same plane
Legs:	slightly apart
Knees:	level and not bowed or knock kneed
Ankles:	normal arch in feet
Feet:	slight outward toeing

TABLE 19–1	SUMMARY OF COMMON POSTURAL DEVIATIONS		
	Lateral View	**Posterior View**	**Anterior View**
Head	Forward	Tilted Rotated	Tilted Rotated Mandible asymmetrical
Cervical spine	Exaggerated curve Flattened curve		
Shoulders	Rounded	Elevated Depressed	Elevated Depressed
Scapulae		Abducted Adducted Winged	
Thoracic spine	Exaggerated curve	Lateral deviation	
Lumbar spine	Exaggerated curve Flattened curve	Lateral deviation	
Pelvis	Anterior pelvic tilt Posterior pelvic tilt	Lateral pelvic tilt Pelvis rotated	
Hip			Medially rotated Laterally rotated
Knee	Genu recurvatum Flexed knee	Genu varum Genu valgum	External tibial torsion Internal tibial torsion
Ankle/foot	Forward posture Flattened longitudinal arch Exaggerated longitudinal arch	Pes planus Pes cavus	Hallux valgus Claw toe Hammer toe Mallet toe

POSTERIOR VIEW

In the standing position and viewed from the **posterior position,** the plumb line should also be aligned to pass through the midsagittal plane of the body, dividing the body into two equal halves (Fig. 19–5). The following body segments listed should be aligned as follows:

Head:	extended, not flexed or hyperextended
Shoulders:	level and not elevated or depressed
Spinous processes:	centered in the midline
Hips:	level with both PSISs in the same plane
Legs:	slightly apart
Knees:	level and not bowed or knock kneed
Ankles:	calcaneus should be straight

Sitting Posture

Good postural alignment while sitting is important because sitting is an activity that can place a great deal of pressure on the intervertebral disk. Studies by Nachemson have shown that disk pressure in the sitting position increases by slightly less than half the amount of disk pressure of standing. To state the obvious, shifting weight

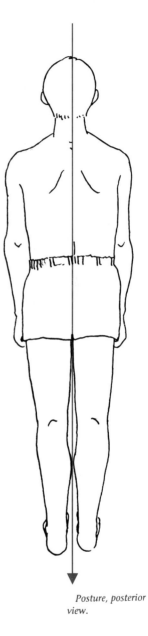

FIGURE 19–4. Posture, anterior view. (From Minor, MA and Lippert, LS: Kinesiology Laboratory Manual for Physical Therapist Assistants. FA Davis, Philadelphia, 1998, p 280, with permission.)

Posture, posterior view.

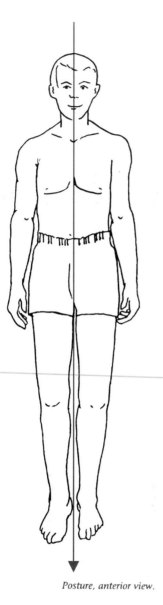

Posture, anterior view.

FIGURE 19–5.   Posture, posterior view. (From Minor, MA and Lippert, LS: Kinesiology Laboratory Manual for Physical Therapist Assistants. FA Davis, Philadelphia, 1998, p 280, with permission.)

on to the front part of the vertebrae will increase the amount of pressure placed on the intervertebral disks. As the person leans forward, disk pressure increases. As a person reaches, and/or picks up a weight, disk pressure further increases as the weight and/or length of the lever arm increases. Figure 19–6 illustrates disk pressure in various positions.

   If the lumbar curve is decreased, such as often happens when sitting with the back unsupported (Fig. 19–7), the pressure on the intervertebral disks and posterior structures increases. A chair with the seat inclined anteriorly, such as the kneeling stool (Fig. 19–8), can decrease disk pressure by tilting the pelvis forward slightly. This helps to maintain the lumbar curve. However, because the back is unsupported, increased and sustained muscle contraction is required to keep the body upright. With sitting postures, a chair that has a lumbar support maintaining the lumbar lordosis will

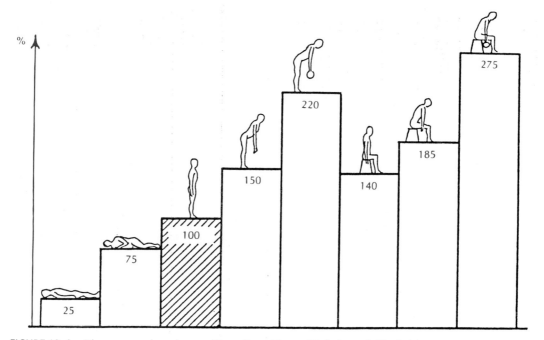

FIGURE 19–6.   Disc pressures in various positions. (From Magee, DJ: Orthopedic Physical Assessment. WB Saunders, Philadelphia, 1987, p 378, with permission; original source, Nachemson, A: The lumbar spine: An orthopaedic challenge. Spine 1:59–71, 1976.)

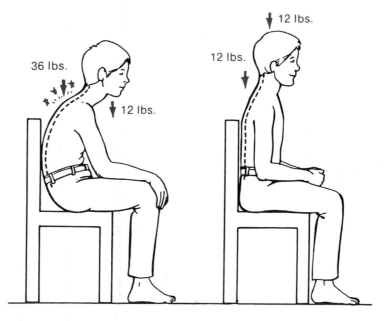

FIGURE 19–7.   Slouched posture increases disc pressure. (From Saunders, HD: For Your Back: Self-help Manual. Viking Press, Minneapolis, 1985, p 21 with permission.)

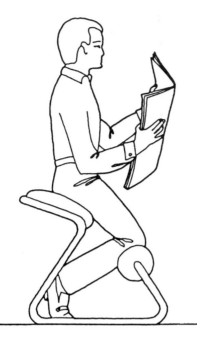

FIGURE 19–8. Kneeling stool reduces disc pressure. (From Oliver, J: Back Care: An Illustrated Guide. Butterworth-Heinemann, Oxford, England, Boston, 1994, p 81 with permission.)

place the least amount of pressure on the disks. Maintaining the vertebral curves, keeping the feet flat on the floor, having the low back supported, and keeping the upper body in good alignment are key elements of good sitting posture (Fig. 19–9).

However, shifting weight on to the front part of the vertebra is not always a problem. Although disk pressure increases in this position, the stresses placed on the posterior part of the vertebra, the facet joints, decreases. Therefore, if a person had a facet joint problem, generally speaking, a flexed position would be more desirable. Conversely, if a person had a disk problem, an extended position would usually be more desirable.

Supine Posture

Lying down is considered a resting position. The least amount of intervertebral disk pressure occurs while lying supine (Fig. 19–10). If you could run a plumb line horizontally, it would intersect many of the same landmarks as in the standing position. Good alignment in this position is also important. A good resting surface should be firm enough to avoid loss of the lumbar curve, yet soft enough to conform and give support to the normal curves of the body. In the sidelying position, the bottom leg is extended and the top leg is flexed. Placing a pillow between the legs can increase comfort by keeping the hips in good alignment. Lying prone is usually not recommended because of the increased pressure placed on the neck. In this position, using a pillow only increases the stresses on the neck.

When actively moving about and changing positions, whether vacuuming the rug, picking up a box from the floor, or raking leaves, keeping the body, especially the trunk, in good postural alignment is important. Most principles of good body mechanics involve avoiding stress to the trunk and maintaining the spinal curves, which involve maintaining good posture.

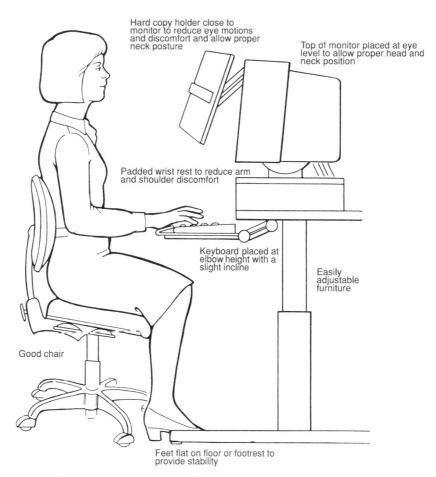

Hard copy holder close to monitor to reduce eye motions and discomfort and allow proper neck posture

Top of monitor placed at eye level to allow proper head and neck position

Padded wrist rest to reduce arm and shoulder discomfort

Keyboard placed at elbow height with a slight incline

Easily adjustable furniture

Good chair

Feet flat on floor or footrest to provide stability

FIGURE 19–9.   Sitting posture. (From MacLeod, D, Jacobs, P, and Larson, L: The Ergonomics Manual. The Saunders Group, Minneapolis, 1990, p 27 with permission.)

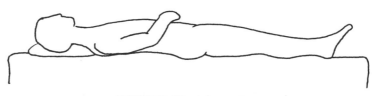

FIGURE 19–10.   Lying posture.

Common Postural Deviations

Table 19–1 is a summary of common postural deviations seen when assessing posture. It is not within the scope of this book to describe the individual causes and effects of postural problems. However, some general statements regarding cause and effect should be made.

Deviation from "good" posture is considered "poor" or "bad" posture. Causes of poor posture can be the result of structural problems. These structural problems may be the result of a congenital malformation such as a hemivertebra. The deviation may be an acquired deformity caused by trauma such as a compression fracture. Postural deviations also may be the result of neurologic conditions causing paralysis or spasticity. Additionally, postural problems may also be functional, or nonstructural, in nature. A person who sits or stands for long periods of time will tend to slouch. This can result in a muscle imbalance.

Generally, if a person tends to maintain a posture in which a curve is increased, the muscles on the concave side will tend to tighten while the muscles on the convex side tend to weaken. For example, you would expect a person with a lumbar lordosis to have tight back extensors and weak abdominal muscles. Also, postures that tend to increase the lordotic curves (cervical and lumbar) will increase the pressure on the more posterior facet joints and decrease the pressure on the more anterior intervertebral disks. Conversely, an increase in the kyphotic curves (thoracic and sacral) will increase the pressure on the intervertebral disks while decreasing the pressure on the facet joints.

REVIEW QUESTIONS

1. If a person had an excessive cervical lordosis, would you expect the cervical extensors or flexors to be tight?

2. Which position(s)—the side, front, or back—would be best to assess the condition in question 1?

3. If a person had an anterior tilt of the pelvis, would you expect the hip flexors or hip extensors to be tight?

4. To assess the condition in question 3, which position(s)—the side, front, or back—would be best?

5. What position should the shoulders be in relation to each other?

6. Which position(s)—the side, front or back—would be best to assess the position of the shoulders in relation to each other?

7. When assessing a person's posture in the lateral standing position and using a plumb line, you should begin by lining up the plumb line with what body structure?

8. For ideal posture (when viewed laterally), where should the plumb line then pass on the following structures:
   a. Knee
   b. Hip
   c. Shoulder
   d. Head

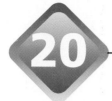

Normal Gait

Walking is moving from place to place on your feet, and *gait* is the style or manner of walking. Each person has a unique style, and this style may change slightly with mood. When you are happy, your step is lighter, and there may be a "bounce" in your walk. Conversely, when sad or depressed, your step may be heavy. For some people, their walking pattern is so unique that they can be identified from a distance even before their face can clearly be seen. Regardless of the numerous different styles, the components of normal gait are the same.

In the most basic sense, walking requires balancing on one leg while the other leg is moved forward. This requires movement not only of the legs but also of the trunk and arms as well. To analyze gait, you must first determine what joint motions occur. Then, based upon that information, you must decide which muscles or muscle groups are acting.

Definitions

Certain definitions must be made to describe gait. **Gait cycle** is the activity that occurs between the time the heel of one extremity touches the floor and the time the same foot touches the floor again (Fig. 20–1). In other words, it occurs between the heel strike of the right leg and the heel strike of the right leg again, including all of the activity in between. The same definition could be given using the left leg. A

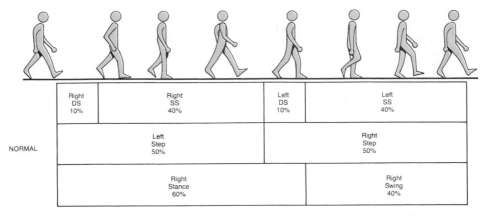

FIGURE 20–1. Phases of the gait cycle. Percentages are approximate and depend on walking speed, (DS = double support; SS = single support). (From Rothstein, JM, Roy, SH, and Wolf, SL: The Rehabilitation Specialist's Handbook. FA Davis, Philadelphia, 1991, p 700, with permission.)

stride length is the distance of the gait cycle; that is, the distance between heel strike of one leg and its subsequent heel strike (Fig. 20–2).

　　Stance phase is the activity that occurs when the foot is in contact with the ground. It begins with heel strike of one foot and ends when that foot leaves the ground. This phase accounts for about 60 percent of the gait cycle (Fig. 20–3). **Swing phase** occurs when the foot is not in contact with the ground. It begins as soon as the foot leaves the floor and ends when the heel of the same foot touches the floor (Fig. 20–4). The swing phase makes up about 40 percent of the gait cycle (see Fig. 20–1).

　　When both feet are in contact with the ground at the same time, there is a period of **double support** (Fig. 20–5). This occurs between heel-off and toe-off of one limb and between heel strike and foot flat on the opposite (contralateral) side. In other words, it is that period when one limb is ending its stance phase and the other limb is beginning its stance phase. Therefore, there are two periods of double support: one when the right leg is ending its stance phase and the other when the left leg is ending its stance phase. Each period of double support takes up about 10 percent of the gait cycle at an average walking speed (see Fig. 20–1). If you increase your walking speed, you spend less time with both feet on the ground. Conversely, you spend more time in double support when you walk slowly.

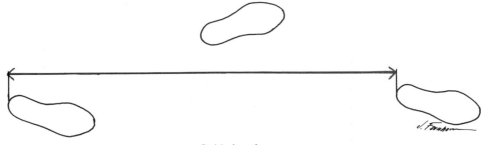

Stride length

FIGURE 20–2. Stride length. (From Norkin, CC and Levangie, PK: Joint Structure and Function: A Comprehensive Analysis, ed 2. FA Davis, Philadelphia, 1992, p 457, with permission.)

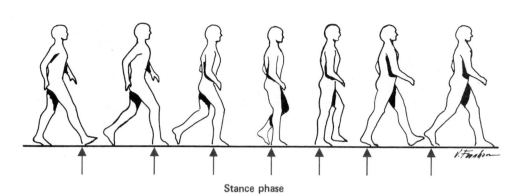

Stance phase

FIGURE 20–3. Stance phase. (From Norkin, CC and Levangie, PK: Joint Structure and Function: A Comprehensive Analysis, ed 2. FA Davis, Philadelphia, 1992, p 451, with permission.)

A period of **nonsupport,** that is, a time during which neither foot is in contact with the ground, does not occur during walking. However, nonsupport does occur during running. This may be the biggest difference between running and walking. Other activities, such as hopping, skipping, and jumping, have a period of nonsupport but lose the order of progression that walking and running have. In other words, these activities do not include all the parts of stance and swing phase as do walking and running.

The period of **single support** occurs when only one foot is in contact with the ground (see Fig. 20–5). Thus, two periods of single support occur: once when the right foot is on the ground and then again when the left foot bears weight. Each single support period takes up about 40 percent of the gait cycle.

As you can see in Figure 20–1, the right and left step times are equal. A **step** includes a period of double support and single support as well as a stance and swing phase. A **step length** is that distance between heel strike of one limb and heel strike of the other (Fig. 20–6). Even with an increased or decreased walking speed, the step percentage of each limb should remain equal. Walking speed, or **cadence,** the number of steps taken per minute, varies greatly. Slow walking may be as slow as 70 steps per minute. However, students on their way to an examination have been

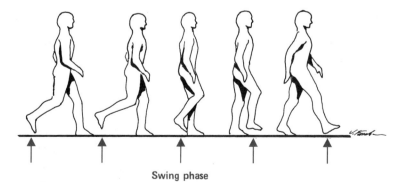

Swing phase

FIGURE 20–4. Swing phase. (From Norkin, CC and Levangie, PK: Joint Structure and Function: A Comprehensive Analysis, ed 2. FA Davis, Philadelphia, 1992, p 452, with permission.)

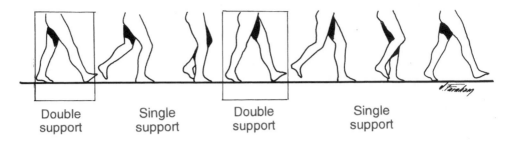

Double support | Single support | Double support | Single support

FIGURE 20–5. Periods of double support and single support. (From Norkin, CC and Levangie, PK: Joint Structure and Function: A Comprehensive Analysis, ed 2. FA Davis, Philadelphia, 1992, p 452, with permission.)

clocked at much slower speeds. Fast walking may be as fast as 130 steps per minute, although race walkers will walk much faster. Regardless of speed, the phase relationship is the same; that is, all parts occur in their proper place at the proper time.

Many sets of terms have been developed from the original, or traditional, terminology to describe the components of walking. In many cases, although the terminology may be accurate, it is often cumbersome. However, terminology developed by the Gait Laboratory at Rancho Los Amigos (RLA) Medical Center has been gaining in acceptance. Perhaps the biggest difference between the two sets of terminology is that the traditional terms refer to *points in time* whereas RLA terms refer to *periods of time*. Although it is best to be familiar with both sets of terms, traditional terminology will be used here. Table 20–1 provides the definitions of traditional terminology as well as the RLA terms. In comparison, one can see that they are similar with a few notable exceptions.

Analysis of Stance Phase

As defined earlier, *stance* is that period in which the foot is in contact with the floor. Traditionally, the stance phase has been broken down into five components consisting of (1) heel strike, (2) foot flat, (3) midstance, (4) heel-off, and (5) toe-off (see Fig. 20–3). Some sources break stance down into only four components, combining heel-off and toe-off into one, calling it "push-off." Because significantly different activities occur during these two periods, it is perhaps best to keep them separated.

Heel strike signals the beginning of stance phase the moment the heel comes

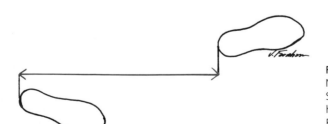

FIGURE 20–6. Step length. (From Norkin, CC and Levangie, PK: Joint Structure and Function: A Comprehensive Analysis, ed 2. FA Davis, Philadelphia, 1992, p 457, with permission.)

TABLE 20–1	**COMPARISON OF GAIT TERMINOLOGY**		
Traditional		*Rancho Los Amigos*	
Term	**Definition**	**Term**	**Definition**
Stance Phase			
Heel strike	Heel contact with ground	Initial contact	Same
Foot flat	Plantar surface of the foot contacts ground	Loading response	Period from just after initial contact until the opposite foot leaves the ground
Midstance	Point at which the body passes over the weight-bearing limb	Midstance	Period from when the opposite foot leaves to ground until body is directly over the weight-bearing limb
Heel-off	Heel leaves the ground, while ball of the foot and toes remain in contact with the ground	Terminal stance	From midstance to initial contact of the opposite foot
Toe-off	Toes leave the ground, ending stance phase	Preswing	From initial contact of the opposite limb to just before the toes leave ground
Swing Phase			
Acceleration	From when the toes leave the ground until the foot is directly under the body	Initial swing	From when the toes leave the ground until maximum knee flexion of the same limb
Midswing	When the non–weight-bearing limb is directly under the body	Midswing	Just after maximum knee flexion until the tibia is in a vertical position
Deceleration	When the limb is slowing down in preparation for heel strike	Terminal swing	From the vertical position of the tibia to just prior to initial contact

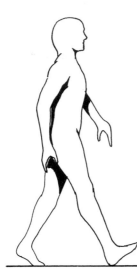

FIGURE 20–7.   Heel strike. (From Norkin, CC and Levangie, PK: Joint Structure and Function: A Comprehensive Analysis, ed 2. FA Davis, Philadelphia, 1992, p 453, with permission.)

in contact with the ground (Fig. 20–7). At this point the ankle is in a neutral position between dorsiflexion and plantar flexion, and the knee begins to flex. This slight flexion provides some shock absorption as the foot hits the ground. The hip is in about 25 degrees of flexion. The trunk is erect and remains so through the entire gait cycle. The trunk is rotated to the opposite side, the opposite arm is forward, and the same-side arm is back in shoulder hyperextension. At this point, body weight begins to shift onto the stance leg.

The ankle dorsiflexors are active in putting the ankle in its neutral position. The quadriceps, which have been contracting concentrically, switch to contracting eccentrically to minimize the amount of knee flexion. The hip flexors have been active. However, the extensors are beginning to contract, keeping the hip from flexing more. The erector spinae are active in keeping the trunk from flexing. The force of the foot hitting the ground transmits up through the ankle, knee, and hip to the trunk. This would cause the pelvis to rotate anteriorly, flexing the trunk somewhat, if it were not for the erector spinae counteracting this force.

"**Foot flat,**" when the entire foot is in contact with the ground, occurs shortly after heel strike (Fig. 20–8). The ankle moves into about 15 degrees of plantar flexion with the dorsiflexors contracting eccentrically to keep the foot from "slapping" down on the floor. The knee moves into about 20 degrees of flexion. The hip is moving into extension, allowing the rest of the body to begin catching up with the leg. Weight shift onto the stance limb continues.

The point at which the body passes over the weight-bearing foot is called **midstance** (Fig. 20–9). In this phase, the ankle moves into slight dorsiflexion. However, the dorsiflexors become inactive. The plantar flexors begin to contract, controlling the rate at which the leg moves over the ankle. The knee and hip continue to extend, both arms are in shoulder extension essentially parallel with the body, and the trunk is in a neutral position of rotation. It is here that the body reaches its highest point in the gait cycle and is in a period of single support.

Following midstance is **heel-off,** in which the heel rises off the floor (Fig. 20–10). The ankle will dorsiflex slightly (approximately 15 degrees) and then begin to plantar flex. This is the beginning of the **push-off** phase, in which the ankle plan-

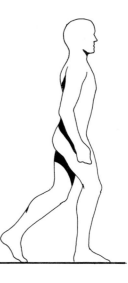

FIGURE 20–8.   Foot flat. (From Norkin, CC and Levangie, PK: Joint Structure and Function: A Comprehensive Analysis, ed 2. FA Davis, Philadelphia, 1992, p 453, with permission.)

tar flexors are active in pushing the body forward. The knee is in near full extension, and the hip has moved into hyperextension. The trunk has begun to rotate to the same side, and the arm is swinging forward into shoulder flexion.

Toe-off is that period just before and including when the toes leave the ground, signaling the end of stance phase and the beginning of swing (Fig. 20–11). The ankle moves into about 10 degrees of plantar flexion, and the knee and hip are flexing.

Analysis of Swing Phase

The swing phase consists of three components: acceleration, midswing, and deceleration (see Fig. 20–4). These components are all non–weight-bearing activities. With

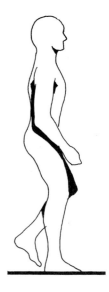

FIGURE 20–9.   Midstance. (From Norkin, CC and Levangie, PK: Joint Structure and Function: A Comprehensive Analysis, ed 2. FA Davis, Philadelphia, 1992, p 453, with permission.)

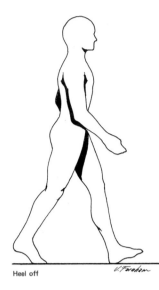

Heel off

FIGURE 20–10. Heel off. (From Norkin, CC and Levangie, PK: Joint Structure and Function: A Comprehensive Analysis, ed 2. FA Davis, Philadelphia, 1992, p 454, with permission.)

acceleration, the limb is behind the body and moving to catch up (Fig. 20–12). The ankle is dorsiflexing, and the knee and hip continue to flex.

At **midswing,** the ankle dorsiflexors have brought the ankle to a neutral position. The knee is at its maximum flexion (approximately 65 degrees) as is the hip (at about 25 degrees of flexion). These motions act to shorten the limb, allowing the foot to clear the ground as it swings through (Fig. 20–13).

In **deceleration,** the ankle dorsiflexors are active to keep the ankle in a neutral position in preparation for heel strike (Fig. 20–14). The knee is extending, and the hamstring muscles are contracting eccentrically to slow down the leg, keeping it from snapping into extension.

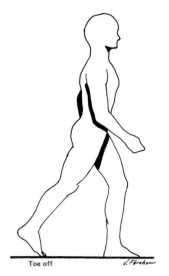

Toe off

FIGURE 20–11. Toe off. (From Norkin, CC and Levangie, PK: Joint Structure and Function: A Comprehensive Analysis, ed 2. FA Davis, Philadelphia, 1992, p 454, with permission.)

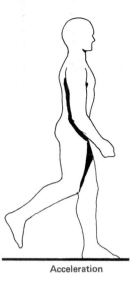

Acceleration

FIGURE 20–12.   Acceleration. (From Norkin, CC and Levangie, PK: Joint Structure and Function: A Comprehensive Analysis, ed 2. FA Davis, Philadelphia, 1992, p 455, with permission.)

Additional Determinants of Gait

To this point, the description of gait has centered mostly on the lower limbs. However, other events are occurring in the rest of the body that must also be considered.

If you were to hold a piece of chalk against the blackboard and walk its length, you would see that the line drawn bobs up and down in wavelike fashion. This is described as the **vertical displacement** of the center of gravity (Fig. 20–15). The normal amount of this displacement is approximately 2 inches, being highest at midstance and lowest at heel strike. There is also an equal amount of **horizontal displacement** of the center of gravity as the body weight shifts from side to side. This displacement is greatest during the single support phase at midstance.

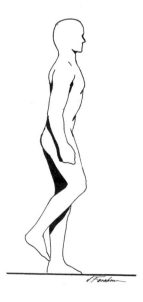

FIGURE 20–13.   Midswing. (From Norkin, CC and Levangie, PK: Joint Structure and Function: A Comprehensive Analysis, ed 2. FA Davis, Philadelphia, 1992, p 455, with permission.)

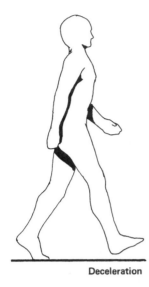

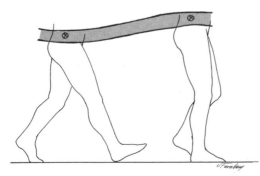

Deceleration

FIGURE 20–14. Deceleration. (From Norkin, CC and Levangie, PK: Joint Structure and Function: A Comprehensive Analysis, ed 2. FA Davis, Philadelphia, 1992, p 456, with permission.)

When you walk, you do not place your feet one step in front of the other but slightly apart. If lines were drawn through the successive midpoints of heel contact on each foot, this distance would range from 2 to 4 inches. This is described as the **width of walking base** (Fig. 20–16).

If you were to walk across the room with your hands on your hips, you would notice that they move up and down as your pelvis on each side drops down slightly. This **lateral pelvic tilt** occurs when weight is taken off the limb at toe-off (Fig. 20–17). This dip would be greater if it were not for the hip abductors on the *opposite* side and the erector spinae on the same side working together keeping the pelvis essentially level. When the pelvis drops on the right side (non–weight-bearing side), the left hip (weight-bearing side) is forced into adduction. To keep the pelvis level, actually dipping slightly, the left hip abductors contract to prevent hip adduction. At the same time the right erector spine muscle, which has an attachment on the pelvis, contracts and "pulls up" on the side of the pelvis wanting to drop (Fig. 20–18).

In addition, step length should be equal in both distance and time. The arms should swing with the opposite leg. The trunk rotates forward as the limb progresses through the swing phase. Arms swinging in opposition to trunk rotation control the amount of trunk rotation by providing counterrotation. The head should be erect, shoulders level, and trunk in extension.

FIGURE 20–15. Vertical displacement of the center of gravity. (From Norkin, CC and Levangie, PK: Joint Structure and Function: A Comprehensive Analysis, ed 2. FA Davis, Philadelphia, 1992, p 461, with permission.)

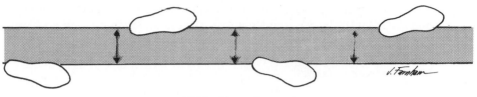

Width of base of support

FIGURE 20–16.   Width of walking base. (From Norkin, CC and Levangie, PK: Joint Structure and Function: A Comprehensive Analysis, ed 2. FA Davis, Philadelphia, 1992, p 458, with permission.)

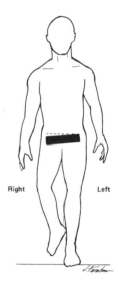

FIGURE 20–17.   Lateral pelvic tilt. (From Norkin, CC and Levangie, PK: Joint Structure and Function: A Comprehensive Analysis, ed 2. FA Davis, Philadelphia, 1992, p 462, with permission.)

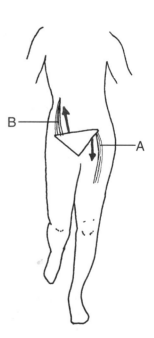

FIGURE 20–18.   Muscles working to minimize lateral pelvic tilt. (*A*) Hip abductors. (*B*) Erector spinae muscle.

When analyzing someone's gait, it is best to view the person from both the side and the front (or back). Step length, arm swing, position of head and trunk, and the activities of the lower limb are usually best viewed from the side. Width of walking base, dip of the pelvis, and position of the shoulders and head should be viewed from the front or back.

Abnormal Gait

Although it is not within the scope of this text to cover gait abnormalities, some of the more common or significant problems are included for an introductory under-standing. Walking abnormally can range from having an early heel rise as a result of tight calf muscles to the waddling gait for a person with muscular dystrophy. There are many methods of classifying abnormal gait. The following is a listing of abnor-mal gaits based on general cause or basis for the abnormality:

Muscular weakness/paralysis
Joint muscle range of motion (ROM) limitation
Neurologic involvement
Pain
Leg length discrepancy

MUSCULAR WEAKNESS/PARALYSIS

Generally speaking, with muscle weakness, the body tends to compensate by shift-ing the center of gravity over, or toward, the part that is involved. Obviously, the portion of the gait cycle affected will be that portion in which the muscles or joint have a major role. In the case of the **gluteus maximus gait,** the trunk quickly shifts posteriorly at heel strike. With the foot in contact with the floor, the hip is maintained in extension during stance phase. This shifting is sometimes referred to as a "rocking horse" gait because of the extreme backward-forward movement of the trunk.

With a **gluteus medius gait,** the individual shifts the trunk to the affected side during stance phase. When the left gluteus medius, or hip abductor, is weak, the right side of the pelvis will drop when the right leg leaves the ground and begins swing phase. This gait is also referred to as a "Trendelenburg" gait.

When there is weakness in the **quadriceps** muscle group, several different com-pensatory mechanisms may be used. If only the quadriceps group is involved, the individual may be able to use the hip extensors and triceps surae to pull the knee into extension at heel strike. This reversal of muscle action has been described in Chapter 17. However, if these muscles are also involved, the person may physically push the knee into extension during stance phase.

If the **hamstrings** are weak, two things may happen. During stance phase, the knee will go into excessive hyperextension, sometimes referred to as "genu re-curvatum" gait. During the deceleration part of swing phase, without the ham-strings to slow down the swing forward of the lower leg, the knee will snap into extension.

Depending on how involved the **ankle dorsiflexors** are, the individual may compensate in several ways. If they are weak, they may not be able to support the weight of the body at heel strike as they eccentrically contract. The result is "foot slap." With the dorsiflexors not being able to slow the descent of the foot, the foot slaps into plantar flexion. Depending on how weak these muscles are, they may or may not be able to dorsiflex the ankle during swing phase. If not, or if the muscles are paralyzed, a "foot drop" or "steppage" gait will result. This is seen first during the swing phase. The knee will have to be lifted higher for the drop foot (plantar flexed) to clear the floor. Secondly, instead of heel strike, there is *toe strike*. The ankle dorsiflexors are not able to bring the ankle into dorsiflexion so that the heel can strike first. Instead, the ankle remains in plantar flexion and the toes strike first.

When the **triceps surae group** (the gastrocnemius and soleus) are weak, there is no heel rise at push off, resulting in a shortened step length on the unaffected side. This is sometimes referred to as a "sore foot limp." Although this gait is noticeable on level ground, it becomes most pronounced when walking up an incline.

A **waddling gait** is commonly seen with muscular and other types of dystrophies. The person stands with the shoulders behind the hips, much like a person with paraplegia would balance resting on the iliofemoral ligament of the hips. Little or no reciprocal pelvis and trunk rotation occurs. Therefore, to swing the leg forward, that entire side of the body must swing forward, hence the waddling nature of the gait. Lumbar lordosis and a steppage gait also are also often present.

JOINT/MUSCLE ROM LIMITATION

In this grouping, the joint ankyloses is unable to go through its normal ROM because either there is bony fusion or soft tissue limitation. This limitation can be the result of contractures of muscle, capsule, or skin.

When a person has a **hip flexion contracture,** the hip is unable to go into hip extension and hyperextension during the midstance and push-off phases. To compensate, the person will increase the anterior pelvic tilt and lumbar lordosis. The involved limb may also have simultaneous knee flexion. If the hip is **fused,** the lumbar spine and pelvis primarily compensate for the hip motion. Decreased lordosis and posterior pelvic tilt will allow the limb to swing forward, while increased lordosis and anterior pelvic tilt will swing the limb posteriorly. This is sometimes referred to as a "bell-clapper gait."

A **knee flexion contracture** will result in excessive dorsiflexion during midstance and an early heel rise during push-off. There is also a shortened step length of the unaffected side. If a **knee fusion** is present, the lower limb will be at a fixed length. That length will depend on the position of the joint. If the knee is in extension, the limb will be unable to shorten during swing phase. Therefore, the limb must swing the leg out to the side. Called a "circumducted gait," the leg begins near the midline at push-off, swings out to the side during swing phase, then returns to the midline for heel strike. It is called an "abducted gait" if the limb remains in an abducted position throughout the gait cycle.

Depending on the severity of a **triceps surae contracture,** several things may result. An early heel rise occurs during push-off, the knee will be lifted higher during swing phase, and the toes will land first during heel strike. The latter is called a "steppage gait."

If an individual has an **ankle fusion,** commonly called a triple arthrodesis because of fusion between the subtalar and transtarsal joints, ankle plantar flexion and dorsiflexion will remain. However, these will be limited. Usually, there is a shortened stride length. The person will have more difficulty walking on uneven ground because the ability to pronate and supinate the foot has been lost.

NEUROLOGIC INVOLVEMENT

As would be expected, the amount of gait disturbance will depend on the amount and severity of neurologic involvement. A **hemiplegic gait** will vary somewhat depending on the presence of spasticity or flaccidity. The person usually shifts the body primarily to the uninvolved side, circumducts the affected limb during swing phase, and lands flat-footed or toe-first at heel strike. The involved upper extremity may be in a flexed pattern and usually without reciprocal arm swing. Step length tends to be lengthened on the involved side and shortened on the uninvolved side.

Ataxic gait from cerebellar involvement is evidenced by a wide base of support (abducted gait), and jerky, unsteady movements. The person usually has difficulty walking in a straight line, and tends to stagger. Reciprocal arm motion also appears to be jerky, and uneven.

A **parkinsonian gait** demonstrates diminished movement. The posture of the lower extremities and trunk tends to be flexed, and the reciprocal arm swing and stride length are greatly diminished. The person walks with a shuffling gait and has difficulty initiating movements. Because of the flexed posture, the center of gravity is also forward. In advanced cases, this forward center of gravity results in a "festinating gait." Because the person's balance is too far forward, a series of short, rapid steps are used to regain balance.

Spasticity in the hip adductors results in a **scissors gait.** This gait is most evident during the swing phase in which the unsupported limb swings against or across the stance leg.

A **crouch gait** is often seen with bilateral involvement of the lower extremities. Excessive lumbar lordosis and anterior pelvic tilt, flexion of the hips and knees, and plantar flexion of the ankles occurs. To compensate, the reciprocal arm swing is exaggerated.

PAIN

When a person has pain in any of the joints of the lower extremity, the tendency is to shorten the stance phase. In other words, if it hurts to stand on it, do not stand on it. A shortened, often abducted, stance phase on the involved side results in a rapid and shortened step length of the uninvolved side. Compensation in the reciprocal arm swing also is evident. Reciprocal arm swinging is shortened as the step length is shortened, exaggerated, and often abducted. This gait is often referred to as **antalgic gait.**

LEG LENGTH DISCREPANCY

We all have legs of unequal length, usually a discrepancy of approximately 1/4 inch between the right and left legs. When the discrepancy is minimal, compensation occurs by dropping the pelvis on the affected side. Although this may not look abnormal, it does place added stress on the low back. Leg length discrepancies of up to 3 inches can be accommodated in this manner.

When the discrepancy is moderate, approximately between 3 and 5 inches, dropping the pelvis on the affected side will no longer be effective. A longer leg is needed, so the person usually walks on the ball of the foot on the involved (shorter) side. This is called an **equinnus gait.**

A severe leg length discrepancy is usually any discrepancy over 5 inches. The person may compensate in a variety of ways. Dropping the pelvis and walking in an equinnus gait plus flexing the knee on the uninvolved side is often used. To gain an appreciation for how this may feel or look, walk down the street with one leg in the street and the other on the sidewalk.

REVIEW QUESTIONS

1. Compare and contrast walking and running.

2. What are the main differences between the traditional terminology and terminology developed by Rancho Los Amigos?

3. What is the phase called that occurs between heel strike and toe-off?

4. What is the time called when both feet are in contact with the ground? Which part of stance phase is each foot in during this time?

5. At what part of which phase is a person's overall vertical height the greatest?

6. During which phase is the person's foot not in contact with the ground?

7. What will happen to the step length and cadence when a person increases their walking speed?

8. If unsteady, how does a person tend to adjust walking?

9. If "foot drop," is present, which phase(s) of the person's gait will be altered?

10. If a person has an unrepaired ruptured Achilles' tendon, which phase(s) of the gait will be altered?

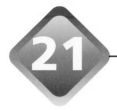

Arthrokinematics

Osteokinematic Motion

Joint movement is commonly thought of as one bone moving on another causing such motions as flexion, extension, abduction, or rotation. These movements, which are done under voluntary control, are often referred to as **classical, physiologic, or osteokinematic motion.** This type of motion can be done in the form of isometric, isotonic, or even isokinetic exercises. When performed actively, muscles move joints through ranges of motion (ROMs). As we move our joints throughout the day, we are actively performing osteokinematic movements. When a physical therapist, or physical therapist assistant, moves a joint through its range of motion, it is usually done to assist in maintaining full motion or to determine the nature of the resistance at the end of the range. The latter is called the **end feel** of a joint.

END FEEL

The three major types of end feel are bony, capsular, and empty end feel. **Bony end feel** is characterized by a hard and abrupt limit to joint motion. This occurs when bone contacts bone at the end of the ROM. An example would be normal terminal elbow extension. **Capsular end feel** is characterized by a hard, leatherlike limitation of motion that has a slight give. This occurs in full normal joint motion of the shoulder and is related to capsular restriction. An empty end feel is characterized by a lack of mechanical limitation of joint range of motion. This occurs when motion is limited by pain and there is complete disruption of soft-tissue constraints. Capsular end feel is not good.

Two additional characteristics can be used to quantify the limitation of joint motion. A rebound movement felt at the end of the ROM characterizes **springy block.** This occurs with internal derangement of a joint, such as torn cartilage. Asymptomatic limited ROM characterizes **soft tissue approximation.** This occurs when the soft tissue of body segments prevents further motion (e.g., at normal terminal elbow flexion). The ability to palpate normal end feel and to distinguish changes from normal end feel is important in protecting joints during ROM exercises.

Arthrokinematic Motion

Another way of looking at joint movement is to look at what is taking place within the joint at the joint surfaces. Called **arthrokinematic motion,** it is defined as the manner in which adjoining joint surfaces move on each other during osteokinematic joint movement. Therefore, osteokinematic motion is referred to as joint motion, and arthrokinematic motion is joint surface motion.

ACCESSORY MOTION TERMINOLOGY

Terminology can be somewhat confusing because various experts use the same terminology somewhat differently. Paris describes **accessory movement** as motions that accompany (are accessory to) the classical movement and are essential to normal full range and painless function (Paris and Patla, 1986). He further divides this motion into (1) **joint play movements,** which are not under voluntary control and occur only in response to an external force, and (2) **component movements,** which take place within a joint to facilitate a particular active motion. An example of joint play exists at the end of all active ROMs. A component movement is the associated anterior glide of the tibia as the knee goes into extension. Kisner, on the other hand, refers to component movements as motions that accompany active motion, but are not under voluntary control (Kisner and Colby, 1990). An example would be shoulder girdle upward rotation. The motion, which cannot be done alone, must accompany shoulder flexion. Kisner describes joint play as motions occurring within the joint that are necessary for normal joint function. They can be done passively by applying an external force but cannot be done actively by the individual. This describes such terms as glide, spin, and roll.

Regardless of how these accessory movements are defined, it is generally agreed that these accessory movements are necessary for joint mobilization. **Joint mobilization** is generally described as a passive oscillatory motion or sustained stretch that is applied at a slow enough speed by an external force that the individual can stop the motion. Gould describes joint mobilization as the attempt to improve joint mobility or decrease pain originating in joint structures by the use of selected grades of accessory movements.

Many physical therapists and physical therapist assistant educators do not consider the skill and technique of joint mobilization to be a part of entry-level education. However, an understanding of arthrokinematic motion and a familiarity of related terminology are considered entry-level knowledge. Further discussion of joint mobilization is beyond the scope of this book. These terms and related concepts are introduced to provide basic understanding of joint movement.

Another term, **manipulation,** is defined as a passive movement applied with a very forceful thrust within a short range that cannot be stopped. It is also applied under anesthesia. This maneuver is well beyond the scope of this text and the practice of the physical therapist assistant.

JOINT SURFACE SHAPE

To understand arthrokinematics, the type of motion occurring at a joint depends on the shape of the articulating surfaces of the bones. Most joints have one concave joint end and one convex joint end (Fig. 21–1). A convex surface is rounded outward much like a mound. A concave surface is "caved" in much like a cave.

All joint surfaces are either ovoid or sellar. An **ovoid joint** has two bones forming a convex-concave relationship. For example, in the proximal interphalangeal (PIP) joint one surface is concave (middle phalanx) and the other is convex (proximal phalanx) (see Fig. 21–1). Most synovial joints are ovoid. Usually in an ovoid joint, one bone end is larger than its adjacent bone end. This permits a greater ROM on less articular surface, which reduces the size of the joint.

In a **sellar** or **saddle-shaped joint,** each joint surface is concave in one direction and convex in another. The carpometacarpal (CMP) joint of the thumb is perhaps the best example of a sellar joint (Fig. 21–2).

TYPES OF ARTHROKINEMATIC MOTION

The types of arthrokinematic motion are roll, glide, and spin. Most joint movement involves a combination of all three of these motions. **Roll** is the rolling of one joint surface on another. New points on each surface come into contact throughout the motion (Fig. 21–3). Examples include the surface of your shoe on the floor during walking, or a ball rolling across the ground. **Glide,** or **slide,** is linear movement of a joint surface parallel to the plane of the adjoining joint surface (Fig. 21–4). In other words, one point on a joint surface contacts new points on the adjacent surface. An ice skater's skate blade (one point) sliding across the ice surface (many points) demonstrates the glide motion. **Spin** is the rotation of the movable joint surface on the fixed adjacent surface (Fig. 21–5). Essentially the same point on each surface remains in contact with each other. Examples of this type of movement would be a top spinning on a table. If the top remains perfectly upright, the top spins in one place. Examples in the body would be any pure (relatively speaking) rotational movement such as the humerus medially and laterally rotating in the glenoid fossa, or the head of the radius spinning on the capitulum of the humerus.

As discussed in Chapter 17, the knee joint motion demonstrates clearly that all three types of arthrokinematic motion are necessary to obtain full knee flexion and

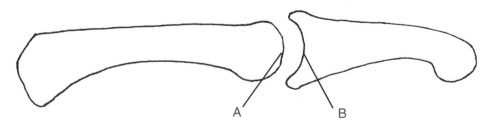

FIGURE 21–1. Convex (*A*) and concave (*B*) joint surfaces of an ovoid joint.

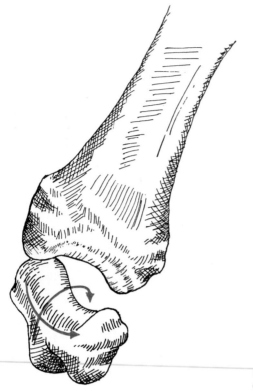

FIGURE 21–2. CMP joint of thumb as an example of a sellar joint.

extension. In this motion during weight bearing, the femoral condyles roll on the tibial condyles. Because of the large range of flexion and extension permitted, the femur would roll off the tibia if the femoral condyles did not also glide posteriorly on the tibia. Because the femoral condyles are different sizes, and the medial and lateral aspects of the knee joint move at different speeds, there must be spin (medial rotation) of the femur on the tibia during the last 15 degrees of knee extension. In a non–weight-bearing activity, the same motions are occurring except that the tibia is moving on the femur, and the spin motion is lateral rotation of the tibia on the femur (see Fig. 17–3).

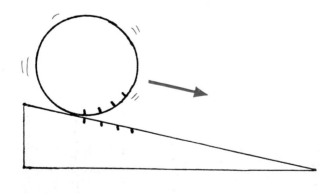

FIGURE 21–3. Roll—movement of one joint surface on another.

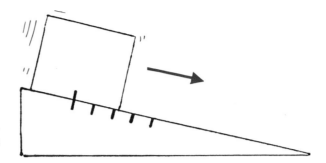

FIGURE 21–4. Glide—linear movement of one joint surface parallel to the other joint surface.

CONVEX-CONCAVE LAW

Knowing that a joint surface is concave or convex is important because shape determines motion. The **concave-convex law** describes how the differences in shapes of bone ends require joint surfaces move in a specific way during joint movement. The law is described as such:

A concave joint surface will move on a fixed convex surface in the same direction as the body segment is moving. For example, the proximal portion of the proximal phalanx is concave and the distal portion of the metacarpal is convex (Fig. 21–6). During finger extension (from finger flexion) the proximal phalanx moves in the same direction as the phalanx itself while moving on the convex metacarpal joint surface. To summarize, the **concave joint surfaces** move in the **same direction** as the joint motion.

A convex joint surface will move on a fixed concave surface in the opposite direction as the moving body segment. For example, the head of the humerus is convex whereas the glenoid fossa of the scapula, in which it articulates, is concave (Fig. 21–7). During shoulder flexion, the convex surface of the humeral head moves in

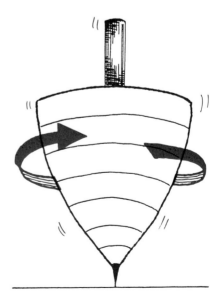

FIGURE 21–5. Spin—rotation of one joint surface on another. The points of contact remain the same on both surfaces.

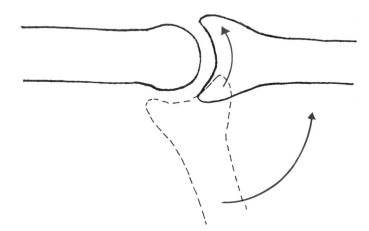

FIGURE 21–6. The concave proximal portion of proximal phalanx moving on the convex distal portion of the metacarpal. The concave joint surface is moving in the same direction as the joint motion.

the opposite direction (downward) from the rest of the humerus, which is moving upward. Thus, the **convex joint surface** moves in the **opposite direction** of joint movement.

JOINT SURFACE POSITIONS (JOINT CONGRUENCY)

The joint surfaces of an ovoid joint or sellar joint are congruent in one position and incongruent in other positions. When a joint is **congruent,** the joint surfaces have maximum contact with each other, are tightly compressed, and difficult to distract (separate). The ligaments and capsule holding the joint together are taut. This is known as the **close-packed position.** It usually occurs at one extreme of the ROM. For example, if you place your knee in the fully extended position you can manually move the patella slightly from side to side and up and down. However, if you flex your knee, such movement is *not* possible. Therefore, the close-packed position

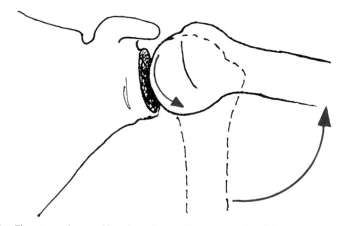

FIGURE 21–7. The convex humeral head moving on the concave glenoid. The convex joint surface moves in the opposite direction of joint motion.

of the patellofemoral joint is flexion. Other close-packed positions are ankle dorsiflexion, metacarpophalangeal flexion, and extension of the elbow, wrist, hip, knee, and interphalanges. Table 21–1 gives a more detailed listing of the close-packed positions of joints. When ligaments and capsular structures are tested for stability and integrity, the joint is usually placed in the close-packed position.

In all other positions the joint surfaces are incongruent. The position of maximum incongruency is called the **open-packed** or **loose-packed position.** Parts of the capsule and supporting ligaments are lax. It is these open-packed positions that allow for the roll, spin, and glide, necessary for normal joint motion. Table 21–2 gives a more detailed listing of the loose-packed positions of joints. Because the ligaments and capsular structures tend to be more relaxed, joint mobilization techniques are best applied in the open-packed position.

Also, in these open-packed positions a certain amount of **accessory motions,** or **joint play,** can be demonstrated. This is the passive movement of one articular surface over another. Because joint play is not a voluntary movement, it requires relaxed muscles and the external force of a trained practitioner to correctly demonstrate it.

TABLE 21–1	CLOSE PACKED POSITIONS OF JOINTS
Joint(s)	**Position**
Facet (spine)	Extension
Temporomandibular	Clenched teeth
Glenohumeral	Abduction and lateral rotation
Acromioclavicular	Arm abducted to 30°
Sternoclavicular	Maximum shoulder elevation
Ulnohumeral (elbow)	Extension
Radiohumeral	Elbow flexed 90°, forearm supinated 5°
Proximal radioulnar	5° supination
Distal radioulnar	5° supination
Radiocarpal (wrist)	Extension with ulnar deviation
Metacarpophalangeal (fingers)	Full flexion
Metacarpophalangeal (thumb)	Full opposition
Interphalangeal	Full extension
Hip	Full extension and medial rotation*
Knee	Full extension and lateral rotation of tibia
Talocrural (ankle)	Maximum dorsiflexion
Subtalar	Supination
Midtarsal	Supination
Tarsometatarsal	Supination
Metatarsophalangeal	Full extension
Interphalangeal	Full extension

*Some authors include abduction.

(From Magee, DJ: Orthopedic Physical Assessment. WB Saunders, Philadelphia, 1987, p 15 with permission.)

TABLE 21–2	LOOSE-PACKED POSITIONS OF JOINTS
Joint(s)	**Position**
Facet (spine)	Midway between flexion and extension
Temporomandibular	Mouth slightly open (freeway space)
Glenohumeral	55° abduction, 30° horizontal adduction
Acromioclavicular	Arm resting by side in normal physiologic position
Sternoclavicular	Arm resting by side in normal physiologic position
Ulnohumeral (elbow)	70° flexion, 10° supination
Radiohumeral	Full extension and full supination
Proximal radioulnar	70° flexion, 35° supination
Distal radioulnar	10° supination
Radiocarpal (wrist)	Neutral with slight ulnar deviation
Carpometacarpal	Midway between abduction/adduction and flexion/extension
Metacarpophalangeal	Slight flexion
Interphalangeal	Slight flexion
Hip	30° flexion, 30° abduction and slight lateral rotation
Knee	25° flexion
Talocrural (ankle)	10° plantar flexion, midway between maximum inversion and eversion
Subtalar	Midway between extremes of range of movement
Midtarsal	Midway between extremes of range of movement
Tarsometatarsal	Midway between extremes of range of movement
Metatarsophalangeal	Neutral
Interphalangeal	Slight flexion

(From Magee, DJ: Orthopedic Physical Assessment, WB Saunders, Philadelphia, 1987, p 14 with permission.)

ACCESSORY MOTION FORCES

When applying joint mobilization, three main types of forces are used. **Traction,** also called **distraction,** or **tension,** occurs when external force is exerted on a joint causing the joint surfaces to be pulled apart (Fig. 21–8). Carrying a heavy suitcase or hanging from an overhead bar causes traction to the shoulder, elbow, and wrist joints. You can demonstrate this on another person by grasping their index finger at the proximal end of the middle phalanx with one thumb and index finger. Next, grasp the distal end of the proximal phalanx with your other thumb and index finger. Move the PIP joint into a slightly flexed position (loose-packed position), and pull gently in opposite directions. This description, and others to follow, is meant to describe the various forces, and is not a description of therapeutic technique. Extreme care must be exercised when performing these motions.

Approximation, also called **compression,** occurs when an external force is exerted on a joint causing the joint surfaces to be pushed closer together (Fig. 21–9). Doing a chair or floor push-up causes the joint surfaces of the shoulder, elbow, and wrist to be approximated. As a general rule, traction can assist the mobility of a joint, and approximation can assist the stability of a joint.

Shear forces occur parallel to the surface (Fig. 21–10). Shear force results in a glide motion at the joint. Using the positions described with distraction, place your

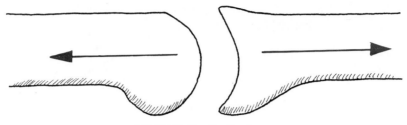

FIGURE 21–8. Traction force.

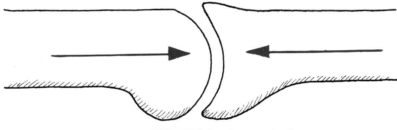

FIGURE 21–9. Compression force.

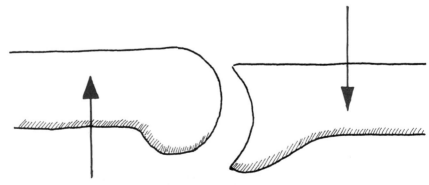

FIGURE 21–10. Shear force.

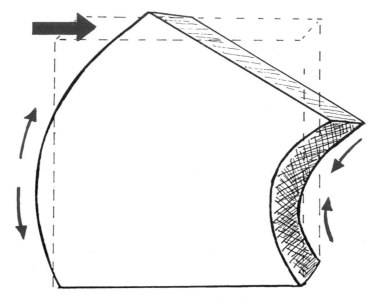

FIGURE 21–11. Bending force.

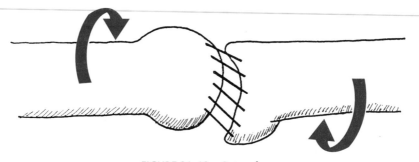

FIGURE 21–12. Rotary force.

thumbs on the dorsal surfaces and your index fingers on the palmar surfaces of the person's finger. With the PIP joint slightly flexed, gently move your two hands in an up-and-down motion. This motion describes anterior/posterior glide of the PIP joint.

Bending and rotary forces are actually a combination of forces. **Bending** occurs when an other-than-vertical force is applied, resulting in compression on the concave side and distraction on the convex side (Fig. 21–11). **Rotary** forces involve twisting, resulting in a combination of compression and shear (Fig. 21–12).

By the nature of the characteristics of a close-packed position, a joint usually is injured when in this position. For example, a knee joint that sustains a lateral force when it is extended (closed-packed position) is much more likely to be injured than when it is in a flexed or semiflexed position (loose-packed position).

REVIEW QUESTIONS

1. Shoulder flexion and extension is a type of arthrokinematic/osteokinematic motion.

2. Shoulder distraction is a type of arthrokinematic/osteokinematic motion.

Referring to the knee joint:

3. The tibia has a concave/convex surface and the femur has a concave/convex surface.

4. The majority of knee motion involves what two types of arthrokinematic motion?

5. Terminal knee extension also involves what type of arthrokinematic motion?

6. From the starting position of sitting on a treatment table with the knee flexed, extend the knee. This demonstrates a concave/convex joint surface moving on a fixed concave/convex joint surface.

7. The motion in question #6 demonstrates the joint surface moving in the same/opposite direction of the joint movement.

Referring to the hip joint:

8. The femur is a concave/convex surface, whereas the acetabulum is a concave/convex surface.

9. Flexing the hip from an extended position describes a concave/convex surface moving on a concave/convex surface.

10. The motion in question #9 demonstrates the joint surface moving in the same/opposite direction of the joint movement.

Bibliography

Basmajian, J and Blonecker, CE: Grant's Method of Anatomy, ed l. Williams & Wilkins, Baltimore, 1989.

Basmajian, J and MaConaill, MA: Muscles Alive: Their Functions Revealed by Electromyography, ed 5. Williams & Wilkins, Baltimore, 1985.

Cailliet, R: Knee Pain and Disability, ed 3. FA Davis, Philadelphia, 1992.

Cailliet, R: Hand Pain and Impairment, ed 3. FA Davis, Philadelphia, 1982.

Cailliet, R: Hand Pain and Impairment, ed 4. FA Davis, Philadelphia, 1994.

Cailliet, R: Low Back Pain Syndrome, ed 4. FA Davis, Philadelphia, 1988.

Cailliet, R: Neck and Arm Pain, ed 3. FA Davis, Philadelphia, 1991.

Cailliet, R: Shoulder Pain, ed 3. FA Davis, Philadelphia, 1991.

Cailliet, R: Soft Tissue Pain and Disability, ed 3. FA Davis, Philadelphia, 1996.

Calais-Germain, B: Anatomy of Movement, ed 1. Eastland Press, 1993.

Carlin, E: Human Anatomy and Biomechanics: Tapes 1–10 [Audio tape]. Audio-Learning, Norristown, 1975.

Cooper, J and Glassow, R: Kinesiology, ed 3. CV Mosby, St. Louis, 1972.

Curtis, BA: Neurosciences: The Basics, ed 1, Lea & Febiger, Malvern, PA, 1990.

Daniels, L and Worthingham, C: Muscle Testing: Techniques of Manual Examination, ed 5. WB Saunders, Philadelphia, 1986.

Donatelli, RA: The Biomechanics of the Foot and Ankle, ed 2. FA Davis, Philadelphia, 1996.

Evjenth, O and Hamberg, J: Muscle Stretching in Manual Therapy: A Clinical Manual, vol. 1: The Extremities, ed 1. Alfta, Sweden, Chattanoga, 1984.

Goldberg, S: Clinical Anatomy Made Ridiculously Simple, ed 1. MedMaster, Miami, 1990.

Goss, CM (ed): Gray's Anatomy of the Human Body, American ed 29. Lea & Febiger, Philadelphia, 1973.

Gould, J and Davies, G (eds): Orthopaedic and Sports Physical Therapy, ed 2. CV Mosby, St. Louis, 1985.

Hall, SJ: Basic Biomechanics, ed 3. WCB McGraw-Hill, Boston, 1999.

Hay, J: Biomechanics of Sports Techniques, ed 1. Prentice-Hall, Englewood Cliffs, 1973.

Hinson, M: Kinesiology, ed 2. WC Brown, Dubuque, 1981.

Hole, Jr. JW: Human Anatomy and Physiology, ed 5. WC Brown, Dubuque, 1990.

Hoppenfeld, S: Physical Examination of the Spine and Extremities, ed 1. Appleton-Century-Crofts, New York, 1976.

Jacob, S and Francone, C: Elements of Anatomy and Physiology, ed 3. WB Saunders, Philadelphia, 1989.

Jenkins, DB: Hollinshead's Functional Anatomy of the Limbs and Back, ed 7. WB Saunders, Philadelphia, 1998.

Jones K and Barker, K: Human Movement Explained, ed 1. Butterworth-Heinemann, Oxford, 1996.

Kapandji, I: Physiology of the Joints: Upper Limbs, vol. 1, ed 2. Livingstone, Edinburgh, 1970.

Kessler, R and Hertling, D: Management of Common Musculoskeletal Disorders: Physical Therapy Principles and Methods, ed 1. Harper & Row, Philadelphia, 1983.

Kendall, FP and McCreary, EK: Muscles Testing and Function, ed 3. Williams & Wilkins, 1983.

King, B and Showers, M: Human Anatomy and Physiology, ed 6. WB Saunders, Philadelphia, 1969.

Landau, BR: Essential Human Anatomy and Physiology, ed 2. Scott, Foresman, Glenview, IL, 1980.

Leeson, C and Leeson, T: Human Structure: A Companion to Anatomical Studies, ed 1. WB Saunders, Philadelphia, 1972.

Low, J and Reed A: Basic Biomechanics Explained, ed 1. Butterworth Heinemann, Oxford, 1996.

Lehmkuhl, LD and Smith, LK: Brunnstrom's Clinical Kinesiology, ed 4. FA Davis, Philadelphia, 1983.

MacConaill, M and Basmajian, J: Muscles and Movements: A Basis for Human Kinesiology, ed 1. Williams & Wilkins, Baltimore, 1969.

MacLeod, D, Jacobs, P and Larson, N: The Ergonomics Manual, ed 1. The Saunders Group, Minneapolis, 1990.

Magee, D: Orthopedic Physical Assessment, ed 1. WB Saunders, Philadelphia, 1987.

Magee, KR and Saper, JR: Clinical and Basic Neurology for Health Professionals, ed 1. Year Book Medical, Chicago, 1981.

Manter, JT and Gatz, AJ: Essentials of Clinical Neuroanatomy and Neurophysiology, ed 8. FA Davis, Philadelphia, 1993.

Melloni, J, et al: Melloni's Illustrated Review of Human Anatomy, ed 1. JB Lippincott, Philadelphia, 1988.

Miller, B and Keane, C: Encyclopedia and Dictionary of Medicine, Nursing, and Allied Health, ed 4. WB Saunders, Philadelphia, 1989.

Minor, MA, and Lippert, LS: Kinesiology Laboratory Manual for Physical Therapist Assistants, ed 1. FA Davis, Philadelphia, 1998.

Minor, M and Minor, S: Patient Evaluation Methods for the Health Professional, ed 1. RestonPublishing, Reston, 1985.

Moore, K: Clinically Oriented Anatomy, ed 2. Williams & Wilkins, Baltimore, 1985.

Netter, FH: Ciba Collection of Medical Illustrations: Musculoskeletal System: Part I, Anatomy, Physiology, and Metabolic Diseases, vol. 8: ed 1. Ciba-Geigy, Summit, NJ, 1987.

Netter, FH: Ciba Collection of Medical Illustrations: Nervous System, Part I, Anatomy and Physiology, ed 1. Ciba Pharmaceutical, West Caldwell, NJ, 1983.

Norkin, C and Levangie, P: Joint Structure and Function: A Comprehensive Analysis, ed 1. FA Davis, Philadelphia, 1983.

Norkin, C and Levangie, P: Joint Structure and Function: A Comprehensive Analysis, ed 2. FA Davis, Philadelphia, 1992.

Norkin, C and White, D: Measurement of Joint Motion: A Guide of Goniometry, ed 1. FA Davis, Philadelphia, 1985.

Oliver, J: Back care: An illustrated guide. Butterworth–Heinemann, 1994, Oxford.

Palastanga, N, Field, D, and Soames, R: Anatomy and Human Movement: Structure and Function, ed 2. Butterworth–Heinemann, Oxford, 1994.

Palmer, M and Epler, M: Clinical Assessment Procedures in Physical Therapy, ed 1. JB Lippincott, Philadelphia, 1990.

Palmer, M and Epler, M: Clinical Assessment Procedures in Physical Therapy, ed 2. JB Lippincott, Philadelphia, 1998.

Paris, SV and Patla, C: E-1 Course Notes: Introduction to Extremity Dysfunction and Manipulation. Institute Press, 1986.

Perry JF, Rohe, DA, and Garcia, AO: The Kinesiology Workbook, ed 2. FA Davis, Philadelphia, 1996.

Pratt, NE: Clinical Musculoskeletal Anatomy, ed 1. JB Lippincott, Philadelphia, 1991.

Rasch, P: Kinesiology and Applied Anatomy, ed 7. Lea & Febiger, Philadelphia, 1989.

Richardson, JK and Iglarsh ZA: Clinical Orthopaedic Physical Therapy, ed 1. WB Saunders, 1994.

Romanes, G (ed): Cunningham's Textbook of Anatomy, ed 10. Oxford University Press, New York, 1964.

Rothstein, JM, Roy, SH, and Wolf, SL: The Rehabilitation Specialist's Handbook, ed 1. FA Davis, Philadelphia, 1991.

Rothstein, JM, Roy, SH, and Wolf, SL: The Rehabilitation Specialist's Handbook, ed 2. FA Davis, Philadelphia, 1998.

Roy, S and Irvin, R: Sports Medicine: Prevention, Evaluation, Management, and Rehabilitation, ed 1. Prentice-Hall, Englewood Cliffs, 1983.

Scanlon, VC and Sanders, T: Essentials of Anatomy and Physiology, ed 3. FA Davis, Philadelphia, 1999.

Sieg, K and Adams, S: Illustrated Essentials of Musculoskeletal Anatomy, ed 2. Megabooks, Gainesville, 1985.

Smith, LK, Weiss, EL, and Lehmkuhl, LD: Brunnstrom's Clinical Kinesiology, ed 5. FA Davis, Philadelphia, 1996.

Soderberg, G: Kinesiology: Application of Pathological Motion, ed 1. Williams & Wilkins, Baltimore, 1986.

Somers, MF: Spinal Cord Injury–Functional Rehabilitation, ed 1. Appleton & Lange, Norwalk, 1992.

Steindler, A: Kinesiology of the Human Body: Under Normal and Pathological Conditions, ed 1. CharlesThomas, Springfield, 1955.

Thibodeau, G: Anatomy and Physiology, ed 1. Times Mirror/Mosby College Publishing, St. Louis, 1986.

Tomberlin, JP, and Saunders, HD: Evaluation, Treatment and Prevention of Musculoskeletal Disorders, Vol 2: Extremities, ed 3. The Saunders Group, Minneapolis, 1994.

Tortora, G: Principles of Human Anatomy, ed 5. Canfield Press, San Francisco, 1990.

Tortora, G and Anagnostakos, N: Principles of Anatomy and Physiology, ed 3. Harper & Row, New York.

Tyldesley, B and Grieve, JI: Muscles, Nerves and Movement: Kinesiology in Daily Living, ed 1. Blackwell Scientific, Oxford, 1989.

Tyldesley, B and Grieve, JI: Muscles, Nerves and Movement: Kinesiology in Daily Living, ed 1. Blackwell Scientific Oxford, 1989.

Vidic, B and Suarez, F: Photographic Atlas of the Human Body, ed 1. CV Mosby, St. Louis, 1984.

Warwick, R and Williams, P (eds): Gray's Anatomy, British ed 35. WB Saunders, Philadelphia, 1973.

Wells, K and Luttgens, K: Kinesiology: Scientific Basis of Human Motion, ed 7. WB Saunders, Philadelphia, 1982.

Williams, M and Lissner, H: Biomechanics of Human Motion, ed 1. WB Saunders, Philadelphia, 1962.

Yokochi, C: Photographic Anatomy of the Human Body, ed 1. University Park Press, Baltimore, 1971.

Answers to Review Questions

CHAPTER 1 ◆ BASIC INFORMATION

1. Anterior.
2. Posterior.
3. Inferior.
4. Proximal.
5. Lateral.
6. *Linear motion:* A person riding a bicycle.
   Angular motion: The lower extremity joint motion of a person pedaling a bicycle.
7. Neck hyperextension.
8. Shoulder medial rotation.
9. Trunk lateral bending.
10. Hip lateral rotation.
11. Anatomical position and fundamental position are the same except for the forearms, which are supinated in anatomical position and in neutral position (between supination and pronation) in the fundamental position.
12. Dorsal surface of dog, posterior surface of person.
13. The football is demonstrating curvilinear motion, while the kicker's leg is demonstrating angular motion.

CHAPTER 2 ◆ SKELETAL SYSTEM

1. The axial skeleton contains no long or short bones, whereas the appendicular skeleton contains no irregular bones. The bones of the axial skeleton are particularly important in providing support and protection; the appendicular skeleton provides the framework for movement.
2. Compact bone is found in the diaphysis of long bones, and cancellous bone is found in the metaphysis and epiphysis. In other types of bone, cancellous bone is found sandwiched between layers of compact bone.
3. Compact bone is heavier than cancellous bone because it is less porous.
4. Most height growth is a result of growth in the epiphysis of long bones.

5. Sesamoid bones protect tendons from excess wear. The patella has the additional function of increasing angle of pull of the quadriceps muscle.
6. a. Foremen, fossa, groove, meatus, sinus.
   b. Condyle, eminence, facet, head.
   c. Crest, epicondyle, line, spine, trochanter, tubercle, tuberosity.
7. a. *Bicipital groove:* Ditchlike depression.
   b. *Humeral head:* Rounded articular projection that fits into a joint.
   c. *Acetabulum:* Deep depression.
   d. *Scapular spine:* Long thin projection to which tendons attach.
   e. *Supraspinous fossa:* Depression or hollow.

CHAPTER 3 ◆ ARTICULAR SYSTEM

1. A joint that allows no motion is referred to as a fibrous joint. The three types of fibrous joints are: synarthrosis, syndesmosis, and gomphosis.
2. A joint that allows a great deal of motion is called a synovial joint or diarthrosis.
3. Diarthrodial joints can be described by the number of axes, the shape of the joint, and the joint motion involved.
4. Tendon.
5. Bursa.
6. Characteristics of a synovial joint:
   a. It involves two articulating bones whose ends are lined with articular (hyaline) cartilage.
   b. There is a space between the two bone ends.
   c. There is a joint capsule.
   d. The inside lining of the capsule has a synovial membrane.
   e. The synovial membrane secretes synovial fluid.
7. Hyaline cartilage is located on bone ends of synovial joints and provides a smooth articulating surface. Fibrocartilage is thicker and is located between bones. Fibrocartilage provides shock absorption and spacing. Examples of fibrocartilage are the menisci of the knee and the discs of the vertebrae.
8. The joint motion involved is elbow flexion; it occurs in the sagittal plane around the frontal axis.
9. The joint involved is forearm pronation; it occurs in the transverse plane around the vertical axis.
10. The joint motion involved is finger (MP) adduction; it occurs in the frontal plane around the sagittal axis.
11. Shoulder = 3, elbow = 1, radioulnar = 1, wrist = 2, MCP = 2, PIP = 1, DIP = 1.

CHAPTER 4 ◆ MUSCULAR SYSTEM

1. Insertion; origin.
2. Reversal of muscle action.
3.   *At the shoulder*   *At the elbow*
    a. Shoulder abduction   a. Elbow extension
    b. Isotonic contraction   b. Isometric contraction
    c. Concentric   c. N/A (no answer needed)

4.   *Shoulder: First 90 degrees*   *Shoulder: Second 90 degrees*
  a. Shoulder flexion   a. Shoulder flexion
  b. Isotonic contraction   b. Isotonic contraction
  c. Concentric (of shoulder flexors)   c. Eccentric (of shoulder extensors)

5. The muscles are agonists in wrist flexion and antagonists in ulnar/radial deviation.

6. The gluteus minimus muscles acts as a hip medial rotator to neutralize the lateral rotator component of the action of the gluteus maximus muscle.

7. Active insufficiency.

8. Eccentric

9. a. Wheelchair push-ups   Closed chain activity
  b. Exercises with weight cuffs   Open chain activity
  c. Overhead wall pulleys   Open chain activity

CHAPTER 5 ◆ THE NERVOUS SYSTEM

1. L2.

2. Gray matter is unmyelinated tissue, and white matter is myelinated tissue.

3. The brain is protected from trauma by:
  a. The bony outer layer called the *skull*.
  b. Three layers of membrane called the *meninges*.
  c. Shock absorption provided by cerebrospinal fluid.

4. The circle of Willis is a set of interconnecting arteries at the base of the brain. It is the source of the arteries that supply the brain. The interconnection of the arteries means that interruption of flow in one artery will not seriously decrease blood supply to all the regions of the brain.

5. Motor neurons that synapse above the level of the spinal cord's anterior horn are upper motor neurons. Those synapsing at the anterior horn or peripherally are lower motor neurons. Pathological conditions occurring to either upper or lower motor neurons have quite different clinical signs.

6. Thoracic nerves directly innervate the muscles near where they arise from the spinal cord. Cervical or lumbar nerves branch and/or divide, forming a plexus and innervate muscle quite distal from the level of the cord from which they originate.

7. Afferent nerve fibers transmit sensory impulses from the periphery toward the brain. Efferent fibers transmit motor impulses from the brain or spinal cord toward the periphery.

8. The involved nerve is the median nerve. The condition is referred to as *ape hand*.

9. The involved nerve is the peroneal nerve. The condition is referred to as *foot drop*.

10. The muscle group involved with claw hand is the intrinsics, which is most innervated by the ulnar nerve.

CHAPTER 6 ◆ BASIC BIOMECHANICS

1. The wrist, because there is a longer resistance arm when the weight is around the wrist than when it is around the elbow.

2. The shorter person has a lower COG.

3. a. 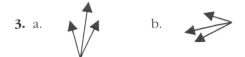 b.

4. First one—scalar = 5 miles (magnitude only).
Second one—vector = 30 feet to the north (magnitude and direction).

5. The person on the left (force) side would go up because the resistance *r* is increased.

6. To balance the seesaw, the person on the left should move back to make the force arm longer.

7. The load would be lighter because shifting the load forward moves the resistance closer to the axis, which shortens the lever arm. If it were possible, making the handles of the wheelbarrow longer would increase the force arm, which would also make the load feel lighter.

CHAPTER 7 ◆ SHOULDER GIRDLE

1. The shoulder girdle includes the articulations between the scapula and clavicle. The shoulder joint includes the scapula and humerus. The shoulder complex includes the scapula, clavicle, humerus, sternum, and rib cage.

2. Use the inferior angle as a point of reference. When it moves away from the vertebral column, the motion is scapular upward rotation. When it moves toward the vertebral column, the motion is scapular downward rotation.

3. Elevation/depression and protraction/retraction are more linear. Upward and downward rotation are more angular.

4. Scapulohumeral rhythm is the movement relationship between the shoulder girdle and shoulder joint. After the first 30 degrees, for every 2 degrees of shoulder joint flexion or abduction, the shoulder girdle rotates upwardly 1 degree. Without this shoulder girdle movement, one cannot normally and completely raise the arm above the head.

5. Because the three different attachments of the trapezius muscle produce three different lines of pull, the three parts have different muscle actions. The rhomboid muscles, however, have the same line of pull, thus the same muscle action. There is no functional difference between the rhomboid muscles.

6. The serratus anterior plus the upper and lower trapezius muscles.

7. *Force couple:* a situation in which two or more muscles pull in different, often opposite, directions to accomplish the same motion.

8. The pectoralis minor muscle.

9. The pectoralis minor attaches to the coracoid process, and serratus anterior attaches to the anterior surface of the scapula.

10. The rhomboid muscles, the lower and middle trapezius muscles, the levator scapula muscle, and the upper trapezius muscle.

CHAPTER 8 ◆ SHOULDER JOINT

1.
   a. In the frontal plane around the sagittal axis: shoulder abduction/adduction.
   b. In the transverse plane around the vertical axis: shoulder medial/lateral rotation, horizontal abduction/adduction.

   c. In the saggital plane around the frontal axis: shoulder flexion/extension.
2. The circular arc of the upper extremity formed by a combination of the shoulder motions-flexion, abduction, extension, and adduction.
3. Subscapular fossa.
4. The supraspinous and infraspinous fossas.
5. With the humerus in the vertical position, the bicipital groove facing anteriorly, and head facing medially, the right humeral head faces toward the left.
6. The supraspinatus, infraspinatus, teres minor, and subscapularis muscles.
7. They hold the head of the humerus in toward the glenoid fossa as it moves within the socket.
8. The subscapularis and coracobrachialis muscles and the short head of the biceps brachii muscle.
9. The teres major and minor, infraspinatus, supraspinatus, and posterior deltoid muscles.
10. The anterior deltoid, pectoralis major, and latissimus dorsi muscles.
11. The biceps brachii muscle and the long head of the triceps muscle.

CHAPTER 9 ◆ ELBOW

1. Forearm pronation and supination.
2. *Joints:* the superior radioulnar joint and inferior radioulnar joint. *Bones:* the radius and ulna.
3. The elbow joint, which consists of the humerus articulating with the ulna and radius.
4.

	Forearm	Elbow
a. *Number of axes:*	1	1
b. *Shape of joint:*	Pivot	Hinge
c. *Type of motion allowed:*	Supination/pronation	Flexion/extension

5. The trochlear notch at the superior end faces anteriorly, the radial notch at the same end faces laterally, and the styloid process at the inferior end is on the medial side.
6.
   a. Lateral, or radial, collateral ligament.
   b. Medial, or ulnar, collateral ligament.
   c. Annular ligament.
7. The biceps and triceps muscles.
8. Radius, because it is the radius moving around the ulna that produces these motions.
9. The biceps, brachialis, brachioradialis, and pronator teres muscles.
10. The triceps and anconeus muscles.
11. The pronator quadratus and biceps muscles.
12. The biceps (to radius) and triceps (to ulna) muscles.
13. Anconeus, triceps, and brachialis muscles.
14. Pronator teres and brachioradialis muscles.

CHAPTER 10 ◆ WRIST

1. The distal end of the radius articulates with the scaphoid, lunate, and triquetrum.

2.
   a. Wrist flexion and extension.
   b. Wrist ulnar and radial deviation.
   c. There are no such wrist motions.

3.

	Radiocarpal joint	Intercarpal joint
a. *Number of axes:*	2	0
b. *Shape of joint:*	Condyloid	Plane or irregular
c. *Joint motion allowed:*	f/e, rd/ud	Gliding

4. Flexor carpi ulnaris, flexor carpi radialis, palmaris longus.

5. Extensor carpi radialis longus and brevis, extension carpi ulnaris.

6. If the pisiform bone and "hook" of the hamate bone are visible, it would be the anterior side.

7. Extensor carpi radialis longus and flexor carpi radialis.

8. Extensor carpi ulnaris and flexor carpi ulnaris.

9. The palmaris longus located on the anterior surface in the middle of the wrist.

10. Flexor carpi ulnaris, palmaris longus (with flexor digitorum superficialis and profundus deep to it), flexor carpi radialis, (abductor pollicis longus, extensor pollicis long and brevis, which are primarily thumb muscles but do cross the wrist) extensor carpi radialis longus and brevis, (extensor digitorum, a finger extensor), and extensor carpi ulnaris.

CHAPTER 11 ◆ HAND

1.
   a. *Finger:* MCP abduction/adduction.
      Thumb: MCP and IP flexion/extension.
   b. *Finger:* MCP, PIP, DIP flexion/extension.
      Thumb: CMP abduction/adduction.
   c. *Thumb:* opposition/reposition.

2. Each finger and the thumb have a metacarpal, proximal, and distal phalange. While each finger has a middle phalange, the thumb does not. Therefore, the thumb has only two joints (MCP and IP), and the fingers have three (MCP, PIP, and DIP).

3. Flexion, abduction, and rotation.

4. It holds the extrinsic tendons close to the wrist.

5. The floor of the carpal tunnel is made up of the carpal bones, and the ceiling is the transverse carpal ligament portion of the flexor retinaculum. The flexor digitorum superficialis and profundus muscles and the median nerve run through the carpal tunnel.

6. An extrinsic muscle has its proximal attachment above the wrist and its distal attachment below the wrist. The extrinsic muscles include the flexor digitorum superficialis and profundus, extensor digitorum, extensor digiti minimi, and extensor indicis muscles.

7. An intrinsic muscle has both attachments below the wrist; intrinsic muscles include the flexor and abductor pollicis brevis, opponens and adductor pollicis, flexor/abductor/opponens digiti minimi, interossei, and lumbricales.

8. Thenar muscles are intrinsic muscles on the thumb side (lateral) of the hand; hypothenar muscles are on the little finger side (medial). Any intrinsic muscle with "pollicis" in its name is a thenar muscle, whereas one with "digiti minimi" is a hypothenar muscle.

9. The indention formed between the tendons of the extensor pollicis brevis and longus is referred to as the "anatomical snuffbox."
10. The lumbrical muscles; they attach proximally to the tendons of the flexor digitorum profundus muscle and distally to the tendons of the extensor digitorum muscle.
11. Abduction/adduction of the thumb occurs at the CMC joint, whereas the abduction/adduction of the fingers occurs primarily at the MCP joints.
12.

a. Holding the handle of a skillet	Variation of cylindrical grip
b. Pulling a little red wagon	Hook grip
c. Picking up a cassette tape	Pad-to-pad prehension
d. Fastening snaps or buttons	Tip-to-tip prehension
e. Carrying a mug by its handle	Lateral prehension
f. Holding a hand of cards	Lumbrical grip
g. Holding an apple	Spherical grip
h. Holding on to a barbell	Cylindrical grip

CHAPTER 12 ◆ TEMPOROMANDIBULAR JOINT

1. Zygomatic and temporal bones.
2. Synonymous terms are mandibular:
   a. Depression.
   b. Elevation.
   c. Retraction or retrusion.
   d. Protraction or protrusion.
   e. Lateral deviation.
3. Mandible and temporal bones.
4. Temporalis.
5. Masseter.
6. Diagastric.
7. Changes direction of the line of pull.
8. Fifth cranial (trigeminal) nerve.
9. Anterior rotation of the mandibular condyle on the disk.
10. The left condyle spins in the mandibular socket while the right condyle slides forward.
11. The thyroid cartilage.

CHAPTER 13 ◆ NECK AND TRUNK

1.
   a. Neck and trunk lateral bending.
   b. Neck and trunk rotation.
   c. Neck and trunk flexion, extension, and hyperextension.
2. The cervical vertebra has a bifid spinous process, and there is a foramen in the transverse process. The thoracic vertebrae have a long slender, downward-pointing spinous process with rib facets on the body and transverse processes; the superior articular processes face posteriorly. The lumbar vertebra has a large spinous process pointing straight back; the superior articular processes face medially.

3. The front/back position of the superior and inferior articular processes.
4. The side-to-side position of the superior and inferior articular.
5. *From the occiput to C7:* nuchal ligament. *From C7 to the sacrum:* supraspinal ligament.
6. Ligamentum flavum.
7. Anterior and posterior longitudinal ligaments.
8. The muscle's line of pull is through or close to the center of the frontal axis of trunk flexion and extension, thus making it ineffective in this motion. To be effective in rotation, the muscle's line of pull would have to be horizontal or diagonal. The quadratus lumborum has a vertical line of pull.
9. The erector spinae.
10. A combination of trunk flexion and rotation to the right brought about by the rectus abdominis left external oblique and right internal oblique.

CHAPTER 14 ◆ RESPIRATION

1. The sternum, ribs, and costal cartilages, and thoracic vertebrae.
2. The bodies and transverse processes of the thoracic vertebrae articulate with the tubercle and neck of the ribs.
3. Elevation and depression bringing about inspiration and expiration.
4. During inspiration the ribs elevate and the diaphragm lowers, and during expiration the ribs depress and the diaphragm muscle elevates.
5. The origin, or more stable attachment, is above the rib cage and in a position to pull the rib cage up.
6. No. While the line of pull does not change from front to back, the muscle moves 180 degrees around the rib cage giving the appearance of changing direction from front to back.
7. The origin, or more stable attachment, has a bony attachment, but the insertion attaches to a central tendon. When the muscle is relaxed, it is dome-shaped. When it contracts, the muscle flattens out, allowing more room in the thoracic cavity.
8. You talk only during expiration when air is moving out through the airway.
9. The accessory muscles of inspiration pull up on the sternum and rib cage while the accessory muscles of expiration pull down.
10. Rib cage movement is compared to bucket handle movement; thoracic cavity movement is compared to movement of a bellows.
11. The person with a C3 injury will not have an innervated diaphragm; therefore, they will need the assistance of a ventilator to breathe. A person with a C5 injury will have a neurologically intact diaphragm and can breath without mechanical assistance.

CHAPTER 15 ◆ PELVIC GIRDLE

1.
   a. anterior/posterior pelvic tilt.
   b. Lateral tilt.
   c. Pelvic rotation.
2. To the left.
3. The hip joints.

4.
    a. Hip flexion.
    b. Hip extension.
    c. Hip abduction on the unsupported side and hip adduction on the weight-bearing side.

5.
    a. Right hip medial rotation/left hip lateral rotation.
    b. Right hip lateral rotation/left hip medial rotation.

6.
    a. Hyperextension.
    b. Flexion.
    c. Lateral bending to opposite side.

7. Back extensors, hip flexors.

CHAPTER 16 ◆ HIP

1.
    a. Two hip bones, the sacrum, and the coccyx.
    b. The fused bones of the ilium, ischium, and pubis.
    c. Acetabulum of the hip bone and head of the femur.
    d. The ilium, ischium, and pubis.
    e. The ischium and pubis.
    f. The ilium and ischium.

2. With the greater sciatic notch posterior and the body of pubis anterior, the acetabulum faces laterally. Therefore, if the acetabular opening is facing to the right in this position, it is a right hip bone.

3. With the femur in the vertical position, the linea aspera and lesser trochanter are posterior, and the head faces medially. Therefore, in this position the head of the right femur faces toward the left.

4.
    a. *Number of axes:* 3.
    b. *Shape of joint:* Ball and socket.
    c. *Type of motion allowed:* Flexion/extension, abduction/adduction, and rotation.

5.
    a. Medial and lateral rotation.
    b. Flexion/extension.
    c. Abduction/adduction.

6. The distal attachment of the iliofemoral ligament; because it splits into two parts forming an upside-down Y.

7. The acetabulum forms a deep socket holding most of the femoral head, and the joint is surrounded by three very strong ligaments.

8. The line of attachment of the ligaments is a spiral. This arrangement causes the ligaments to become taut as the joint moves into extension and to slacken with flexion, thus limiting hyperextension without impeding flexion.

9. The rectus femoris, sartorius, gracilis, semitendinosus, semimembranosus, biceps femoris (longhead), and tensor fascia latae muscles.

10. The sartorius muscle is involved in hip flexion, abduction, and lateral rotation; the tensor fascia latae muscle is involved in flexion and abduction.

11. When you lift your right foot off the floor, the left gluteus medius and minimus contract to keep the right side of the pelvis from dropping.

12. A force couple; the hip abductors are pulling down while the trunk extensors are pulling up.

CHAPTER 17 ◆ KNEE

1.

	Knee joint	Patellofemoral joint
a. *Number of axes:*	1	0
b. *Shape of joint:*	Hinge	Irregular
c. *Type of motion:*	Flexion/extension	Gliding

2. Knee flexion and extension occur in the sagittal plane around the frontal axis.
3. The Q angle is formed by the intersection of the line between the tibial tuberosity and middle of the patella and the line between the asis and the middle of the patella. The greater the angle, the higher the stress on the patellofemoral joint during knee flexion and extension.
4. The anterior cruciate ligament prevents the tibia from moving anteriorly on the femur while the posterior cruciate ligament does just the opposite.
5. The medial collateral ligament keeps the medial side of the knee from separating while the lateral collateral does just the opposite.
6. Femur and tibia.
7. The quadriceps group.
8. The hamstring group and the sartorius, gracilis, gastrocnemius, and popliteus muscles.
9. Because it initiates knee flexion, moving the knee out of the "locked" position of extension.
10. The hamstring muscle group.
11. The rectus femoris muscle.
12. None—gotcha!
13. The distal attachments of the sartorius, gracilis, and semitendinosus muscles.
14. Weakened knee extension (quadriceps = L2–L4) and no knee flexion (hamstrings = L5–S2)
15. Closed kinetic chain.
16. Yes, they both are.

CHAPTER 18 ◆ ANKLE JOINT AND FOOT

1.
   a. 1
   b. Hinge.
   c. Dorsiflexion, plantar flexion.
   d. Tibia and talus (primarily).
2. The subtalar joint involves the talus and calcaneus; the transverse tarsal joint involves the talus and calcaneus with the navicular and cuboid bone.
3. The function of the interosseous membrane, which is located between the tibia and fibula, is to hold the two bones together and to provide a large area for muscle attachment.
4. The deltoid ligament, made up of the tibionavicular, tibiocalcaneal, and posterior tibiotalar ligaments.
5. The lateral ligament, made up of the posterior and anterior talofibular and calcaneofibular ligaments.

6. The longitudinal arch is made up of the calcaneus and the navicular, cuneiform, and first three matatarsal bones. Its function is to provide some shock absorption when the foot hits the ground.
7. The transverse arch, made up of the cuboid and three cuneiform bones, also provides some shock absorption.
8. Tibialis posterior, flexor digitorum longus, and flexor hallucis longus muscles.
9. Tibialis posterior, tibialis anterior, peroneus longus muscles.
10. Peroneus longus and peroneus brevis muscles.
11. Peroneus brevis and tertius muscles.
12. Tibialis anterior and peroneus longus muscles; together, the peroneus longus and tibialis anterior muscles are sometimes referred to as the stirrup of the foot because the peroneus longus muscle vertically descends the leg laterally before crossing the foot medially to join the tibialis anterior muscle. The tibialis anterior muscle vertically descends the leg medially to meet the peroneus longus muscle, forming a U or stirrup.
13. No, the strongest plantar flexors are the gastrocnemius and soleus, which are innervated at the S1–S2 levels. The posterior deep group is innervated at the L5–S1 level primarily.

CHAPTER 19 ◆ POSTURE

1. Cervical extensors.
2. The side view.
3. Hip flexors.
4. The side.
5. Level and not elevated or depressed.
6. From the front or back.
7. Slightly in front of the lateral malleolus.
8. Knee—slightly posterior to the patella.
   Hip—through the greater trochanter.
   Shoulder—through the tip of the acromion process.
   Head—through the ear lobe.

CHAPTER 20 ◆ GAIT

1. Both have the same components and sequence of events. Walking has a period of double support while running does not. Running has a period of non-support that walking does not have.
2. Traditional terminology refers to single points in a time frame while RLA terminology refers to periods in a time frame.
3. Stance phase.
4. Period of double support; between heel-off and toe-off of one foot and heel strike and foot flat on the opposite foot.
5. During midstance of the stance phase.
6. Swing phase.
7. Step length lengthens, and cadence increases.
8. Walk with feet father apart to widen the base of support.
9. Heel strike of stance phase and midswing of swing phase.
10. Push-off off stance phase.

CHAPTER 21 ◆ ARTHROKINEMATICS

1. Osteokinematic.
2. Arthrokinematic.
3. Concave, convex.
4. Roll, glide.
5. Spin.
6. Concave, convex.
7. Same direction.
8. Convex, concave.
9. Convex, concave.
10. Opposite direction.

Index

Note: boldface numbers indicate illustrations